Contents

List of contributors   vii

Preface   ix

1   What is cancer?   1
Pauline Richardson

2   Promoting health and preventing cancer   13
Wendy Boothroyd

3   Body awareness in the prevention and early detection of cancers   29
Norma Sutherland

4   Screening for cancer   48
Penny Craddock

5   Chemotherapy and the administration of cytotoxic drugs into established lines   77
Julia Luken and Janice Middleton

6   Radiotherapy: its nature and scope   113
Philippa Green and Shaun Kinghorn

7   Surgery and the cancer patient   146
Annie Topping

8   Biological and hormonal therapy   174
Jaqualyn Moore

9   Communication   204
Susie Wilkinson

10   Ethical pathways in cancer and palliative care   224
Kevin Kendrick

11   An introduction to hospice and palliative care   245
Alison Barnes

12   Symptom control in advanced cancer   262
Tracey Pilsworth, Dot Pye and Anita Roberts

13   Caring for the dying patient in the community   304
Christine Searle

14   Support for the family in bereavement   323
     Val Smith

15   Rehabilitation: adding quality to life   350
     Jill David

16   Educational opportunities in cancer care   376
     Eileen Gape

17   Where to get help   394
     Jan Viret

     Index   415

Contributors

Alison Barnes
Regional Nurse Manager, Marie Curie Cancer Care, London, UK

Wendy Boothroyd
Director of Education, Marie Curie Cancer Care, Education Department, London, UK

Penny Craddock
Practice Nurse Tutor, Marie Curie Cancer Care, London, UK

Jill David
Research Officer (education), Marie Curie Cancer Care, Education Department, London, UK

Eileen Gape
Tutor, BUPA Hospital, Cardiff, UK

Philippa Green
Clinical Nurse Specialist, Northern Centre for Cancer Treatment, Newcastle General Hospital, Newcastle upon Tyne, UK

Kevin Kendrick
Senior Lecturer, Philosophy and Health Care Ethics, School of Health Care, Liverpool John Moores University, Liverpool, UK

Shaun Kinghorn
Nurse Teacher, Conrad House Marie Curie Centre, Newcastle upon Tyne, UK

Julia Luken
Clinical Nurse Specialist, Royal South Hants Hospital, Southampton, UK

Janice Middleton
Clinical Nurse Specialist, Royal South Hants Hospital, Southampton, UK

Jaqualyn Moore
Clinical Nurse Specialist, The Royal Marsden Hospital, Fulham Road, London, UK

Tracey Pilsworth
Trainee Lecturer–practitioner, Harestone Marie Curie Centre, Caterham, UK

Dot Pye
Deputy Matron, Liverpool Marie Curie Centre, Woolton, Liverpool, UK

Pauline Richardson
Tutor, Beaconfield Marie Curie Centre, Belfast, UK

Anita Roberts
Inservice Training Officer, Liverpool Marie Curie Centre, Woolton, Liverpool, UK

Christine Searle
Tutor, Holme Tower Marie Curie Centre,
Penarth, UK

Val Smith
Tutor, Fairmile Marie Curie Centre, Edinburgh, UK

Norma Sutherland
Tutor, Hunters Hill Marie Curie Centre, Springburn, Glasgow, UK

Annie Topping
Senior Lecturer in Nursing and Health Studies, University of Huddersfield, Huddersfield, UK

Jan Viret
Tutor, Harestone Marie Curie Centre, Caterham, UK

Susie Wilkinson
Director of Studies, Liverpool Marie Curie Centre, Woolton, Liverpool, UK

Preface

Over the years Marie Curie Cancer Care has provided an education service to nurses in aspects of cancer prevention, detection and patient care. This is achieved through short courses, which include screening for cancer, the administration of cytotoxic drugs, communication with the cancer patient, palliative care and the care of the dying patient. These courses are offered at a number of centres in the UK and are available to all nurses. Marie Curie staff working in the hospice centres and Marie Curie nurses who work part-time caring for patients in their own homes can attend appropriate courses free of charge.

The aim of this text is to provide background information which will support all these courses and act as an introduction to cancer care for nurses who find themselves caring for cancer patients and their families. It is structured to cover all the topics associated with cancer, from prevention to palliative care and bereavement, and as such will act as a resource on those subjects for nurses working in other fields of care. By including subjects covered by the whole range of courses it is hoped that the individual reader will be encouraged to increase, by reading, his or her background knowledge of cancer, its treatment and patient care.

By broadening their knowledge, nurses will be better able to support their clients – educating them in cancer prevention, encouraging them to take up screening opportunities, supporting them and their families during treatment and palliation.

Jill David
London, UK

What is cancer? 1

Pauline Richardson

INTRODUCTION

People often refer to cancer as the big 'C' and think of it as a single disease, which it is not. The word 'cancer' is a generic term used to describe as many as 200 malignant diseases which arise in different tissues and cause different illnesses. There are therefore at least as many types of cancer as there are cell types in the body. Each of these has its own characteristics of incidence, spread and survival rates, but all share one common characteristic: that there is uncontrolled division of malignant cells, generally from a single primary site (Taylor, 1992). The multiplication of the cancer cells is not necessarily fast but is inappropriate (Currie, 1989).

To monitor changes in the incidence (new cases), types of cancers occurring and mortality from cancer, data have been collected over many years by national and international researchers. Their data come from sources such as death certificates, regional cancer registries, health authorities, hospitals and health research bodies who all collect their own data. Although errors can be introduced at all levels and the data collected by different groups may contain different facts, an overall picture can be built up of national and international patterns of cancer incidence and mortality (Muir, 1992). A number of fact sheets giving data on the incidence of cancers and cancer deaths in the 12 member states of the European Community is now available from the Cancer Research Campaign. These show some interesting national variations in the incidence of cancers, particularly those of the lung and breast, even between European countries (Europe Against Cancer, 1993). Similarly, data exist which show differences in the incidence of cancers according to social class (Kogevinas, 1992) and to occupation (Vainio, 1992). In the UK the number of people for whom the primary cause of death is cancer is recorded by the Registrar General and annual statistics on deaths are available from the Office of Population Censuses and Surveys (OPCS). Analysis of these figures shows that approximately one in three of the population in the UK will develop a cancer at some time in their life and that cancer is the identified cause of one-fifth of all deaths. Although cancer can occur at any age, and some forms, notably acute lymphoblastic leukaemia, are primarily seen in children, the figures demonstrate that cancer is a disease of the aged. The number of deaths from cancer rises steadily from the age of 40, with well over half the deaths from cancer occurring in the over-65-year age group (OPCS, 1992). The increase is rapid, with the cancer rate for those in the 65–69-year group being almost twice that of people aged 55–59 years (McCaffrey Boyle and Engelking, 1993).

International statistics on cancer rates compiled by the World Health Organization (WHO) show that cancer is a world-wide disease but that the rates for individual cancers vary from country to country. Some of these cancers can be related to international differences in behaviour and culture, for example dietary fat and breast cancer, smoking and occupational hazards (Doll and Peto, 1986).

THE HISTORICAL PERSPECTIVE

Cancer is a universal disease which has been known and written about for thousands of years. Whatever its earliest beginnings, cancer was known in most of the ancient civilizations. Signs of cancer have been found in skeletal remains dating back some thousands of years. By the sixth century BC cancer was sufficiently common to have been named and classified by the Greeks.

Their classification of cancers was initially attempted by philosophical enquiry, but later using more scientific measures they attempted to systematize their knowledge of cancer. The use of the word 'cancer', derived from *carcinos*, the word for crab, indicates a comparison between the behaviour of crabs and cancer and an appreciation of the hidden nature, irrational spread and infiltration of the disease. To Hippocrates (460–380 BC) the origin of all tumours was *atrablis* or black bile, which together with blood, phlegm and yellow bile constituted the four body humours. This was later expanded by Galen (AD129–199). Galen's system of tumour classification persisted with various adjustments until the beginning of the nineteenth century, when Bichat, a French pathologist, categorized 21 tissue systems of the body, each of which was ascribed its own vital force. Harmony between these vital forces was believed to produce health, while disharmony accounted for disease.

The work of Bichat, with that of other pathologists and histologists of the time, led to further attempts during the late nineteenth century to make a more modern classification system of cancers. By the beginning of the twentieth century the basis of our modern system had developed and this bore no resemblance to the approach taken by the Greeks. Further developments have taken place in this century, particularly since the 1950s, in light of the considerable increase in the understanding of cellular structure, function and biochemistry. More recently developments in technology have increased the ability to identify cellular changes and visualize tumours, and computers can assist diagnosis.

Whatever the scale of present-day knowledge and how deeply it is based in scientific research, the attitudes of the public and indeed many health care professionals to cancer remains largely uninformed and superstitious (Box, 1984). Their attitudes are based on the perpetuation of beliefs held, but disproven, before the beginning of this century. One commonly held belief is that cancers are infectious and can be caught like a cold or 'flu'. This simply is not true. Statistical evidence has established beyond reasonable doubt that cancer is not, in the general acceptance of the term, an infectious disease (Doll and Peto, 1986). In other words, people who are in close contact with those who have a cancer do not themselves have a higher risk of developing cancer.

Perpetuation of this belief, fuelled by the fact that cancer is a common disease, is something which can unfortunately lead to a great deal of distress – for example, when the person who has cancer feels that friends or relatives no longer visit because they fear that they might 'catch' the disease. The psychological deprivation engendered by this may serve to increase any fears and anxieties already held by the person with cancer. This in turn can lead to a decrease in self-esteem, feelings of worth and closeness with family and friends just at the time when the person is in the greatest need of comfort, help and support. Fear is further nurtured by the conspiracy of silence which often surrounds cancer. Questions about the nature and cause of cancers may be difficult to answer, particularly if you are yourself unsure of the facts. A recent publication, *Cancer Information at your Fingertips*, is a useful guide to the sort of questions which patients and their relatives ask and can act as a resource when answering their questions about cancer, its nature and treatment (Speechley and Rosenfield, 1992).

The ancient myths and mythicisms which have persisted over the centuries are only slowly being transformed. Surveys of public attitudes to cancer show that there are common misconceptions about cancer; for example, respondents in all the surveys reviewed by Box (1984), which dated from 1953 to 1973, believed that cancer killed more people than heart disease, although the number who believed that 'early treatment increased the chance of cure' rose slightly and those that believed 'cancer was never completely cured' fell over the 20-year time span. The fact that these beliefs still exist and that individuals reported that they did not always believe what health care professionals said, for example 'they say you must not smoke, but they smoke', are important reminders of how influential culture and the behaviour of others can be.

This century has seen an escalation in attempts to understand and treat cancer; new treatments receive publicity but their effects take some time to become apparent. Research and scientific developments have led to major advances in the classification, biology, detection and treatment of cancers. Campaigns such as 'Europe Against Cancer', which initiated the 10-point 'European Code Against Cancer' (see Chapter 2), aim to raise public awareness to the avoidable causes of cancer. More recently they have targeted general practitioners in a campaign to encourage them as professionals to give up smoking (Europe Against Cancer, 1993). Publicity for screening has raised awareness of the benefits of early detection, and groups such as the British Association of Cancer United Patients and their families and friends (BACUP) provide a telephone advice service for information and support for patients and the general public. There is, however, still a lot of work to be done.

The main reaction still aroused by cancer is fear. Not only fear of the disease itself, but also fear of the treatment (disfigurement and discomfort) and fear of the consequences of the disease in terms of outcome. The fear of the disease is engendered and increased by the fact that the disease does not have a uniform occurrence, affecting some but not others despite similar environmental, familial or ethnic conditions. Many smokers develop lung cancer, supporting the research which has appeared since the first publication by Doll and Hill in 1950 showing that smoking greatly increases the risk of lung cancer. In spite of this, in any group of individuals there is always someone who knew a person 'who smoked all their life but never got cancer'; the relative risks are clear but do not determine who will develop cancer (Europe Against Cancer, 1993). There are also some women who have a strong familial history of breast cancer who get the disease, while others in the same family are spared. Indeed it would appear that the only people who can be certain of not dying from cancer are those who die first from another disease! These inconsistencies are misleading to the public, who do not understand statistical evidence, and may help those with high-risk behaviours to justify their resistance to change.

For those who have been diagnosed as having cancer their biggest fear may be the perceived threat to their survival. This very real threat, as the individual sees it, may or may not be actual. Many cancers if diagnosed and treated at an early enough stage do not pose any immediate threat to life. The five-year survival rates for most cancers have increased since the 1950s (Doll and Peto, 1986) and are above 50% for breast, bladder, cervix and uterus, 85% for testicular cancer and 90% for skin cancers, excluding malignant melanoma (Consumers' Association, 1986). McCaffrey (1991) states that 'cancer boasts an overall cure rate greater than many other chronic illnesses and it has been predicted that cure rates will rise to 67% by the first decade of the twenty-first century'. The uncertainties of cure and survival alone are difficult to cope with; added to this are the patient's feelings of anxiety, anger, hope and despair, helplessness, and their lack of control over what is happening to them (Moorey, 1988). We all like to feel that we have some measure of control over what is happening in our lives. Patients frequently see that measure of control eroded by the 'something' growing within their body over which they have no means of restraint.

While cancer does bring great physical, psychological and practical problems, the scale of these problems can be minimized by knowledge of the facts in terms of what to expect, the treatments available and where to get help and support (Webb, 1988). Many publications are available for patients, their families and friends on cancer in general, specific cancers and their treatments. Some are listed at the end of this chapter; others will be found listed in the appropriate treatment chapters that follow and in the final chapter, 'Where to get help'.

CANCER: THE DISEASE PROCESS

Cancer, as stated above, is not one single disease but a group of over 200 diseases. Cancers can develop in any tissue of the body where an abnormal cell multiplies to produce an expanding mass of disorganized tissue known as a tumour. This tumour is usually a clone of cells that has enlarged by successive divisions from that one original deviant cell (Currie, 1989). Cancer is therefore a disease of the cell and is caused by whatever led it to become abnormal. Any consideration of the cause of the disease must therefore start at a cellular level.

All cells have the same basic structure of a nucleus which is surrounded by a nuclear membrane within cytoplasm and contained within the external cell membrane. The genetic information for the cell, which has to be replicated prior to being passed to the two daughter cells at cell division, is stored in the nucleus as deoxyribonucleic acid (DNA), whose long strands are coiled up to form the chromosomes. Information for cell activity is transferred from the nucleus to the cytoplasm by messenger ribonucleic acid (RNA).

NORMAL CELLS VERSUS CANCER CELLS

Normal cells

The tissues of the average adult are made up of over 100 different cell types, all with their individual programmed life spans. Some types of cell do not reproduce in the adult, for example cells of the heart muscle, brain cells and voluntary muscle cells. All other types of cell do reproduce but at vastly different rates which depend on need. The cells of the skin and gut are constantly being worn out and replaced, whereas in the kidney the requirement is so low it is practically undetectable. Throughout the body the timing of the formation of new cells is coordinated with the loss of existing cells. There are established mechanisms which are important in the control of cell activity. Normal cells have a balanced metabolism which is controlled by enzymes; cell maturation, the specialization into which they differentiate and their progress from immature to mature are pre-determined. They display the property of contact inhibition, where cells are able to recognize cells with similar characteristics as 'self' and those which do not as 'non-self'; they will not infiltrate 'non-self' cells.

Cancer cells

Cancer cells are cells which are out of control; they grow and multiply when they should not. Their metabolic requirement is uncontrolled, so that they keep demanding more energy. They lose the ability to differentiate and so cannot function as mature cells. Contact inhibition is also lost and the cancer cells can infiltrate into other tissue types; this leads to the spread of the cancer locally and eventually to its colonization of distant organs.

The extent to which the cancer cells have undergone a loss of differentiation is an important factor in determining their histogenesis. Tumours are given specific names depending on their tissue or cell origin. Some may have lost all resemblance to their tissue of origin and are known as anaplastic or undifferentiated. Others may still closely resemble the normal tissue in which they originated and are said to be well differentiated. Cancers exhibit a whole range of differentiation, from those which closely resemble the original tissue to those which bear no resemblance at all.

CLASSIFICATION OF TUMOURS

An abnormal growth of tissue is known as a **tumour**; this may be either benign or malignant. These terms are best described by listing the differences between these tumours.

- Malignant tumours have the ability to invade (infiltrate into) and destroy adjacent tissues. They can also spread to and grow in other tissues by cells which break off and are transported in the lymph or blood. Infiltration can lead to haemorrhage and organ failure, and the demands on energy to cachexia and an increased susceptibility to infection.
- Benign tumours grow by expansion; they occupy space and are, depending on the space occupied, potentially damaging. They can cause damage by destroying surrounding tissue or by exerting pressure on local nerves and blood vessels. In this way they also can be life

threatening, for example a benign brain tumour. Tumours can also secrete biologically active hormones (phaeochromocytoma). The growth rate of benign tumours is generally slower than that of malignant tumours which continue to grow even in starving people, leading to cachexia.

IDENTIFICATION OF TUMOUR TYPE

Four criteria are generally used in the identification of malignant tumours (cancers):

1. the anatomical site of the primary tumour, and metastases;
2. the tissue type and its histology;
3. the grade of malignancy;
4. the extent of tumour progression, based on size, degree of invasion and metastatic spread.

NAMES OF TUMOURS

With reference to the nomenclature of the various tumours, the simple use of the suffix '-oma' only following the tissue type usually indicates a benign tumour. For example, a lipoma is a benign tumour of fatty (adipose) tissue, while a liposarcoma is a malignant tumour of the same tissue. However, there are exceptions and to avoid confusion the word 'malignant' is used as a prefix for exceptions – for example, 'malignant melanoma'.

   The names of other malignant tumours or cancers are based on their histogenesis and are derived from the four main tissue types of the body, namely epithelium, connective tissue including lymphatic and blood cell-forming (haemopoietic) tissues, muscle and nerve tissue. In addition some tumours are also know by the name of the individual who first described the condition, for example Hodgkin's disease. The names of tumours and their classification can differ from country to country. In order to make figures comparable, particularly in clinical trials and other comparative situations, the WHO International Classification of Diseases in Oncology (Percy *et al.*, 1990) is the system most widely accepted.

THE PROCESS OF CHANGE

Most cancers originate from a single deviant cell. In the process of change from normal to malignant, the cell and its descendants will have accumulated several mutations (identified changes) in different genes. A single mutation is unlikely to result in malignancy. In the later stages of change the cell may be recognized as having increasing degrees of pre-malignant change. In some cases these can be identified during screening (cervical smear test) and can be treated (see Chapter 4).

At the cellular level the genes whose mutations are most likely to result in cancers which have, to date, been identified fall into two groups: oncogenes and suppressor genes.

Oncogenes

Normal genes whose mutation can cause the cell to become malignant are called **proto-oncogenes**; to date about 30 genes of this type have been identified in mammals (Prescott and Flexer, 1986). In the normal cell they perform an essential variety of cellular functions. If these proto-oncogenes are altered, often very simply, they can become oncogenes. The resulting oncogenes are similar to the genes that are active along the pathways which control cell growth. This suggests that the oncogene proteins interact with growth-controlling systems of the cell and so drive the cell towards malignancy. An oncogene is therefore a gene whose product is involved in inducing cancer (Taylor, 1992).

Tumour suppressor genes and anti-oncogenes

In normal cells tumour suppressor genes and anti-oncogenes are growth-regulating genes. Mutation or loss of these genes can result in the loss of normal regulatory function and restraint in cell growth, which then proceeds unrestricted (Taylor, 1992).

The process of change and its development at the cellular level to produce a tumour is called carcinogenesis. This is a multistage process which does not take place within the confines of a given time span. Exposure to a carcinogen (a cancer-inducing agent) does not immediately, and may in fact never, lead to the production of a tumour. The stages of change that occur are known as initiation, promotion and progression.

Initiation

This is the first step in the natural history of tumour development and reflects a permanent and irreversible change in the cell. The cell at this stage is exposed to a mutagen or transforming virus (the carcinogen). This exposure alters the DNA, which in turn leads to a switching on of oncogenes and/or the switching off of tumour suppressor genes and anti-oncogenes. The altered cell divides and a clone of initiated cells develops which may persist for some time without further growth or grow only slowly. In some individuals further development does not occur and a malignant tumour never develops.

Promotion

There are two ways in which promotion can occur. In one, further genetic alterations over a period of time lead to tumour development. In the other, interaction of the cell with environmental agents promotes tumour development; these include chemicals and viruses. In some cases both these processes are believed to be active, the promoting agents increasing the risk of cancer development by altering the rate at which normal cell proliferation occurs. This in turn increases the chance of genetic errors.

Progression

At this stage the tumour has malignant characteristics, including increased cell multiplication rate and the ability to invade neighbouring tissues. Cells which break off can form metastases by travelling in the blood or lymphatic system to distant organs.

CAUSES OF CANCER

There are many different factors involved in the development of cancers. It is clear that at some stage carcinogens and/or promoting agents must be present. These factors which influence the process of carcinogenesis are of varying origins. Viral, environmental and genetic factors are all agents which have been identified as having a possible part to play in one or all of the initiation, promotion and progression stages of a cancer's development (Doll and Peto, 1986). Examples of carcinogens and the stages at which they are believed to act are shown in Table 1.1.

Epidemiological studies would suggest that at least 80% of cancer incidence is broadly attributable to environmental factors. One of the earliest suggestions for this comes from the work of Dr John Hill in 1761, who established a link between snuff and nasal cancer (Hill, 1761). Later in that century, the physician Percival Pott (1775) identified the relationship between exposure to soot and the incidence of epithelioma of the scrotum in chimney-sweeps. This was therefore the earliest identified occupational cancer. Two centuries later, Sir Ernest Kennaway (Kennaway and Hieger, 1930) identified the actual chemicals present in coal tar which can cause cancer. The difficulty in identifying occupational cancers, and indeed many environmentally induced cancers, is that there is frequently a long time delay between exposure and the onset of cancer – for example in the case of asbestos-related mesotheliomas (Doll and Peto,

Table 1.1   Stages of carcinogenesis induced by specific agents

Class	Examples	Stage
Chemicals	Tobacco smoke, urethane, alfatoxin	Initiation
		Promotion
		Progression
	Phenobarbitone, dietary fat, calories	Promotion
	Prolactin, oestrogens, androgens	Promotion
	Asbestos, benzine, potassium arsenite	Progression
Radiation	Ionizing radiation	Initiation
	Ultraviolet B and C radiation	Progression
Biological	Papova, retro and Epstein–Barr viruses	(Promotion)
		Progression
	Herpes and hepadna viruses	Progression
Genetic	Transgenesis	(Promotion)
		Progression
	Selective breeding	Initiation
		Promotion
		Progression

1986). For the individual hoping to make a claim, liability may be difficult to prove.

Gradually over the last century understanding of cancer and its causes has been extended and developed. Its causes can now be identified as originating from environmental, chemical, viral and hereditary factors or any combination of these. The main problem for health educators is to persuade individuals and governments to reduce the identifiable risks of cancer such as smoking, alcohol consumption and a poor diet, particularly when these risks are pleasurable to the individual and profitable in terms of raising taxes. As health care professionals it is our duty to promote health, be aware of current research-based data and to be able to present that to our clients whenever possible. This process is enhanced by good communication skills, which include the setting of an example of healthy behaviour to the public.

REFERENCES

Box, V. (1984) Cancer: myths and misconceptions. *Journal of the Royal Society of Health*, 104(5), 161–6.

Cancer Research Campaign. 'Cancer in the European Community' fact sheets.

Consumers' Association (1986) Understanding Cancer. Which? Books. A Consumer Council Publication.

Currie, G. (1989) Cancer prevention and the new biology, in *Reducing the Risk of Cancers* (eds T. Heller, B. Davey and L. Bailey), Hodder & Stoughton, London.

Doll, R. and Peto, R. (1986) *The Causes of Cancer*. Oxford University Press, Oxford.

Europe Against Cancer (1993) *Europe Against Cancer Code: A Booklet for General Practitioners*. Print and Micrographic Services, 3M Health Care Ltd, Loughborough.

Hill, J. (1761) *Cautions Against the Immoderate Use of Snuff*. Baldwin & Jackson, London.

Kennaway, E.L. and Hieger, I. (1930) Carcinogenic substances and their fluorescent spectra. *British Medical Journal*, **i**, 1044–6.

Kogevinas, M. (1992) Social inequalities and cancers, in *Preventing Cancers* (eds T. Heller, L. Bailey and S. Pattison), Open University Press, Milton Keynes.

McCaffrey, D. (1991) Surviving cancer. *Nursing Times*, **87**(32), 26–30.

McCaffrey, D., Boyle, D. and Engelking, C. (1993) Cancer in the elderly: the forgotten priority. *European Journal of Cancer Care*, **2**(3), 101–7.

Moorey, S. (1988) The psychological impact of cancer, in *Oncology for Nurses and Health Care Professionals*, Vol. 2: *Care and Support* (eds R. Tiffany and P. Webb), Harper & Row, Beaconsfield.

Muir, C. (1992) Reliability of cancer data, in *Preventing Cancers* (eds T. Heller, L. Bailey and S. Pattison), Open University Press, Milton Keynes.

Office of Population Censuses and Statistics (1992) *Annual Mortality Statistics*.

Percy, C., Van Holton, V. and Muir, C. (eds) (1990) *International Classification of Diseases for Oncology*. World Health Organization, Geneva.

Pott, P. (1775) *Chirurgical Observations Relative to the Cataract, the Polypus of the Nose, the Cancer of the Scrotum, the Different Kinds of Ruptures, and Mortification of the Toes and Feet*. Hawkes, Clark & Collins, London.

Prescott, D.M. and Flexer, A.S. (1986) *Cancer: The Misguided Cell*. Sinauer Associates, Sunderland, MA.

Speechley, V. and Rosenfield, M. (1992) *Cancer Information at your Fingertips*. Cass, London.

Taylor, M. (1992) A simplified biology of cancers, in *Preventing Cancers* (eds T. Heller, L. Bailey and S. Pattison), Open University Press, Milton Keynes.

Vainio, H. (1992) Occupational cancer prevention, in *Preventing Cancers* (eds T. Heller, L. Bailey and S. Pattison), Open University Press, Milton Keynes.

Webb, P. (1988) Teaching patients and relatives, in *Oncology for Nurses and Health Care Professionals*, Vol. 2: *Care and Support* (eds R. Tiffany and P. Webb), Harper & Row, Beaconsfield.

FURTHER READING

Gowing, N. and Fisher, C. (1988) The general pathology of tumours, in *Oncology for Nurses and Health Care Professionals*, Vol. 1: *Pathology, Diagnosis and Treatment* (eds R. Tiffany and P. Pritchard), Harper & Row, Beaconsfield.

Heller, T., Davey, B. and Bailey, L. (1989) *Reducing the Risks of Cancers*. Hodder & Stoughton, London.

Hinwood, B. (ed.) (1993) *A Textbook of Science for the Health Professions*. Chapman & Hall, London.

RESOURCES

BACUP. Cancer Information Service booklets. From: BACUP, 3 Bath Place, Rivington Street, London EC2A 3JR.

British Medical Association (1987) *The BMA Guide to Living with Risk*. Penguin, London.

Cancer Research Campaign. Healthy Lifestyles series.

Health Education Authority. *Cancer Education: A Resource List*. From: HEA Information Dept, Hamilton House, Mabledon Place, London WC1H 9TX.

Imperial Cancer Research Fund. *Cancer: Cutting your Risk* (video). From: Plymouth Medical Films, Palace Vaults, 33 New Street, Barbican, Plymouth PL1 2NA.

Muir, C. (1992) Reliability of cancer data, in *Preventing Cancers* (eds T. Heller, L. Bailey and S. Pattison), Open University Press, Milton Keynes.

Royal Marsden Hospital patient information booklets. From: Haigh & Hochland, International University Booksellers, The Precinct Centre, Manchester M13 9QA.

Taking Action over Cancers. A Community Education Study Pack. The Open University, Milton Keynes.

Ulster Cancer Foundation/NI Health Promotion Agency. *Cancer in the Workplace: Health Promotion and Care Programmes*.

Promoting health and preventing cancer 2

Wendy Boothroyd

WHAT IS HEALTH PROMOTION?

If we are to attempt to answer this question and to plan and evaluate what we do when we are actively engaged in health promotion, we need first to consider what health is.

The most widely quoted definition of health is that presented in the Constitution of the World Health Organization (WHO, 1946):

> Health is a state of complete physical, mental and social well-being, and not merely the absence of disease or infirmity.

This definition has been much criticized, mainly because it is so idealistic. It does, however, help us to focus on two important points. First, health is defined positively as the presence of well-being and not just the absence of ill-health. Second, the definition is holistic, including mental and social, as well as physical components. It could be broadened further by the inclusion of fitness alongside well-being and the inclusion of emotional and spiritual dimensions in the holistic concept.

Health means different things to different people and insights into the way individuals regard health may be gained by discussing with colleagues, family, friends and clients what being healthy means to them.

The following, by no means exhaustive, list (Simnett, 1991) may help you to a better understanding of what health means to you.

Being healthy means:

- following my doctor's orders;
- being able to cope with the pressures of life;
- enjoying a satisfying sexual relationship;
- feeling in harmony with nature and the universe;
- being able to cope with changes in my life, such as bereavement;
- being objective and seeing things in perspective;

- accepting myself and the different sides of my personality;
- taking regular exercise;
- having access to medical treatment when I need it;
- rarely getting colds, and then only getting mild symptoms;
- being the ideal weight for my height;
- living until I am in my eighties;
- developing my potential throughout my life;
- never having a major illness or accident;
- being open and able to trust people;
- getting on well with my parents and family;
- being able to do what is expected of me, at home and at work;
- liking myself most of the time;
- not having any bad habits, such as smoking or taking drugs;
- being able to relax and enjoy my hobbies;
- being able to recognize and express my feelings while staying in charge;
- eating 'healthy' food.

As you read each statement, consider whether it represents an important aspect of your health and consider what you would add to and/or leave out of the list.

It is important that health promoters have an understanding of their own concepts of health as well as of the beliefs of their clients. Without this understanding, effective communication about health issues is unlikely to occur.

In 1984, the WHO proposed a concept of health as:

> The extent to which an individual or group is able, on the one hand, to realize aspirations and satisfy needs; and on the other hand, to change or cope with the environment. Health is, therefore, seen as a resource for everyday living, not the objective of living; it is a positive concept emphasizing social and personal resources, as well as physical capacities.

In this complex definition, health is seen as a positive resource which enables us to adapt, change and cope in an ever-changing world and helps us to fulfil our potential.

Seedhouse (1986) attempts to analyse the meaning of health and its implications for health care from a philosophical perspective. He maintains that health is fundamental to the quality of human life and to the achievement of human potential.

Health is influenced by many factors. Some individuals can control some of the factors which are important for good health, for example, by adopting a healthy lifestyle which optimizes good health, suits them and ensures a feeling of well-being. However, many factors which influence health are outside our control, except by collective action. Table 2.1 categorizes some of the factors influencing the health of the individual and of the nation.

Table 2.1   Factors influencing health

Individual and family level	Community level	Societal level
Individual lifestyle	Employment	Government
	Income	Law
	Housing	Economic strategies
Family lifestyle	Environment	Policies on health and social services
	Social services	Human rights
	Leisure facilities	
Personal network	Education	
	Health services	Policies on food, alcohol, tobacco, drugs
	Transport	Global politics
	Networks and	Environment and natural resources
	support	Communications networks
	Local policies	

The *Alma-Ata Report on Primary Health Care* (WHO, 1978) stated that:

> Health promotion seeks to enable individuals and communities to increase control over the determinants of health and thereby improve their health.
>
> It is, therefore, concerned not only with enabling the development of lifestyles and individual competence to influence factors determining health, but it is also concerned with environmental intervention to reduce factors preventing or prohibiting healthy lifestyles.

Tannahill (1985) developed a model to assist those involved in 'doing' health promotion to define and plan their interventions (Figure 2.1). Downie *et al.* (1990) recommended a definition of health promotion based on this model:

> Health promotion comprises efforts to enhance positive health and prevent ill-health, through the overlapping spheres of health education, prevention and health protection.

This model may be used to explore the roles individuals and communities adopt with regard to health promotion both personally, professionally and politically.

- **Prevention** includes such services as immunization, hypertension case-finding and cervical screening.
- **Health protection** is concerned with policies and legal and fiscal measures to protect health, such as a non-smoking policy in a health centre or an increase in tax on cigarettes.

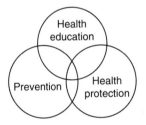

Figure 2.1   A model of health promotion (Tannahill, 1985).

- **Health education** involves the development of health-related life skills such as assertiveness, problem-solving and decision-making.

The areas of overlap include:

- **preventive health education,** which incorporates communications about healthy lifestyles and exploration of the reasons why preventive services are available and uptake of them beneficial;
- **preventive health protection,** which includes public health measures such as fluoridation of water supplies to prevent dental caries;
- **health education aimed at health protection,** which involves educating both the public and policy-makers about the reasons why health protection measures are desirable and securing support for them.

This model of health promotion reinforces the notion that the concept of health promotion involves both individual levels of action and action at the policy level. An example of this would be the policy to have a national programme for cervical screening, to provide this preventive service through primary health care and to offer financial incentives for general practitioners who have high levels of uptake by their patients. However, at an individual level, women need to be informed about the screening programme, its aims and how they might benefit, before making a decision on how to respond to the invitation.

The screening service should be sensitive to the concerns of the women using it and delivered in such a way as to encourage return visits as necessary. Sensitive communication of the results is important in promoting the mental health of the patient. The intervention should also be used as an opportunity to educate about related health issues.

PREVENTION AND PREVENTIVE HEALTH EDUCATION

Prevention can be differentiated into three levels: primary, secondary and tertiary (Baric, 1990).

- **Primary prevention** is concerned with preventing the onset of a disease; anti-smoking educational programmes, and the promotion of behaviours which avoid, limit and/or protect against sun exposure are interventions in this category which prevent lung and skin cancers respectively.
- **Secondary prevention** is concerned with the prevention of the further development of disease and mammography is an intervention in this category. This screening procedure detects cancers at an early stage and coupled with effective treatment prevents the progression of the disease.
- **Tertiary prevention** is concerned with clients who have been treated for disease and with minimizing their mental and physical disabilities,

assisting rehabilitation, raising competence and utilization of support systems. Self-help and support groups for cancer survivors fall into this category.

EFFECTIVE PATIENT HEALTH EDUCATION

Health education in health care settings frequently involves interviews with patients for 'diagnostic' purposes. These explore the health education needs of the patients and perhaps their families also. The needs are then analysed and followed up with communication of information and advice designed to bring about changes in behaviour which will maximize well-being and prevent the onset of, or progression of, disease. The reinforcement of that communication by several members of the health care team, by leaflets, posters and by group discussion, all help to increase the effectiveness of the health education intervention and to maximize patient compliance.

Tones (1977) points out that if health education is to be truly educational it must employ ethical methods which provide the client with genuine understanding without attempts at indoctrination or emotional manipulation. Clients must be aware of the range of options open to them. Hill *et al.* (undated) emphasize that, although health educators should not adopt coercive strategies, they should make use of the research available on compliance in order to be effectively persuasive in giving advice that, if heeded, is likely to benefit the patient's health and sense of well-being.

The long-standing medical model of health education assumes that giving people information results in their acquiring new knowledge which in turn influences their attitudes and eventually their behaviour, leading to improved health.

This is too simplistic and unreliable. Cust (1979) points out that blocks can occur at any point in the chain. Information about the hazards of smoking can lead to people acquiring new knowledge only if they are willing and able to understand the information. The new knowledge may then influence their attitudes to health and their desire to adopt new, healthier behaviours. There are, however, many smokers who are fully conversant with the hazards of their habit but who still regard smoking in a positive way. Those whose attitudes change may succeed in giving up smoking and improve their health, but inevitably there are some who, although they wish to change their behaviour, are unable to do so.

The health belief model (Becker, 1974) involves the identification of the main factors people take into account when they are deciding to take action about their health. It is the individual's **beliefs** about their susceptibility to a disease, the seriousness of the disease, the effectiveness of the change and the relative costs and benefits of the change which will influence their decision to adopt a recommended change in behaviour. The presence of a prompt or trigger (such as a health education message from a nurse) may also assist in promoting healthy changes.

USING THE HEALTH BELIEF MODEL

Patients' beliefs may or may not be correct, but it is those beliefs which will determine their health-related behaviour (Hill *et al.*, undated).

SUSCEPTIBILITY

Patients are unlikely to act in ways which will prevent disease unless they believe they are in some way vulnerable. It is therefore important to ask them about their beliefs.

Patients who smoke could be asked, 'What do you think are the risks you are taking by continuing to smoke?' If their reply indicated that they were aware of the risks of cancer and cardiovascular disease, it is evident that they already believe themselves to be susceptible. A reply such as 'Oh, my father smoked 20 a day and lived until he was 80; I think I'll take after him' indicates that the patient doesn't believe he or she is at risk.

In order to bring about change, this inaccurate belief needs to be challenged with appropriate information.

SERIOUSNESS

Patients are unlikely to act in ways which will prevent disease unless they believe the disease to be serious. Most people believe cancer to be serious, but with some other diseases, including cardiovascular diseases, people may play down the seriousness and have inaccurate beliefs about cures or the course of the illness. Patients who smoke may regard a heart attack as a 'good way to go' and may not understand the serious morbidity problems associated with cardiovascular diseases.

EFFECTIVENESS

If you are suggesting a patient discontinue a habit or change aspects of his or her lifestyle, he or she needs to believe that your prescribed course of action will be effective. A patient may say about smoking, 'It's a bit late to give up now'. In order to encourage change, this inaccurate belief must be challenged and positive information presented. You might, for instance, say that the incidence of lung cancer and cardiovascular disease among people who give up smoking is dramatically less than among those who continue to smoke and that, as an ex-smoker, they would breathe more easily.

COSTS AND BENEFITS

Whenever changes are contemplated, there are losses and gains to be taken into consideration. You can help your patients by exploring the costs related to the change and by emphasizing the benefits of the change.

To continue with the example of the patient who smokes, there may be worries expressed about the loss of cigarettes as a way of coping with stress and the potential unhappiness caused by weight gain. Support for your patients to help them find positive ways of coping with stress and to prevent weight gain is essential if they are to be successful in making the change from smoker to non-smoker.

CHANGE

Helping people to change their behaviour is not an easy task and it is helpful to understand the process of change. At first patients may have no interest in changing their risky lifestyle. They then may start to think about change. They are aware of the potential benefits of change and the risks of their current behaviour, but are not yet ready to attempt to change it. The next stage is the one where they take action. The benefits outweigh the costs and they adjust their behaviour and perhaps their lifestyle in order to accommodate the change. Finally, they achieve a stable state where the change has been accomplished and the new behaviour/lifestyle is maintained over time. Progression through this process of 'unfreezing' old behaviours, changing and finally 're-freezing' into a new pattern of healthier behaviours is often not steady. Patients may relapse and adopt their old behaviours again. If this happens, they need support and reassurance that they have not failed completely but have re-entered the phase of thinking about change and, when ready, can try again.

EFFECTIVE COMMUNICATION

Health education may be defined as:

> Communication activity aimed at enhancing positive health and preventing or diminishing ill health in individuals and groups,

through influencing the beliefs, attitudes and behaviour of those with power and of the community at large. (Downie *et al.*, 1990)

In the health care setting, you are most likely to be communicating with individuals and/or small groups, and Hill *et al.* (undated) provides a check-list for doing this effectively:

- Avoid **jargon** – patients may fail to understand you because you use professional expressions instead of layperson's language.
- Uncover **ignorance** – patients sometimes don't know things you expect them to know and may be reluctant to ask.
- Don't **overload** – if you say more than two things to a patient it is likely that something will be forgotten. It is up to you to assist their memory.
- Do **prioritize** – tell them the most important thing first.
- Do **emphasize** – if something is important, say so and use expression to stress it.
- Do **categorize** – put your points into categories which will help memory.
- Do **repeat** your key points and get your patient to do so as well.
- Use **short** words and sentences.
- Be **specific** with the advice you give – it makes it easier to follow.

CANCER EDUCATION

Let's try some word association. When you read the word 'cancer', what word or phrase comes into your mind? Were your thoughts negative or positive?

Cancers are a group of diseases feared by many and usually associated in people's minds with pain and death. Our feelings and beliefs about cancer develop not only from our knowledge about the subject, but also from our personal experiences of the disease. Approximately one in three people in the UK develop cancer during their lifetimes and one in four die of it, so that most people's lives are affected by cancer either personally or through significant others.

- Do **you** believe cancers can be prevented?
- Do **you** believe cancers can be diagnosed early enough to save lives?
- Do **you** believe cancers can be successfully treated?
- What do you **feel** about cancer treatments – surgery? radiotherapy? chemotherapy?
- What does cancer **cure** mean to you?

How people **feel** about cancer and what they **believe** to be true about cancer can have considerable influence on their behaviour with regard to many aspects of cancer prevention, early detection, treatment, rehabilitation and palliation.

Communicating about cancer may therefore be a more difficult task than communicating about some other health issues because of the negative feelings and beliefs that this disease may trigger in both nurse and patient. It is therefore important for nurses acting as health educators to elicit their own and their patients' feelings and beliefs and so reduce the barriers to effective communication.

EUROPE AGAINST CANCER PROGRAMME

In Europe as a whole there has been an overall increase in cancer incidence, and if this were to continue the one in three risk to the population of the UK would be the average throughout Europe by the year 2000. The Europe Against Cancer programme aims to reverse this trend and ensure that there are 15% fewer deaths from cancer by the year 2000.

In June 1985 the heads of state or government of the European Community agreed in principle on a European Programme Against Cancer. In January 1986 the Committee of Cancer Experts was set up to advise the European Commission on the formulation of the programme. The programme covers four areas: cancer prevention, health information and education, training of health personnel, and cancer research.

The first action plan of 1987–9 ended in 1989 with a European Year of Information on Cancer. Under the second action plan for 1990–4 this public awareness campaign continues, particularly in the context of Europe Against Cancer week, organized each year in the second week of October (Commission of the European Communities, 1990).

The European Code Against Cancer has been drawn up by the Committee of Cancer Experts and approved by the health ministers of the 12 member states and by all the cancer associations. The 10-point code states:

Certain cancers may be avoided –

1. Do not smoke. Smokers, stop as quickly as possible and do not smoke in the presence of others.
2. Moderate your consumption of alcoholic drinks, beers, wines or spirits.
3. Avoid excessive exposure to the sun.
4. Follow health and safety instructions at work concerning production, handling or use of any substance which may cause cancer.

Your general health will benefit from the following two points of the code, which may also reduce the risk of some cancers –

5. Frequently eat fresh fruits and vegetables and cereals with high fibre content.

6. Avoid becoming overweight and limit your intake of fatty foods.

More cancers will be cured if detected early –

7. See a doctor if you notice a lump or observe a change in a mole, or abnormal bleeding.
8. See a doctor if you have persistent problems, such as a persistent cough, a persistent hoarseness, a change in bowel habits or an unexplained weight loss.

For women –

9. Have a cervical smear regularly.
10. Check your breasts regularly, and if possible, undergo mammography at regular intervals above the age of 50.

Nurses are key workers in health promotion and, in order for the Europe Against Cancer programme to achieve its aim, it must be integrated into your field of activity. On a cautionary note, it is important to remember that the Europe Against Cancer programme is a disease-orientated programme based on medically orientated models of health education and health promotion and that, as such, it has intrinsic flaws. Behaviour change is advocated for reasons of risk reduction and disease prevention rather than for the positive values of the new behaviours themselves.

When incorporating the European code into any programme it is therefore essential to examine each of the messages and explore with and emphasize to the patient the positive values of the behaviour changes advocated. Austoker (1992) expands on each area of the code with reference to primary care.

SMOKING

Smoking is the single most important cause of cancer; Doll and Peto (1981) estimate that 30% of all cancer deaths are attributable to tobacco usage. These include most lung cancer deaths and a proportion of deaths from cancers of the mouth, pharynx, larynx, oesophagus, bladder, pancreas, kidney and cervix.

Approximately 400 000 Europeans die each year from smoking-related cancers (Peto, 1988). *The Health of the Nation* document (1992) in the UK sets as one of its objectives: 'to reduce ill-health and death caused by lung cancer – and other conditions associated with tobacco use – by reducing smoking prevalence and tobacco consumption throughout the population'. The target set is: 'to reduce the death rate for lung cancer by at least 30% in men under 75 and 15% in women under 75 by 2010 (from

60 per 100 000 for men and 24.1 per 100 000 for women in 1990 to no more than 42 and 20.5 respectively)'.

Nursing interventions may include implementing:

- smoke-free legislation and the creation of smoke-free work-places;
- smoking cessation counselling, anti-smoking education and structured smoking cessation programmes;
- anti-smoking educational programmes designed for employees in the work-place and for children in school;
- protocols into routine practice which incorporate gathering information about smoking behaviour and following up with advice and referral.

Nurses' attitudes may influence patients' smoking behaviour and for this reason it is important that you provide a positive role model by being a non-smoker and by creating non-smoking environments in your work-places.

ALCOHOL

Alcohol is carcinogenic in humans, and including its synergistic effect with smoking is responsible for up to 10% of all cancer deaths in Europe (Doll, 1989). Cancers produced by alcohol are those of the mouth, pharynx, oesophagus, larynx, liver and possibly of the breast and rectum. The risk of moderate alcohol consumption in the well-nourished, non-smoker is, however, small. Moderate consumption seems also to be associated with a reduced risk of cardiovascular disease. The health promotion messages with regard to alcohol consumption can therefore be related to sensible levels which, in units of alcohol, are no more than 21 units per week for men and 14 units per week for women – a unit of alcohol being a glass of wine, a half pint of beer or lager and a standard measure of spirits such as whisky or gin.

Nursing interventions should include assessment of clients' alcohol consumption and advice, counselling and referral of drinkers identified as being at risk.

SUN

Skin cancer is primarily caused by exposure to sunlight. There are three basic types of skin cancers: basal cell carcinoma, squamous cell carcinoma and melanoma. The non-melanoma types (basal and squamous) are highly curable, having a survival rate of over 95% with early detection and appropriate treatment. Malignant melanoma is the rarest of the skin cancers and is curable when detected early; however, advanced melanoma has a high mortality rate. Over the past decade there has been a dramatic increase in the incidence of and mortality from melanoma in the UK.

The Health of the Nation document (1992) sets as one of its objectives 'to reduce ill-health and death caused by skin cancers – by increasing awareness of the need to avoid excessive skin exposure to ultra-violet light'. The target set is 'to halt the year-on-year increase in the incidence of skin cancer by 2005'.

Skin cancer is preventable by avoiding, limiting or protecting against sun exposure. Prevention begins with educating patients about measures to decrease sun exposure:

- Avoid exposure between 10.00 a.m. and 3.00 p.m. when ultraviolet rays are most intense.
- Wear a hat, protective clothing and sun-glasses.
- Before exposure, apply a sunscreen with a sun protection factor of 15 or more and reapply at regular intervals.

The nurse's role in helping to prevent skin cancer should be to encourage patients to modify sun-seeking behaviour. The nursing assessment should identify individuals who are at greatest risk:

- hair blond or red;
- skin fair which burns and has poor tanning ability;
- large number of naevi and a tendency to freckle.

Advice should be given with regard to prevention and also to encourage patients to undertake skin surveillance and early reporting of any suspicious lesion. Patients should be advised to alert a doctor if an existing mole changes in size, shape or colour or if there is inflammation, oozing, crusting, bleeding or itchiness.

DIET

The evidence on diet and cancer is not conclusive but accumulating data indicate that modifications in the diet may reduce the risk of cancer by one-third (Doll, 1989). Dietary advice with regard to the avoidance of obesity (by reducing total calorie consumption, particularly consumption of fats) and the desirability of increasing consumption of fruit, vegetables and fibre is, however, justified.

Dietary intervention by nurses should be based on general guidelines for healthy eating, which is appropriate for the prevention of cardiovascular disease as well as cancer.

In providing dietary advice through nursing interventions there is a requirement for:

- consistent, accurate messages;
- simple information, advice and support;
- advice tailored to the needs of the individual;
- simple, well-illustrated leaflets to supplement verbal advice.

Referral for group support may be helpful for some patients.

EARLY DETECTION

In general terms, the earlier a cancer is detected, the greater is the chance of the patient being cured following appropriate treatment. Patients are often reluctant to 'bother' their doctor with symptoms, and nurses have a part to play in educating patients to be aware of their bodies and alert to changes which should be brought to medical attention if they persist for two weeks or more:

- a change in bowel or bladder habits;
- a sore that doesn't heal;
- unusual bleeding or discharge;
- a thickening or lump in the breast, testicle or elsewhere;
- indigestion or difficulty in swallowing;
- change in a wart or mole;
- nagging cough or hoarseness.

SCREENING

One of the objectives listed in *The Health of the Nation* is 'to reduce ill-health and death caused by breast and cervical cancer'. For these two types of female cancer, national screening programmes are in operation which aim to reduce rates of death from these diseases.

The targets set in England are:

To reduce the death rate for breast cancer in the population invited for screening by at least 25% by the year 2000 (from 95.1 per 100 000 population in 1990 to no more than 71.3 per 100 000).

To reduce the incidence of invasive cervical cancer by at least 20% by the year 2000 (from 15 per 100 000 population in 1986 to no more than 12 per 100 000).

Breast cancer is the most common type of cancer in women. One in 12 women will develop breast cancer at some time in their life. Breast screening by mammography followed by appropriate treatment of screen-detected cancers has been shown to reduce breast cancer mortality in women over 50 years of age. In the UK, screening is offered to women aged 50–64 every three years. Nurses have an important part to play in encouraging women to take up their invitations to be screened and discussing the benefits of screening. Women who are more knowledgeable about cancer and cancer screening are more likely to attend.

Women of all ages should be encouraged to be 'breast aware' and take opportunities to feel and observe their breasts whilst washing and dressing so as to become familiar with what is normal for their breasts. Any changes from this normal state should be brought to the attention of their doctor. It is particularly important that women who are entered into the screening programme remain breast aware through the intervals between screens.

Cervical cancer is less common than breast cancer and is largely preventable in women who attend regularly for screening (every three or five years). The smear test detects pre-cancerous changes in the cells of the cervix and therefore when these are treated they have no opportunity to develop into malignant cells.

Cervical smear tests are undertaken largely by practice nurses or general practitioners. The challenge to the nurse includes:

- providing educational materials to encourage patients to respond to invitations to be screened;
- to provide a sensitive service which will increase patient satisfaction and encourage return visits;
- to follow up laboratory results in ways which will reduce patient anxiety;
- to support the patient through the screening process and any follow-up procedures.

Nursing assessment should also include assessment of patients at increased risk of cervical cancer:

- genital infection
- smoking
- multiple sexual partners
- intercourse before age 20
- poor hygiene.

Where appropriate, advice with regard to reducing risk by modification of behaviour, such as the use of barrier-type contraceptives (condoms and diaphragms), should be given.

PROMOTING HEALTH AND PREVENTING CANCER

Nurses have an important role to play in promoting health and preventing cancer, and your effectiveness could be increased by the setting of appropriate health education targets and identifying ways of measuring performance. For example, a nurse who was concerned to address the issue of smoking could set the target: to increase the proportion of smokers who have received advice about smoking cessation.

Performance could be measured by:

- assessing all patients' smoking behaviour by direct questioning and recording whether they were smokers or non-smokers;
- discussing the benefits of non-smoking with smokers and offering a leaflet about giving up.

Follow-up after an interval would enable measurement of acceptability of advice and action taken by the smoker. This then enables the nurse to assess the appropriateness or not of the target and continue with or modify the approach. Target-setting, performance measurement and evaluation should be an integral part of all activities aimed at promoting health and preventing cancer.

REFERENCES

Austoker, J. (1992) *Cancer Prevention in Primary Care. Report to the NHS Management Executive.* Cancer Research Campaign, Oxford.

Baric, L. (1990) *Health Promotion and Health Education. Module I: Problems and Solutions.* Barns Publications, Altrincham, Cheshire.

Becker, M.H. (1974) *The Health Belief Model and Personal Health Behaviour.* Slack, New Jersey.

Commission of the European Communities (1990) *European File: Europe Against Cancer, Second Action Plan 1990–94.*

Cust, G. (1979) A preventive medicine viewpoint, in *Health Education, Perspectives and Choices* (ed. I. Sutherland), George Allen & Unwin, London.

Doll, R. (1989) *The Prevention of Cancers: Spreading the Message*, in *Reducing the Risk of Cancers* (eds T. Heller, B. Davey and L. Bailey), Hodder & Stoughton, London.

Doll, R. and Peto, R. (1981) *The Causes of Cancer.* Oxford University Press, Oxford.

Downie, R.S., Fyfe, C. and Tannahill, A. (1990) *Health Promotion Models and Values.* Oxford University Press, Oxford.

Hill, D., Heffernan, M. and Ley, P. (undated) *Effective Patient Health Education.* International Union Against Cancer, Geneva.

Peto, R. (1988) The future effects caused by smoking, in *Tobacco or Health: The Way Ahead*, Proceedings of the First European Conference on Tobacco Policy. WHO Regional Office for Europe, Copenhagen.

Rodmell, S. and Watt, A. (1986) *The Politics of Health Education: Raising the Issues.* Routledge & Kegan Paul, London.

Seedhouse, D. (1986) *Health: The Foundations for Achievement.* Wiley, Chichester.

Simnett, I. (1991) *The Nature, Agents and Competencies of Health Promotion.* Certificate in Health Education Open Learning Project, Health Education Authority, London.

Tannahill, A. (1985) What is health promotion? *Health Education Journal,* **44,** 167–8.

The Health of the Nation: A Strategy for Health in England (1992) HMSO, London.

Tones, B.K. (1977) *Effectiveness and Efficiency in Health Education: A Review of Theory and Practice.* Occasional Paper, Scottish Health Education Group, Edinburgh.

World Health Organization (1946) *Constitution.* WHO, New York.

World Health Organization (1978) *Alma-Ata Report on Primary Health Care.* WHO, Geneva.

World Health Organization (1984) *Health Promotion: A Discussion Document on the Concept and Principles.* WHO, Copenhagen.

RESOURCES

Resources for health promotion and cancer prevention are available from the following:

Health Education Authority, Hamilton House, Mabledon Place, London WC1H 9TX.

Health Education Board for Scotland, Health Education Centre, Woodburn House, Canaan Lane, Edinburgh EH10 4SG.

Health Promotion Agency for N. Ireland, 18 Ormeau Avenue, Belfast BT2 8HS.

Health Promotion Wales, Ffynnon-Las, Ty Glas Avenue, Llanishen, Cardiff CF4 5DZ.

Body awareness in the prevention and early detection of cancers 3

Norma Sutherland

THE DEVELOPMENT OF BODY AWARENESS

NORMAL GROWTH AND DEVELOPMENT

From the moment of birth, babies become aware of their bodies through experiences which may be of discomfort (cold, hunger and pain) or pleasure (warmth, contact with their mother and suckling). Infants learn to have discomforts alleviated by letting those around them know, in no uncertain terms, that they have a problem.

During normal growth and development the baby learns by exploring the world within reach, including his own body (Head, 1920). He learns what is pleasurable, repeats actions which he enjoys and learns how to get others to respond to him. Smiling, gurgling, sucking fingers, touching clothing, gnawing hands and grabbing anything available are all part of this voyage of discovery and are readily acceptable to parents and society in general.

Although a natural extension of this exploration, handling of the genitals or playing with excreta, by contrast, arouse anxiety in the same loving parents who have readily accepted their baby's other attempts at finding out about himself and the world around.

As he grows the child thus starts to receive two different sets of messages: one which tells him that 'this is OK' and another which tells him that 'this is not OK'. Sorenson (1973) points out that small children have been spanked and threatened with all sorts of dire consequences if they masturbate and can begin to develop feelings of guilt associated with sexuality and the genital area which will affect their future attitudes.

When they reach the stage of adolescence, young people become more aware of their body, its shape and size, and tend to compare themselves with their friends as counterparts. There is a need to conform with the peer group in terms of fashion and behaviour. They become concerned about being 'right' and have worries about their appearance, some of which may appear trivial to the adults around them. These may consist of excruciating anxiety about being the right height, too fat or thin, and girls worry about their breasts being too small or large. Boys worry about their sexual development because their genitalia have not developed at the same rate as their peers' or because they have no axillary or pubic hair. They just want to disappear when it comes to changing or showering at PE classes (Masters *et al.*, 1992).

As they grow through the pubertal changes, young people may also experiment with their bodies in ways which are perfectly normal and natural. However, if their upbringing has been restrictive and oppressive in the field of sexuality they may also develop a burden of guilt and fear which persists into adulthood.

The ancient Greek philosophy of Plato, especially in its subsequent development where the body is disparaged, has been absorbed into the culture over the centuries (Ferguson and Wright, 1988). Thus pleasure associated with the body and its functions has been disapproved of and has festered the thinking of many in society today. In spite of our permissive society the teaching of those ancient Greeks persists, so that even the normal development tasks of finding out about oneself have become guilt- and fear-ridden. Because of these misunderstandings some Christians have perpetuated this by teaching the philosophy in a somewhat tyrannical form, using threats and suggesting madness as a possible outcome of masturbation. Although this has not been recorded as a cause of insanity, the taboo remains, with all the consequent implications for health.

Through awareness of the body the individual develops an image of his body. This image develops throughout life and, as described above, changes with the influences of family, peers and society at large. The image built up has been described as having three main components: body reality, body ideal, and body presentation (Price, 1990). Body reality is the body as it exists, subject to its genetic make-up, the effects of living and ageing. The body ideal is the picture held by individuals of how they would like the body to look and perform, and body presentation is the effort employed to balance the reality and ideal images of the body. To do this the individual adapts through grooming, dress and the use of props. This is mostly for public consumption and is laden with symbolic value (Price, 1990). Thus many factors influence the development of the individual's body image.

CULTURAL EFFECTS

The culture in which the individual is brought up has a role in the development of body awareness. This can cause conflicts for people who are born into one culture and live within the society of another. For instance, in Western culture there is an emphasis on being slim. 'Slim' is considered to be more attractive than being 'fat', with the result that the overweight can be the butt of humiliating jokes and are said to be less successful in gaining promotion than their slim counterparts. This is especially true in the case of women. In the book *Fat is a Feminist Issue*, Susy Orbach (1978) puts forward the theory that women in Western society subconsciously resist the stereotype of 'the attractive slim little woman at home' by making themselves fat through over-indulgence in food. In other parts of the world being overweight or having a fat wife is considered to be desirable and is a sign of family prosperity.

While some cultural differences such as dress, diet and behaviour are governed by religious beliefs and rules, others are the subject of national identity, passing fashion or social class and thus change as the individual matures, changes jobs, marries or accesses different cultural areas.

PEER GROUP INFLUENCES

Most people are influenced by their friends and their peer group; this is the normal way to acquire new interests and integrate with the social group. In this setting they come to believe that some things are appropriate while others are not. Some may be pressurized to be involved in practices which are harmful to their bodies but which in the group setting appear to be 'good', social or pleasurable.

For the adolescent who has a desire to conform with the group, behaviour can be influenced by the norms of others (Ajzen and Fishbein, 1980) or by imitation of the behaviour of others (Bandura, 1986).

MEDIA INFLUENCE

The media is a very powerful influence: the attitudes and behaviour of the individuals portrayed on television, the big screen, at concerts and on radio impress the receiver with their lifestyle, appearance and behaviour. Here, too, commercial influences enhance these stereotypes by using actors in television and magazine advertising to promote their products and to convince society that they really cannot live adequately without the current in-vogue product.

INFLUENCES TO TAKE UP HARMFUL PRACTICES

Throughout life developing body awareness and image, sexuality, peer group and media pressure all interact to influence the susceptible individual to take up practices which can be harmful to health and in this instance increase the risk of cancer. Many factors are involved in reducing this risk, most importantly health promotion (see Chapter 2), governments, companies and the community. The ways in which this can be achieved are described in *Reducing the Risk of Cancers* (Heller *et al.*, 1991).

TOBACCO

Many people take up smoking as adolescents; at this time they may be persuaded to take up the habit by peer pressure or the media. They may do it out of rebelliousness, risk-taking or to seek attention (Vries *et al.*, 1992). Whatever the reason, advertising by tobacco companies must take some responsibility for promoting the habit in an attractive light. Women and young girls are particularly influenced by this type of advertising, seeing that by virtue of smoking they can be slim, confident, popular and full of sex appeal. While the number of smokers is in decline in other age groups it is increasing in young women and girls. As many as 25% of adolescents are smoking by the time they leave school (Murray *et al.*, 1983). The influence of peer group is also seen in female-dominated professions, where a higher proportion of women smoke than is seen in the general population (Harvey *et al.*, 1986). This was also found to be true for nurses working in the hospice setting (David, 1992). In some cultures where smoking is seen as an exclusively male habit boys express their transition from childhood to manhood by taking up the habit. In this and other settings the smoking habits of the parents are a direct influence on those of the children (Hyssala *et al.*, 1992).

The effects of passive smoking (Health Education Authority *et al.*, 1991) are also now coming to light as the influence of atmospheric tobacco smoke on the health of non-smoking individuals is researched. It has now been demonstrated that passive smoking can cause respiratory disease in children and lung cancer in adult non-smokers (Jarvis, 1992). As many as 300 deaths a year are now attributable to passive smoking (Russell *et al.*, 1986).

ALCOHOL

The use of alcohol is also publicized as an aid to self-confidence and a demonstration of grown-up behaviour. This can influence young adults at a time when they wish to appear 'cool', thus encouraging them to try it out and take up the habit for themselves. The number of young people receiving help for drinking problems has increased over recent years, as has under-age drinking. With alcohol implicated in the development of some cancers this is a cause for concern (Gillis, 1988). Drinking is an acceptable social activity in Western cultures, where it is associated with togetherness and shared experiences by young couples (Hyssala, 1992). Those who do not partake are seen as abnormal and those who do are entrapped by the enjoyable experience.

EXPOSURE TO THE SUN

A sun tan is generally considered to give the individual a healthy look. It is also a status symbol in that the tan indicates a holiday in sunny climes or on the ski slopes. It is hardly surprising then that when on holiday people try their best to get a tan as quickly as possible in spite of recommendations to the contrary. In the media and in fashion magazines heroes and models are shown as bronzed and beautiful, suggesting to the young that this is the model they should aspire to. Skin cancer is the commonest form of cancer; it is also the cancer most easily prevented, diagnosed and treated (Quinlan, 1992).

IMPLICATIONS FOR HEALTH

BODY IMAGE AND SELF-ESTEEM

An individual's view of him- or herself (body image) is closely linked to feelings of self-worth and self-esteem. Thus, a healthy body image is felt by the individual to be an attribute which will enhance his self-image (Price, 1990). As a contrast, feeling less than perfect physically may lead the individual to resort to doing things which will make him feel better. He hopes that society will then look at him with a kindly eye. Large amounts of money are therefore spent by people who wish to look good, because looking good makes them feel better and more acceptable to others (Johnson, 1990). Most human beings enjoy company and being invited to socialize, hence they do things which make them part of the group. Some of these things seem strange to some people but are relevant to the people involved. For example: imagine the mother who considers herself to be fairly liberated but is confronted by her younger son sporting a yellow and red Mohican tuft. It was hardly surprising that she, in her own words, 'literally flipped'; however, for her son his appearance made him one of the group.

ENCOURAGING POSITIVE HEALTH

Most people have some idea of how healthy they are. This may be influenced by how they see themselves and how they perceive their activities. When it comes to their risk of disease, in this case cancer, they are less able to define the risks or practise positive health activities such as attending for check-ups or screening. In a review of public attitudes to cancer Box (1984) states that in the USA up to 36% of people go for health checks, while in the UK general practitioners do not encourage this practice. Hopefully attitudes are changing. The same review reports a lack of knowledge about the early warning signs of cancer and a pessimistic attitude to survival.

Younger individuals are less concerned about their health, which they generally equate with physical fitness (David, 1994). This ongoing research suggests that they see their risks of developing cancer as low and are not concerned that they practise habits which are dangerous to their health. These attitudes can affect the individual's uptake of positive health practices such as quitting smoking, using sunscreen or reducing drinking, and make it difficult to encourage self-examination and attendance at screening clinics.

ACCEPTABILITY OF SCREENING

Screening or an examination by another person may not be acceptable to the individual who has been brought up to think that touching the sexual organs is 'not nice'. In addition to this, the publicity of facts like 'women who have multiple partners are at greater risk of cervical cancer' (Kogevinas, 1992) could deter women who are at the greatest risk from attending for screening. The uptake of screening services can also be made more difficult if those who are intended to benefit are full of unfounded displeasure, guilt and fears related to their bodies. This applies to both men and women, so that care and sensitivity are always required by those who staff clinics and screening units.

SELF-CARE

Understanding of the development of body image and self-esteem will help in the promotion of self-care to vulnerable groups and individuals or to those who are responsible for them (Price, 1990). Helping people to feel good about themselves may help to overcome resistance to positive health promotion messages. This subject is well covered by Ewles and Simnett (1985) (see Further reading list).

PROMOTING GOOD HEALTH

There is now a body of knowledge which supports the view that a healthy lifestyle, including good eating habits, exercise and positive attitudes to life, can be protective against some forms of cancer (Iverson, 1992). Men and women who go on strict diets and then regain the weight they have lost soon afterwards are more predisposed to cancer than those who maintain appropriate body weight through good eating habits.

This does not mean that we should become a nation of faddy eaters. Far from it. We should be aware, however, of foods that are tasty and provide us with satisfaction from hunger as well as being good for us (Nutrition Matters, 1990). Books about diets abound, as do slimming clubs, health clubs and some rather weird and wonderful groups who promise to make people slim but whose main function is to make a profit.

A major problem is that people go on a diet then come off a diet. Instead they should be changing to a more healthy style of eating long term; this is beneficial, and while there may be treats these should not be the mainstay of eating (Iverson, 1992).

Helping men and women to approach lifestyle changes in a positive way is a challenge for the nurse, and no less so when the nurse is also one of the people trying to change. Identifying causes of stress and learning how to use positive coping strategies can help (SHEG, 1989).

An appropriate use of complementary therapies such as herbalism, aromatherapy and relaxation may assist in the reduction of anxiety and promote a feeling of well-being during a change in lifestyle.

CONTROL AND HEALTH

Supporting clients in their own positive health practices but still leaving them in control has been shown to be much more effective than telling them where they have gone wrong and what they ought to do instead. Effective ways of achieving this are through self-monitoring (Bertera and Cuthie, 1984) and personalized health information (Glynn and Manley, 1989). Family economics, personal preferences and being empowered to make decisions and exercise choice in the selection of food will also have an effect on the food chosen by the younger generation while growing up. Patterns of eating which used to be passed down from generation to generation are gradually being eroded; as eating out becomes more popular different types of food are consumed – some for convenience, others for pleasure (Wheelock, 1992).

Obesity is linked to the incidence of cancer of the uterus, and the intake of dietary fat to cancers of the breast in women (Carroll, 1985), to endometrial cancer (Hill and Thompson, 1984) and to cancer of the bowel. There are also indications that salt plays a part in stomach cancer. On the positive side, increases in consumption of fruit and vegetables which provide dietary fibre have a protective effect (Wheelock, 1992).

If eating food is used to give comfort during periods of stress, then assisting people to find other coping strategies which are more beneficial and less of a threat to health is important. When positive coping skills are in place then it is helpful to find if there are problems which would benefit from being shared and aired. In a society which brings boys up to 'be good and don't cry' it may be difficult for men to admit to not being able to cope. Building a relationship of trust is important and may take some time. Meanwhile if they have been taught positive coping strategies they are doing something good for themselves instead of using food, alcohol or cigarettes to excess.

Examples of coping are rest and relaxation, and the 'three P' exercises. These three Ps are: 'pink, perspiring and panting'. Any exercise which can be done safely and which causes the three Ps is good for coping and produces a 'feel-good' sensation. Some psychiatric units are now using exercise in the treatment of depression because of its 'feel-good' factor. In the management of stress the exercise should be of a non-competitive nature, otherwise competition forces the sufferer on to a treadmill of stress (*SHEG Guide to Women's Health*).

CANCER PREVENTION AND SELF-AWARENESS

For the individual, awareness of his or her normal body appearance, behaviour and interaction with the environment is the key to identifying changes. The individual also needs to be aware of the changes which occur normally with age.

SKIN CANCERS

Since the 1930s it has become fashionable to have a tan. More of the body is exposed and people who did not in the past expose themselves to the sun are doing so. Skin cancers have increased most particularly in women. Although associated with exposure to the sun it is not necessarily exposure to Mediterranean sun, as was found by MacKie and Aitchinson (1982) in their study in Scotland. The most worrying fact is the high proportion of melanomas. Projects in Australia, The Netherlands and the USA aim to identify skin cancers at an early stage by taking screening services to the beaches or holding skin cancer fairs, where advice can be given and identification made (MacKie, 1992).

A tanned skin may look nice and healthy but it is in fact a damaged skin. Exposure to the sun also increases the ageing process in the skin and care is needed to reduce these effects (Body Shop, 1993). For children care is particularly important because exposure to the sun in childhood increases the risk of skin cancer at a later age (MacKie, 1992).

Precautions

When on holiday or when working in the sun it is important to protect the skin using sun-blocks or lotions with skin protection factors (SPF). The protection offered by these preparations varies but is related to the increase in time that the individual can be exposed to the sun without burning; for example, an SPF of 10 allows the user to stay out in the sun 10 times longer than if no application were made. To tan safely it is recommended that a high protection of SPF 15 or more (depending on skin type and conditions) be used initially and the protection reduced gradually over a period of days or weeks. Some individuals will never be able to reduce the SPF however long they are in a sunny climate. It should also be remembered that exposure is just as damaging when it is not hot: skiing, walking in a cool breeze or sitting in the shade are all equally risky and protection should be used either in the form of a skin protection lotion or long-sleeved clothing.

People with a fair skin (red-heads) are most at risk, as are young children. Their skin should be liberally spread with repeated applications of high-protection lotion or sun-block (SPF 25) as long as they are exposed and they should wear a T-shirt in the sun or shade. A hat should be worn to protect the face and back of the neck, although compliance can be difficult! If children have been in the water sun-block should be reapplied and it is important to follow the manufacturer's instructions.

The Australian health authorities, dismayed by the numbers of people who have skin cancer and being aware that early exposure has had a large part to play in causation, have introduced the slogan 'SLIP, SLOP, SLAP', which stands for: 'SLIP on a T-shirt; SLOP on the sunscreen; SLAP on a hat'.

The dangers of exposure to sunlight are not confined to the natural form. Sun-beds and artificial tanning lamps should also be used with caution, as the ultraviolet A emission produced by these lamps places the user at risk of developing melanoma (MacKie, 1992). It is essential to wear the goggles provided and not to stay on the sun-bed longer than is recommended by the manufacturer.

Checking for skin changes

Self-awareness is vital to the early detection of skin cancers – found early, many can be cured. Skin self-examination (SSE) takes only a few minutes (Friedman *et al.*, 1985). When examining the skin the individual needs to be aware that not every change is indicative of skin cancer. Knowing and looking at one's own skin is the first and most important stage. Familiarity with its normal appearance, position and number of moles and freckles on the skin helps in the identification of changes. Finding that a mole has changed in appearance, in colour, shape or size, or that there is a discharge or bleeding or newly grown hairs are signs that medical advice should be sought (Quinlan, 1992).

Some people put off seeking advice because they are frightened by the possibility of cancer and hope that the problem will go away. Time wasted before seeking diagnosis can make a difference to the prognosis and for 'at risk' individuals the importance of early detection should be stressed. Government awareness of this problem has led to the encouragement of screening clinics for skin cancers in some countries and more recently in the UK. Marie Curie Cancer Care now includes examination of the skin in its screening courses for practice nurses (Marie Curie Cancer Care, 1994).

BREAST CANCER

Breast cancer is the most common cancer in women and it is estimated that one in 12 women in the UK will develop breast cancer (Cancer Research Campaign, 1988). Advances in treatment have brought some improvement in survival but the most crucial factor is the stage at which the cancer is diagnosed. Breast self-examination (BSE) is the best way of detecting the early signs.

The majority of women of reproductive age are aware that there are monthly changes in their breasts. It is important for women to be aware of these changes, particularly when they have lumpy breasts with lumps which fluctuate over the month. In this younger age group very few lumps turn out to be malignant but it is still important to have them checked because of the danger of breast cancer in younger women (Austoker and Evans, 1992). Remembering the discussion above about the growth and development of body awareness, people's attitudes to touching and examining their breasts are likely to vary considerably. In some instances women may feel that to carry out BSE is 'bad' and some may not even like looking at their breasts in the mirror (Scottish Health Education Group: *Well Woman*), while some may not have an appropriately private or suitable mirror to look in. In addition women who are visually impaired will also have problems.

When teaching BSE it is important to consider these problems and call upon creative thinking in suggesting solutions to problems which women may have.

Teaching BSE

There are several useful leaflets (HEA; SHEG; Tomlinson and Scott, 1992) available for distribution which have either line drawings or photographs which depict the routines recommended for examining the breasts. These are useful to support teaching but are not in themselves sufficient.

Women may become anxious that they are 'not doing it right' or are not sure that what they are feeling is normal. It makes sense therefore to demonstrate the technique and show the individual what is and is not normal. This can then be supported by a leaflet such as the latest one from the Breast Care and Mastectomy Association which takes this approach (BCMA, 1993). A visit to the well women's clinic is the ideal time to teach this skill and to explain to the woman the best method for her. During the examination the practitioner can draw the woman's attention to what is normal for her and give reassurance.

Alternative teaching methods include groups where discussion and the sharing of ideas can take place. This type of session can help to get the message across and if well handled can also provide the health professional with information about the current state of women's knowledge of general health issues. It will provide an opportunity to deal with myths about how cancer is 'transmitted' and how it can be prevented. For women who cannot face the possibility of someone else touching their breasts this is a good opportunity.

Videos can be helpful to support teaching in groups or for individuals; however, it should be remembered that the models used have pleasant-looking breasts of very average size and this could be 'off putting' for women with large or pendulous breasts. In addition this group would probably appreciate advice on how to go about examining their breasts. Before embarking on teaching BSE to clients it is an advantage for the nurse to take a proper course in breast screening; this will give confidence and ensure that clients receive the best possible advice (see Chapter 4). For women who are post-menopause, examination by mammography is more effective because the breast tissue is less dense.

Mammography

A mammogram is a specialized X-ray picture which shows up the breast tissue. Possible malignant changes can be detected at a very early stage, often before they can be felt manually even by skilled practitioners. Because the picture obtained by taking the X-ray is clearer in older women and because the over-fifties are more at risk, mammograms are offered to women of this age in the UK every three years. Taking the mammogram is quick and simple, although for some women it can cause discomfort when the breast is squashed against the X-ray plate to get a clear picture. The procedure and the reason for this action need to be explained because women who have been hurt could be unwilling to attend for the next screening. However, under the UK programme of screening for the over-fifties care has been taken to write encouraging invitations, be flexible with appointments and to explain the procedure.

Detecting breast changes

When women are taught BSE it is important that they know how breast cancer presents (Devitt, 1983) and what changes they should report. These include:

- changes to the shape and contour of the breast;
- changes in appearance of the skin – puckering or dimpling;
- discharge from a nipple;
- new or unusual lumps – women with naturally lumpy breasts may find this difficult and will appreciate help in doing this.

Nurses need to remember that women may associate their breasts with their femininity and the potential loss of a breast or surgical intervention may be seen as robbing them of their femininity. Self-esteem and body image are intrinsically tied together and although a woman may realize that she needs medical help, she may be slow to seek it because of the possible consequences. Difficulties in accessing a medical consultation may also deter her: busy surgeries with appointment systems where patients have to tell the receptionist 'what is the matter' can easily put off a woman already embarrassed and made sensitive by her problem.

This is when the woman needs a listening ear and the advice of an understanding nurse. It is a time when there are decisions to be made and it is better to base these on fact than on old wives' tales.

TESTICULAR CANCER

For many years screening has been concerned mostly with women's health issues and it is only in the past 10–12 years that men's health issues have been addressed and well man clinics established. Screening tests at these clinics tended to concentrate on executive health problems like high blood pressure but other areas, including testicular self-examination (TSE), are now included.

Testicular cancer is largely age-related, affecting adolescent and young males up to the age of 35 years, although it may occur at an older age (Blackmore, 1991). As with breast cancer, when detected early testicular cancer can be treated and has a high cure rate.

Persuading young men of the need and teaching them to carry out TSE could be a problem. Having been chastised as young children for 'playing with themselves' they are now being actively encouraged to examine in detail their 'naughty bits'. Old taboos still remain and health promotion in this area should include information to parents and carers so that they understand what needs to be done and why TSE is being encouraged.

People who teach TSE should be competent and ready to answer all the questions which the opportunity offers. Leaflets are available which can be used as adjuncts to one-to-one or group teaching (Johnson, 1992, 1993). There is also an excellent video produced by Europe Against Cancer which explains and demonstrates TSE. The examination is best undertaken after a warm bath, when the skin of the scrotum is soft and more easily manipulated. Each testicle should be examined in turn for unusual lumps or textures. Explanation of the anatomy of the scrotum and testis needs to be explained so that boys can identify the epididymis and not be alarmed that it is a lump.

The need to report abnormalities quickly should be stressed and fears that treatment may cause sterility addressed. The belief that orchidectomy may lead to not being a 'real man' is a real problem but when compared with normal young men patients who have had this operation and been supported sympathetically are no more likely to suffer at a later date (Blackmore, 1988). The possibility of sperm banking can also be explained; this can support those who are loath to seek help because they fear sterility, which is not, however, always a side-effect of treatment (Blackmore, 1991).

CHANGES IN BODILY FUNCTION

There are other signs and symptoms worthy of note in relation to body awareness. Any change in function could be an indicator of disease. It is easy to develop awareness of things which can be seen or physically touched or felt such as moles and lumps. If we are to provide clients with a cancer screening service which is complete, informative and beneficial we need to be able to help them become aware of other potential indicators of cancer.

Bleeding

Any unexplained bleeding from any source needs to be investigated. Bleeding from the bladder or bowel is not normal, nor is it normal for blood to be coughed up or to appear in vomit; all these symptoms should be reported to a doctor. The cause of the bleed may not necessarily be cancer, however; infections or haemorrhoids which cause bleeding should nevertheless be investigated. Any unusual bleeding from the vagina, such as bleeding between periods and any bleeding after menopause, requires urgent investigation.

Regular attendance at cervical screening clinics should be encouraged to detect pre-malignant changes which can be treated. The nature of the examination does inhibit some women and recent publicity about errors in the procedure may have reduced confidence in the technique. This has, however, led to renewed efforts to ensure the quality of this service which will be of benefit to all (see Chapter 4).

Cough and hoarseness

The symptoms of lung cancer are often non-specific, so that the condition is well advanced before more definite signs and symptoms are experienced (Smits, 1991). Cough is a presenting symptom in 80% of cases, together with dyspnoea, sputum and possible haemoptysis (Smits, 1991). Any persistent cough which does not appear to be caused by infection and particularly when it is accompanied by hoarseness or loss of weight merits immediate investigation. The individual may not feel unwell and may put the cough down to smoking habits and put off seeking advice because he fears being told to give up smoking. Such delays can be dangerous and referral should be encouraged.

Bowel changes

Colorectal cancer is the second most common cancer in the UK, accounting for 12% of deaths, and is more common in the elderly (Topping, 1991). A change in bowel habit is often the first sign that there is something wrong; this can take the form of either diarrhoea or constipation. Although these can be brought about by a change in diet (increased fibre intake), occurring without any apparent cause they are a cause for concern.

The loss of fresh blood per rectum is easily recognized; changes in the colour of stools as well as their frequency are also indicators of bowel disease. Darkened stools can indicate small bowel cancer.

Changes in body weight

Of all the symptoms associated with cancer, weight loss is probably the one most frequently linked with the disease by the general public. Initially, weight loss may be welcomed but in time it becomes an embarrassment to the individual as clothes do not fit or people make comments about how thin they are. Similarly a perceived weight gain or increased girth, which is mistaken for 'middle-aged spread' and commented upon as such, can be the presenting feature in ovarian cancer. These kinds of comments, although unkind, may be helpful in that they send people to the doctor before they become unwell. Body image plays an important part in self-esteem and if people feel that they look unusual they will normally attempt to do something to combat this and become socially acceptable again. It is better to visit the doctor and be told that the problem is a dietary one than to wait too long, only to discover that the condition might have been treatable if diagnosed earlier.

To get these health messages across, it would be helpful to encourage behaviours which promote health. Iverson (1992) and colleagues have formulated a programme of 20 principles which characterize successful behaviours in health promotion. These include moves to educate the population at large, develop effective low-cost programmes, and identify characteristics of behaviour which initiate positive actions and the characteristics of non-participants in health care programmes. They suggest new initiatives, education in schools and the use of mass media as well as the development of individual programmes. Their suggestions are wide ranging and consider that everyone has a part to play. To this end it would be useful if all places of work had some occupational health input and if leaflets and books on health screening could be available in the work-place.

HELPING PEOPLE TO BECOME BODY AWARE

Before attempting to encourage other people to become body aware it is important to be well prepared, and to ensure that we have the knowledge to guide them and to support our arguments for self-examination.

These skills include:

- a knowledge and understanding of cancer;
- the prognosis of the individual cancers and their presenting symptoms;
- competency in teaching BSE, SSE and TSE;
- knowledge of the early signs of cancers, for example when a mole needs investigation;
- understanding of the social taboos which may inhibit self-examination;
- a knowledge of health promotion materials currently available.

In addition it is important, as an individual about to embark on teaching a subject involving very personal matters, that we examine our own feelings to discover any personal 'hang-ups' we may have with our own body image.

Most of the other chapters in this book are relevant to developing these skills, in particular Chapter 1 on the nature of cancer, Chapter 2 on promoting health, Chapter 4 on screening and Chapter 9 on communications. Additional material is also included in the references, resources and further reading lists.

REFERENCES

Ajzen, I. and Fishbein, M. (1980) *Understanding Attitudes and Predicting Social Behaviour*. Prentice Hall, Englewood Cliffs, NJ.

Austoker, J. and Evans, J. (1992) Breast self-examination, in *Preventing Cancers* (eds T. Heller, L. Bailey and S. Pattison), Open University Press, Milton Keynes.

Bandura, A. (1986) *Social Foundations of Thought and Action: A Social Cognitive Theory*. Prentice Hall, New York.

Bertera, R.L. and Cuthie, J.C. (1984) Blood pressure self-monitoring in the workplace. *Journal of Occupational Medicine*, **26**, 183–8.

Blackmore, C. (1988) The impact of orchidectomy upon the male with testicular cancer. *Cancer Nursing*, **2**(1), 33–9.

Blackmore, C. (1991) Nursing patients with testicular cancer, in *Oncology for Nurses and Health Care Professionals*, Vol. 3: *Cancer Nursing* (eds R. Tiffany and D. Borley), Harper Collins, London.

Body Shop (1993) *Be Safe under the Sun*. The Body Shop, West Sussex, UK.

Box, V. (1984) Cancer myths and misconceptions. *Journal of the Royal Society of Health*, **104**(5), 161–6.

Breast Care and Mastectomy Association of Great Britain (1993) *Breast Awareness*. BCMA, London.

Cancer Research Campaign (1988) *Breast Cancer*. Cancer Research Campaign, London.

Carroll, K.K. (1985) Diet and breast cancer: experimental approaches, in *Diet and Human Carcinogenesis* (eds J. Joosens, M. Hill and J. Geboers), Excerpta Medica, Amsterdam.

David, J. (1992) A survey of hospice staff smoking behaviour and their opinions on smoking at work. *European Journal of Cancer Care*, **1**(5), 19–21.

David, J. (1994) Personal communication.

Devitt, J. (1983) How breast cancer presents. *Cancer Medical Association Journal*, **129**, 43–7.

Ewles, L. and Simnett, I. (1985) *Promoting Health*. Wiley, Chichester.

Ferguson, S. and Wright, D. (eds) (1988) *New Dictionary of Theology*. IVP, London.

Friedman, R.J., Rigel, D.S. and Kopf, A.W. (1985) Early detection of malignant melanoma: the role of the physician – examination and self-examination of the skin. *CA-A Journal of Physicians*, **35**(3), 130–51.

Gillis, C. (1988) The epidemiology of human cancers, in *Oncology for Nurses and Health Care Professionals*. Vol. 1: *Pathology, Diagnosis and Treatment* (eds R. Tiffany and P. Pritchard), Harper & Row, Beaconsfield.

Glynn, T.J. and Manley, M.W. (1989) *How to Help your Patients Stop Smoking*. National Cancer Institute, Bethesda.

Harvey, S., MacLeod Clark, J. and Kendall, S. (1986) Nurses and smoking education: a literature review. *Nurse Education Today*, **6**, 237–43.

Head, H. (1920) *Studies in Neurology*. Oxford University Press, Oxford.

Health Education Authority. *A Guide to Examining your Breasts*. HEA, London.

Health Education Authority, Health Education Board of Scotland and ASH (1991) *Passive Smoking: Questions and Answers*. HEA, London.

Heller, T., Davey, B. and Bailey, L. (eds) (1991) *Reducing the Risks of Cancers*. Open University Press, Milton Keynes.

Hill, M.J. and Thompson, M.H. (1984) Role of endogenous carcinogens, in *Risk Factors and Multiple Cancer* (ed. B. Stoll), Wiley, London.

Hyssala, L., Rautava, P., Sillanpaa, M. and Tuominen, J. (1992) Changes in the smoking and drinking habits of future fathers from the onset of their wives' pregnancies. *Journal of Advanced Nursing*, **17**, 849–54.

Iverson, D.C. (1992) Programme principles associated with successful health education and health promotion interventions, in *Preventing Cancers* (eds T. Heller, L. Bailey and S. Pattison), Open University Press, Milton Keynes.

Jarvis, M.J. (1992) Passive smoking, in *Preventing Cancers* (eds T. Heller, L. Bailey and S. Pattison), Open University Press, Milton Keynes.

Johnson, M.H. (1992) Promoting testicular self-examination. *Journal of Cancer Care*, **1**(1), 55–6.

Johnson, M.H. (1993) Promoting testicular self-examination. *Journal of Cancer Care*, **2**(1), 20–1.

Johnson, R. (1990) Restructuring: an emergency theory on the process of losing weight. *Journal of Advanced Nursing*, **15**(11), 1289–96.

Kegevinas, M. (1992) Social inequalities and cancers, in *Preventing Cancers* (eds T. Heller, L, Bailey and S. Pattison), Open University Press, Milton Keynes.

MacKie, R. (1992) Malignant melanoma: the story unfolds, in *Preventing Cancers* (eds T. Heller, L. Bailey and S. Pattison), Open University Press, Milton Keynes.

MacKie, R.M. and Aitchinson, T.C. (1982) Severe sunburn and subsequent risk of primary malignant melanoma in Scotland. *British Journal of Cancer*, **46**, 955–61.

Marie Curie Cancer Care (1994) *Marie Curie Cancer Education Diary*. Marie Curie Cancer Care, London.

Masters, W.H., Johnson, V.E. and Kolodny, R.C. (eds) (1992) *Human Sexuality*. Harper Collins, London.

Murray, M., Swan, A.V., Johnson, M.R.D. and Bewley, B.R. (1983) The development of smoking during adolescence: the MRC/Derbyshire smoking study. *International Journal of Epidemiology*, **12**, 3–9.

Nutrition Matters (1990) *Healthy Eating*. Quaker Oats Nutrition Centre, Milton Keynes.

Orbach, S. (1978) *Fat is a Feminist Issue: A Self-Help Guide for Compulsive Eaters*. Berkley, New York.

Price, B. (1990) A model for body-image care. *Journal of Advanced Nursing*, **15**, 585–93.

Quinlan, L. (1992) Skin cancer prevention. *Journal of Cancer Care*, **1**(4), 227–8.

Russell, M.A.H., Jarvis, M.J. and West, R.J. (1986) Use of urinary nicotine concentrations to estimate exposure and mortality from passive smoking in non-smokers. *British Journal of Addiction*, **81**, 275–81.

Scottish Health Education Group. *Breast Self-examination*. Edinburgh Breast Screening Clinic and SHEG, Edinburgh.

Scottish Health Education Group (1989) *Finding out about Stress*. SHEG, Edinburgh.

Scottish Health Education Group. *Well Woman: A Guide to Women's Health*. SHEG, Edinburgh.

Smits, A. (1991) Nursing patients with lung cancer, in *Oncology for Nurses and Health Care Professionals*. Vol. 3: *Cancer Nursing* (eds R. Tiffany and D. Borley), Harper Collins, London.

Sorenson, J. (1973) cited in Masters, W.H., Johnson, V.E. and Kolody, R.C. (eds) (1992) *Human Sexuality*. Harper Collins, London.

Tomlinson, J. and Scott, I. (1992) Breast self-examination (BSE). *Journal of Cancer Care*, **1**(2), 125–6.

Topping, A. (1991) Nursing patients with tumours of the gastrointestinal tract, in *Oncology for Nurses and Health Care Professionals*. Vol. 3: *Cancer Nursing* (eds R. Tiffany and D. Borley), Harper Collins, London.

Vries, H. de, Kok, G. and Dijkstra, M. (1992) Young people and their smoking behaviour, in *Preventing Cancers* (eds T. Heller, L. Bailey and S. Pattison), Open University Press, Milton Keynes.

Wheelock, V. (1992) Food policy and cancers, in *Preventing Cancers* (eds T. Heller, L. Bailey and S. Pattison), Open University Press, Milton Keynes.

FURTHER READING

Atrobus, M. (1987) The neglected sex. *Nursing Times*, **83**(4), 31–3.

Brown, M.S. (1977) *Normal Development of Body Image*. Wiley, London.

Calnan, M. (1986) Maintaining health and preventing illness: a comparison of the perceptions of women from different social classes. *Health Promotion*, **1**(2), 167–77.

Coughlan, A. (1993) Gut fights fat. *New Scientist*, **139**(1886), 6.

Darbyshire, P. (1987) Danger man. *Nursing Times*, **83**(48), 30–2.

Denny, E. and Jacob, F. (1990) Defining health promotion. *Senior Nurse*, **10**(10), 7–9.

Dilnot, A. and Kell, M. (1987) How women suffer. *New Society*, **81**(1286), 22–3.

Editorial: 'In Brief' (1990) Fatty genes. *New Scientist*, **126**(1719), 27.

Europe Against Cancer (1993) *European Code Against Cancer: A Booklet for General Practitioners*. Print and Micrographic Services, 3M Health Care Ltd, Loughborough.

Hardy, L.K. (1982) *Health: Self-appraisal – A Manual for Nurse Teachers*. Scottish Health Education Group, Edinburgh.

Hunt, S. and McLeod, M. (1987) Health and behavioral changes: some lay perspectives. *Community Medicine*, **9**(1), 68–76.

MacKie, R.M., McHenry, P. and Hole, D. (1993) Accelerated detection with prospective surveillance for cutaneous malignant melanoma in high-risk groups. *Lancet*, **341**(8861), 1618–20.

Macleod Clark, J., Haverty, S. and Kendall, S. (1990) Helping people to stop smoking: a study of the nurse's role. *Journal of Advanced Nursing*, **15**(3), 357–63.

Martell, R. (1993) Don't be so passive. *Nursing Standard*, **7**(50), 18.

Martin, J.P. (1990) Male cancer awareness: impact of employee education program. *Oncology Nurses Forum*, **17**(1), 59–64.

Martus, L. (1987) Thinking fat: self schema for body weight and processing of weight-relevant material. *Journal of Applied Social Science*, **17**, 50–71.

McCorkle, R. (1988) Women with cancer, in *Oncology for Nurses and Health Care Professionals*. Vol. 2: *Care and Support* (eds R. Tiffany and P. Webb), Harper & Row, Beaconsfield, pp. 282–5.

Parijs, L.G. von (1986) Public education in cancer prevention. *Bulletin of the World Health Organization*, **64**(6), 917–27.

Ruzek, S. and Hill, J. (1986) Promoting women's health: redefining the knowledge base and strategies for clarifying. *Health Promotion*, **1**(3), 301–9.

Spence, S.H. (1991) *Psychological Therapy*. Chapman & Hall, London.

Willis, J. (1993) Dying of embarrassment. *Nursing Times*, **89**(27), 22–3.

RESOURCES

Chest and Stroke Association. *We're Dead Against It* (video, VHS). Health Care Productions Ltd, 166 Cleveland Street, London W1P 5DN.

Europe Against Cancer. *Looking Good after Surgery* (video, VHS). From Concorde Films, 201 Felixstowe Road, Ipswich IP3 9BJ.

European Bureau for Action on Smoking Prevention (1993) *A Report on Passive Smoking*. European Community, Brussels.

Health Education Authority. *Cancer: How to Reduce your Risks*.

Health Education Board for Scotland. *Breast Self-examination* (paused tape/slide presentation with clear illustrations).

Health Education Council in collaboration with BBC and the Cancer Co-ordinating Group of the United Kingdom and Republic of Ireland (1986) *Can you Avoid Cancer?* HEA, London.

Leicester Health Authority. *Prevention and Early Detection of Cancer* (video, VHS). Useful for lay audience, illustrates breast and testicular self-examination. Available in Scotland from SCET, Glasgow, and in the rest of the UK from Concorde Films, 201 Felixstowe Road, Ipswich IP3 9BJ.

4 Screening for cancer

Penny Craddock

INTRODUCTION

After coronary heart disease, cancers are the most common cause of mortality in the UK. In 1989 cancers accounted for 25% of all deaths and 26% of the total life years lost under the age of 65 years. In women, cancers account for some 37% of life years lost. As part of the 'Health for All by the Year 2000' strategy, the European Region of the World Health Organization (WHO) have set a target of reducing cancer deaths in people aged under 65 by at least 15% by the year 2000, compared with 1980 (Bourn, 1992).

Cancers are all different and the scope for reducing the ill-health and death they cause varies enormously. Evidence suggests that a high proportion of deaths from cancer in the Western world might be avoidable, but inadequate knowledge leads to practical dilemmas regarding the prevention of cancer.

Primary prevention involves suggesting to symptomless people radical changes in lifestyle that have no guarantee of saving or prolonging life. In the area of secondary prevention, which involves screening and early detection, doubts exist as to whether such programmes lead to higher cure rates and not just longer survival after diagnosis. Screening tests therefore have to be carefully evaluated in order to assess the advantages and costs that will inevitably be incurred. These costs are not just financial but also physical, psychological, economic and political.

WHAT IS SCREENING?

Screening is:

> the practice of investigating apparently healthy individuals with the object of detecting unrecognized disease or people with an exceptionally high risk of developing disease, and intervening in ways that will prevent the occurrence of disease or improve the prognosis when it develops. (Farmer and Miller, 1983).

Key points in screening (Adapted from Knight and Taylor, 1992.)

1. 'Apparently healthy individuals'. Individuals invited to be screened are apparently healthy; they are not ill and are not being offered screening because they are symptomatic.
2. 'Detecting unrecognized disease'. Screening is a means of detecting disease before there are recognizable symptoms and before a person is aware of them. For many diseases, by the time there are recognizable signs and symptoms the disease process may be too far advanced to be treated successfully. The majority of people do not perceive themselves as having a disease unless they have symptoms, and are therefore unlikely to seek medical advice.
3. 'Exceptionally high risk of developing disease'. Selective screening is used for individuals who are apparently at a higher risk of developing the disease. However, it is often impossible or impractical to identify individuals with a greater risk of developing a certain disease, so mass screening may be employed. Mass screening involves testing large numbers of people for the presence of a disease without specific reference to their individual risk of having or developing the disease.
4. 'Intervening in ways that will prevent the occurrence of disease or improve the prognosis when it develops'. Screening enables an intervention in the natural history of a disease with the intention of preventing the occurrence of the disease or improving the prognosis when it develops. Evidence that intervening produces benefit in terms of preventing disease or improving prognosis needs to be provided before a screening programme is implemented. Not all screening procedures are beneficial and there are situations where the detection of a disease may only extend the time the person is aware of it and not ultimately prolong life.

    Screening falls short as an ideal method of cancer control, because to be cost effective and of any real value large numbers of usually well people have to be subjected to a medical procedure from which most will gain no obvious benefit and by which some will actually be harmed.

    Cancers grow at different rates so it is unlikely screening can be favourable for all cases. It has also been suggested that the early cellular changes identified histologically do not always progress to invasive cancer, which implies that not all early abnormalities are progressive.

    It is therefore essential to evaluate every screening test to ensure the advantages significantly outweigh the costs that will be incurred.

CRITERIA FOR SCREENING

Criteria devised by Wilson and Jungner for the WHO in 1968 are used as a basis to assess the viability of screening tests. In practice, screening tests for cancer fail to satisfy many of these criteria but clear evidence of a substantial reduction in mortality would be necessary to justify screening. The 10 general principles of screening set out by Austoker (1990) are discussed below:

1. **The condition screened for should pose an important health problem.** There would be no support for setting up a screening programme for a disease that was not considered to be an important health problem. The value of screening for certain cancers is constantly being evaluated.

2. **The natural history of the condition should be well understood.** The natural history of cancer development is not well understood, so that the behaviour of lesions detected by screening may differ from those diagnosed with symptoms. Individual cancers may have different rates of progress through successive changes and it is therefore unlikely that screening can favourably influence all cases (Chamberlain, 1991).

3. **There should be a recognizable latent or early stage.** The identification of pre-invasive states by screening may confer considerable benefit by reducing the incidence of invasive cancer and subsequent mortality. Detection of a disease at a pre-clinical stage was crucial in the decision to establish a national breast-screening programme (Forrest, 1986).

4. **Treatment of the disease at an early stage should be of more benefit than treatment started at a later stage.** Intervention should produce benefit, thus the value of screening is limited to detection of those tumours which are going to progress and in which early treatment is capable of arresting their course.

5. **There should be a suitable test or examination.** The decision about which screening method to employ is determined by its ability to detect a high proportion of asymptomatic disease at a stage when prognosis can be improved by earlier treatment. The criteria for assessing screening methods are that they should:

    ● be simple;
    ● be easy to apply;
    ● have a high sensitivity and specificity;
    ● be reproducible;
    ● be cost effective;
    ● have a low risk-to-benefit ratio.

6. **The test or examination should be acceptable to the population.** Acceptability or otherwise of a screening test (e.g. cervical smears or mammography) is very much a personal decision. Education about the

screening programme is therefore an essential factor in encouraging individuals to attend.

7. **For diseases of insidious onset screening should be repeated at intervals determined by the natural history of the disease.** The sensitivity of a screening test is the ability to detect a disease. The specificity of a test is the ability to exclude people who do not have a disease. The total incidence of cancers arising with symptoms in the interval between screens (interval cancers) must be kept as low as possible. The interval between routinely repeated screens is determined by the rate at which detectable but pre-symptomatic disease progresses to the symptomatic stage when it would normally present.

8. **There should be adequate facilities available for the diagnosis and treatment of any abnormalities detected.** It is extremely important when organizing a screening programme that adequate facilities for diagnosis and treatment are available. A positive test result can be very distressing and it is essential that positive results can be investigated with the minimum of delay.

9. **The chance of physical or psychological harm should be less than the chance of benefit.** It is important that health professionals are aware of the advantages and disadvantages of screening, which can be both physical and psychological. Individuals accepting screening should be able to make a decision based on informed choice (Tables 4.1 and 4.2).

10. **The cost of case-finding (including diagnosis and subsequent treatment) should be economically balanced against the benefit it provides** (Table 4.3). Economic appraisal is a general term for a set of techniques which are used to compare the relative efficiency of

Table 4.1   Physical benefits and disadvantages of breast screening

Benefits	Disadvantages
Life years gained for those with curable cancer	Morbidity of the screening test
	Extended morbidity if prognosis is unaltered
Avoidance of morbidity of radical treatment	
	'Over-diagnosis' resulting in women receiving unnecessary treatment for lesions which might otherwise have regressed
	Unnecessary diagnostic morbidity for false positives

Reproduced from Austoker, *Breast Cancer Screening: Practical Guide for Primary Care Teams*; published by Cancer Research Campaign, Oxford, 1990.

Table 4.2   Psychological benefits and disadvantages of breast screening

Benefits	Disadvantages
Reassurance in those where cancer is not present	Fear of being found to have cancer when invited for screening
Reassurance that the disease is at a very early stage	False reassurance of false negatives
Possible psychological advantages of avoiding radical treatment	Anxiety in those found to have a positive test
	Extended psychological morbidity if prognosis is unaltered
	Anxiety about prognosis in those with non-progressive neoplasia
	Anxiety about prognosis in those with incurable cancer

Reproduced from Austoker, *Breast Cancer Screening: Practical Guide for Primary Care Teams*; published by Cancer Research Campaign, Oxford, 1990.

Table 4.3   Cost benefits and disadvantages of breast screening

Benefits	Disadvantages
Avoid expense of treatment of advanced cancers	Screening expenses
	Extra diagnostic expenses in false positives
Extra years of productivity	Cost of additional cases treated
	Cost of treating cases earlier and longer follow-up
	Personal expenditure in attending screening and assessment centres
	Repeated invitations to non-attenders

Reproduced from Austoker, *Breast Cancer Screening: Practical Guide for Primary Care Teams*; published by Cancer Research Campaign, Oxford, 1990.

alternative ways of using society's scarce resources. For the policy-maker (Table 4.4) the decision is somewhat easier if the cost per QUALY (quality-adjusted life year) gained by the screening programme can be compared with the cost per QUALY of alternative uses of the resources (Chamberlain, personal communication).

Table 4.4 Political, scientific and organizational benefits and disadvantages of breast screening

Benefits	Disadvantages
Potential for improved understanding of the natural history of early cancer through large-scale studies	Inadequate population registers to enable effective coverage of the target population
Potential for improving treatment of pre-invasive conditions through national clinical trials	Diversion of scarce resources to the breast screening programme rather than to support more cost-effective primary prevention programmes (e.g. anti-smoking campaigns for lung cancer and cardiovascular disease)
Opportunity to improve diagnostic and therapeutic services for breast cancer	

Reproduced from Austoker, *Breast Cancer Screening: Practical Guide for Primary Care Teams*; published by Cancer Research Campaign, Oxford, 1990.

EVALUATION OF SCREENING FOR CANCER

The International Union against Cancer (UICC) project on the Evaluation of Screening for Cancer (Miller *et al.*, 1990) reports on trials from around the world on the evaluation of screening for individual sites or groups of sites. The recommendations are in general related to the application of screening as a public health policy, and discussion revolves around the research that is considered necessary before such policies on screening can be implemented.

Apart from breast and cervical cancer, which will be dealt with later, other sites evaluated led the members of the UICC project to conclude for other cancers, including lung, bladder, oral, endometrial, colorectal, prostate and melanoma of the skin:

> that screening should not be considered as public health policy for these sites. (Miller *et al.*, 1990)

However, trials continue world-wide in a constant effort to identify screening methods that could lead to a reduction in mortality from various cancers.

The following are extracts from some of the Miller *et al.* (1990) trials.

Screening for lung cancer

Chest X-ray and sputum cytology at varying intervals have been suggested as screening tests for lung cancer. However, there is no evidence that screening for lung cancer can reduce lung cancer mortality but there is evidence that screening with chest X-rays plus sputum cytology does improve stage at diagnosis.

Screening for colorectal cancer

Current controlled trials in a number of centres using faecal occult blood testing (FOBT) at varying intervals of between one and three years are producing useful data but each trial alone will not be definitive and most will still take several more years.

Screening for stomach cancer

Stomach cancer is one of the most common cancers in the Western Pacific, Central and South Americas and Eastern Europe. Screening for stomach cancer for those aged 40 and over began in Japan in 1960 using barium X-ray. From 1960 to 1988 over 2.5 million persons were screened and 5350 cases of stomach cancer were detected. Data from Japan suggest that stomach cancer screening can reduce mortality. Recommendations are that screening should continue in high-risk areas but that screening for stomach cancer cannot yet be recommended as public health policy in other countries.

Screening for cancer of the prostate

Screening for prostate cancer is confronted by a number of questions from the sensitivity and specificity of the screening tests to the ethics of screening for the disease. Post-mortem studies have shown many times more latent prostate cancers than will ever surface in life, so over-diagnosis and over-treatment is a distinct possibility. Screening on a large scale is therefore not recommended.

These examples demonstrate that not only are screening trials being undertaken throughout the world but that the issues raised are not simple or straightforward.

THE UNITED KINGDOM COORDINATING COMMITTEE ON CANCER RESEARCH (UKCCCR)

The UKCCCR provides a forum for the coordination of the activities of bodies funding cancer research in the UK and for collaboration in joint projects. The UKCCCR is funded by the Imperial Cancer Research Fund, Cancer Research Campaign and the Medical Research Council, with further membership from the Leukaemia Research Fund, Marie Curie

Memorial Foundation, Institute of Cancer Research, Tenovus Fund and the Ludwig Institute.

The UKCCCR has a network of subcommittees covering several cancer sites and, under their supervision, is conducting five treatment trials:

1. the Anal Cancer Trial;
2. AXIS (Adjuvant X-ray Infusion Study) Trial in colorectal cancer;
3. the UKHAN (UK Head and Neck) Trial;
4. the PCI (Prophylactic Cranial Irradiation) Trial in lung cancer;
5. the DCIS (Ductal Carcinoma In-Situ) Trial in cancer detected through the National Breast Screening Programme.

It is also conducting three trials relating to breast cancer screening:

1. the one- versus two-view Mammography Trial;
2. a trial looking at commencing screening in women at age 40;
3. the Frequency of Screening (one-yearly versus three-yearly) Trial.

The subcommittee also consider general matters relating to cancer research and will convene workshops or produce reports where appropriate. A central trials committee is overseeing the preparation of the UK Cancer Trials Register and has established a working group investigating ways to educate patients about the importance of clinical trials.

SCREENING SERVICES AVAILABLE

The foregoing illustrates that research continues into the viability and value of screening tests as public health policy. Certain 'at risk' individuals are included in screening programmes such as that offered by the Imperial Cancer Research Fund (ICRF) in many centres in the UK. Scientists are looking at the hereditary element which exists in some forms of cancer. This work has two major benefits: identifying families 'at risk' so that any disease is found at an early, curable stage; and examining the genetic basis of these rare forms of cancer in the hope they may provide clues to the commoner cancers. Some families appear to have a long history of certain types of cancer, for example bowel, stomach or breast cancers. There is obvious concern amongst family members as to their own risk of developing these cancers and if there is an inherited risk.

Screening for families with a history of bowel cancer would be by colonoscopy, which involves examining the whole of the inside of the large bowel looking for evidence of polyps. When polyps are found they are often not malignant but may be a type which indicate a high risk of developing bowel cancer. Routine screening would continue for the patient and his or her direct family. People with a family history of bowel cancer are on average about three times more likely to develop the disease than the general population (ICRF, 1992a). Women who have a close relative, for example mother or sister, with breast cancer are at a slightly increased risk; only about 5% of breast cancers are due to inherited susceptibility genes. These families usually have a large number of people with breast cancer and the daughters of affected women have a 50% risk of inheriting the gene and a much higher lifetime risk of developing breast cancer.

The gene may also be passed by fathers to their daughters and in this case the daughter's risk will be the same as if she inherited the gene from her mother. Occasionally a male with the gene will develop breast cancer. Patients found to be at risk are given information and counselling to help them come to terms with their risk and they are offered regular screening checks where possible, so that if a cancer should develop it will be identified early and treated at a more curable stage.

Current screening for breast cancer uses conventional mammography which, evidence has shown (Cancer Research Campaign (CRC) Factsheet 7.1, 1991), is useful for older women but not so helpful for screening the more dense breasts of women under 50 years. If a woman has a long family history of breast cancer then regular screening may be recommended. The ICRF is involved in comparing the results of conventional mammograms with those of computer-enhanced mammograms, which it is hoped will give a clearer picture of abnormal growths in the younger woman at an earlier stage.

SCREENING FOR FEMALE CANCERS

Deaths from cancer in the UK for 1989 included:

- 15 300 female deaths from breast cancer;
- 2170 female deaths from cervical cancer;
- 4275 female deaths from ovarian cancer;
- 1030 female deaths from uterine cancer.

This accounted for some 37% of life years lost (CRC Factsheet 3.3, 1989).

OVARIAN CANCER

Ovarian cancer is the fifth commonest cancer in women, with over 5000 new cases occurring in the UK each year. The overall prognosis is poor. More than two-thirds of patients die from the disease. This is mainly due to its late diagnosis in the majority of patients. The symptoms of early ovarian cancer are not easily recognizable and the disease often presents at a stage when it has already metastasized. There is good evidence to suggest that if the disease is picked up in its early stages, the five-year survival rate could be improved to more than 90% (Young *et al.*, 1990). It accounts for 6% of all cancer deaths and is the cause of more deaths in women than all other gynaecological malignancies combined (CRC Factsheet 17, 1991).

Recent research has been directed towards finding a method of diagnosing the disease at an early stage. The features of the disease which make screening an attractive proposition are the much larger survival when the disease is confined to the ovary compared to when it is more advanced, and the fact that most cases present clinically with abdominal symptoms when it has already spread into the peritoneum and beyond (Cuckle and Wald, 1991).

Ovarian cancer screening tests

There are several tests which have been evaluated for screening for ovarian cancer. These include bi-manual pelvic examinations, abdominal ultrasound and serum CA125 levels (Jacobs and Oram, 1990; Campbell *et al.* 1989; Bourne *et al.*, 1989). Additional new techniques are being developed, including other monoclonal antibodies and markers (serum and urinary), vaginal ultrasound, flow studies and radioimmunoscintography. Few studies have been published to date, and those reported have been on self-selected populations.

To date no single screening test for ovarian cancer has combined high enough levels of sensitivity and specificity to be considered suitable for use in population screening.

The following report from the UKCCCR highlights the problems faced with screening for ovarian cancer.

UKCCCR: Ovarian cancer screening report – November 1989

Summary of findings
On current evidence the benefit of screening for ovarian cancer is unproved. Screening outside population-based studies is inadvisable since it may cause anxiety but may not, in fact, benefit the woman. Furthermore, if screening is offered widely (through private practice) it may prejudice the opportunity for proper randomized studies. On current evidence, no single test is sufficiently specific or sensitive to be used as a screening service. Further research would be necessary to evaluate the most effective combination of tests, the optimum frequency and the effect of menopausal status. Death rates from ovarian cancer are roughly one-third those of breast cancer so that randomized trials of screening would need to be three times as large if the same degree of effect were to be detected.

Recommendations
1. Screening for ovarian cancer is of unproved benefit, and should not, in the light of current knowledge, be offered as a routine test.

2. Further studies would be necessary before it could be stated whether ovarian cancer screening is effective in reducing deaths from this disease or what is the optimum combination and frequency of tests.
3. Further studies are required to identify high-risk groups. Families identified as being at high-risk should be referred to centres with a specific interest in genetic aspects of the disease.
4. Screening of a high-risk group could provide results more quickly and less expensively than screening of a large population of average risk.
5. Any proposed study of a large population would have to be properly structured from the outset, piloted for patient acceptability and carefully monitored and would require extensive funding.
6. There is a need for basic research into the malignant potential of benign and borderline ovarian tumours.
7. Every effort should be made to stage ovarian cancer accurately at diagnosis. Patients suspected of having the disease should have a laparotomy performed by a gynaecologist, preferably one with a special interest in this condition.

CERVICAL CANCER SCREENING

More is known about the natural history of cervical cancer, the protective effect of screening based on cytology and the mechanisms through which the protection appears than for any other cancer. Screening for cervical cancer is effective in reducing the incidence and mortality from the disease and is therefore recommended as public health policy. Organized programmes offering screening from the age of 20–25 years every three to five years until the age of 60–64 years provide maximal effectiveness.

Incidence

In the UK during 1985, 4496 new cases of invasive cervical cancer were registered; 84% of new cases occurred in women aged 35 and over. About 9000 women were registered with pre-malignant conditions; the vast majority (87%) were in younger women, under the age of 45 years (Austoker and McPherson, 1992). The number dying of the disease is going down. Between 1985 and 1991 there was a 15% decrease in cervical cancer deaths in England and Wales (ICRF, November 1992c).

Survival

Survival after diagnosis and treatment is directly related to stage at the time of diagnosis, and survival is much higher in women who are diagnosed and treated at an early stage. Routine screening therefore has a valuable role to play in identifying abnormalities at an early stage.

Screening

Organized screening programmes have been in operation in parts of Europe and North America for over 20 years. Screening began in Britain in 1964 and it has been largely ineffective. The majority of women who develop invasive cervical cancer have never been screened and failure to follow up abnormal smears and in some cases a long interval between screens (more than five years) has added to the problem. However, in January 1988 the Department of Health and Social Security (DHSS) issued guidelines which aimed at reducing mortality from cervical cancer by regularly screening all eligible women in order to identify and treat conditions that might otherwise develop into cancer (DHSS, 1988).

In 1990 the renamed Department of Health (DOH) introduced a system of target payments designed to encourage general practitioners to promote screening. The DOH set an explicit target for coverage and provided payment to general practitioners (GPs) who achieved 50% or 80% of this target – the remuneration being far greater for over 80% coverage. The cost of this scheme in 1990–1 was £39 million (Bourn, 1992). By 1992 over 80% of women in the 20–64 age range targeted by the cervical screening programme had had a smear test in the previous 5½ years (ICRF, November 1992c).

The International Agency for Research into Cancer estimates that screening women aged 20–64 years at three-year intervals will reduce the incidence of cervical cancer by 91% compared with a reduction of 84% if screening takes place at five-year intervals. Department policy is that women should be recalled at least every five years but the actual frequency of screening in individual health districts is decided at local level based on health needs and circumstances.

Obviously in order for a screening programme to be effective it is essential that a large proportion of the eligible population should be screened regularly and this depends upon identification, invitation and encouragement to attend.

Identification

The Family Health Services Authority (FHSA) issues on a regular basis to all practices lists of women aged 20–64 who should be screened. A problem has been encountered with the accuracy of the FHSA registers of patients on GP lists with particular reference to addresses. This applies particularly to highly mobile populations: an Inner London district

(Parkside) found in 1989 that 50% of cervical screening invitations were inaccurate (Bourn, 1992).

Invitations

The wording of invitations sent to women asking them to attend for cervical screening is obviously important and certain information should be included:

- a female doctor/practice nurse available to take smears in a private setting;
- the reason for the test;
- the optimum time for taking a smear test;
- how results will be obtained.

A carefully worded invitation letter can attract women who otherwise would not attend for screening; the converse is also true.

Encouraging women to attend for screening is fundamental to the success of the programme and consideration must be made of the needs of not only the ethnic minority groups but also of those women who do not understand the importance of cervical screening. There are many women who are unscreened because they are not aware how important cervical screening is or that it can potentially identify **pre-cancerous** abnormalities which when treated early can prevent cancer developing.

Quality of the screening service

The effectiveness of the cervical screening programme depends not only on ensuring that a high proportion of eligible women at risk are screened regularly but also on the quality of service provided. Quality is important at all stages of the screening process:

- taking the smear;
- interpretation of the smear;
- following up women with abnormal smears.

Taking the smear

In 1988 the Intercollegiate Working Group on Cervical Cytology Screening issued a report that produced guidance on these aspects of the screening process. The British Society for Clinical Cytology produced a video and booklet giving guidance on the technique of smear-taking directed at all those involved in this area. In addition, various national courses have been established, which will be detailed later (see 'Education and training', below).

The test involves the doctor or nurse scraping a sample of cells off the surface of the cervix with a softwood spatula. Various spatulas of different shape and material have been developed since Ayre (1944) first advocated a spatula for direct sampling of the cervix. The Ayre spatula and more latterly the Aylesbury spatula are those most commonly used in the UK at the present time. The Aylesbury spatula was designed in 1987 by a consultant cytopathologist with a consultant obstetrician and gynaecologist from Stoke Mandeville Hospital in order to improve the cellular quality of cervical smears. The head of the Aylesbury spatula was designed with a projecting end to fit neatly into the external os and extend 1–2 cm up the endocervical canal, and the head was angled, thus enabling better sampling of the whole of the cervix (Wolfendale *et al.*, 1987). A cytobrush can be used in addition to a spatula as it enables sampling of the endocervix when the os is tight or stenosed and it is not possible to insert the tip of the spatula. The cells are then smeared onto a slide and sent to a cytology laboratory for examination and analysis. The laboratory staff examine the slide under a microscope, scanning the slide for any pre-cancerous changes in the cells. These can vary from minor changes which do not require immediate action to marked changes which may lead to an increased risk of cervical cancer developing if not treated.

In most cases the result of the laboratory examination will be negative (i.e. normal). In these cases women will be recalled when they are next due for a smear test under local screening policy (i.e. in three to five years). However, in around 10% of cases women will be called back because the original smear was inadequate or because the cell changes identified need to be kept under observation.

Where the laboratory has identified more severe changes women will be referred for further investigation by colposcopy. Colposcopy involves a doctor examining the cervix using a magnifying instrument which enables the identification of areas of abnormal cells. The doctor may then decide to remove a small piece of tissue from the abnormal area for further testing (a biopsy). A diagnosis of the degree of abnormality can then be made – classified as cervical intraepithelial neoplasia (CIN) stages I to III. If treatment is required it can be carried out on an out-patient basis, or as a short surgical operation in hospital.

Interpretation of the smear

Following recent problems, the role of the laboratory and the need for adequate quality control procedures is obvious. It is important that a national standard for interpretation is maintained. Variations do exist in the results of smears; 90% of smears are classified as normal but there are regional variations in the levels of abnormal and positive results reported, ranging from 2.6% to 8.1%. Differences in the classification of abnormalities or in interpretation may account for the range of reported results but it does serve to highlight the complexity of cervical cytology.

Results

Reporting smear results from the laboratory to the GP and then to the patient is a vital aspect of good practice, and guidance and fail-safe systems have been introduced nationally (Austoker and McPherson, 1992).

Treatment and follow-up

The treatment and follow-up of cervical abnormalities is also an essential aspect of these fail-safe guidelines and it is of paramount importance to ensure the patient is informed and counselled at each stage of the procedure, from being told the result of the smear test, to attending a colposcopy clinic and to having treatment and follow-up. This can be a very anxious period for the women involved and trials have been undertaken to assess the extent of this anxiety (Wilkinson *et al.*, 1990; Marteau *et al.*, 1990). It has been suggested that investigation and treatment of cervical intraepithelial neoplasia are psychologically traumatic. Good education and counselling from the onset may prevent future psychiatric and psychological morbidity and improve compliance with treatment.

The introduction to *The Positive Smear* (Quilliam, 1992) is a salutary reminder of the many issues surrounding smear tests:

> When a woman has a positive smear, she faces issues around her sexuality, her fertility and her mortality.

THE ROLE OF THE PRIMARY CARE TEAM IN CERVICAL SCREENING

The role played by the primary care team in cervical screening cannot be underestimated. Each member of the team from receptionist to GP has a valuable part to play.

The encouragement of women to attend for regular cervical screening largely depends on the general practices providing an acceptable service. This service starts with identifying the women to be screened and inviting them to attend in such a way as to be sensitive to their needs and to their understanding of the procedures involved as well as to the possible outcome. The quality of smear-taking is important not just in terms of taking an adequate smear but also in relation to the attitude of the smear-taker in acknowledging the woman's possible anxiety or reluctance. Ensuring the results of the smear test are communicated to the woman without undue delay, and that the necessary advice and counselling are available to support women who have abnormal results requiring follow-up, investigation or treatment is essential. In order to ensure the cervical screening programme in the UK meets the needs of the public it is necessary to have not only a technically and administratively efficient service but also one that takes into account the emotional and psychological needs of women of all ages. This service is based in general practice and thus the role of the primary care team is vital to its success.

BREAST CANCER SCREENING

The Secretary of State for Health announced the government's decision to introduce a national breast screening programme by mammography, in February 1987. The DHSS, responsible for defining the aims and objectives of the programme, issued guidance to local health authorities based on the Forrest Report (1986) and set regional health authorities the target of having screening centres in operation by 31st March 1990 and that all eligible women should have recieved an invitation to be screened by the end of 1993.

Incidence

Breast cancer is the major form of cancer among women in the UK, accounting for:

- 26 000 new cases diagnosed per year;
- 16 000 deaths per year;
- 19% of all female cancer deaths;
- 5% of total female deaths;
- the most common cause of death in women aged 35–54 (CRC Factsheet 7, 1991).

The majority of breast cancer cases occur in older women (Figure 4.1). The UK has the highest breast cancer mortality rate world-wide (Figure 4.2). The cause of breast cancer is not understood; therefore there is no possibility of primary prevention at the present time. It is thought that at least two-thirds of women who develop breast cancer will eventually die from it. The average five-year survival rate is 64% in England and Wales and it has been shown that the survival rate is directly related to stage at the time of diagnosis (Figure 4.3).

Why screen for breast cancer?

Evidence from randomized controlled trials of breast cancer screening in New York and Sweden have shown reductions in mortality of about

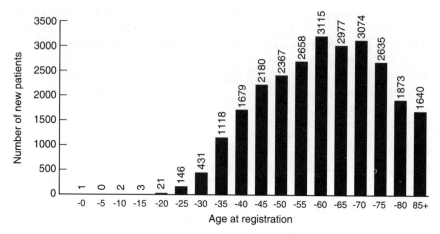

Figure 4.1 Incidence of breast cancer in the UK, 1986. Reproduced from Cancer Research Campaign Factsheet 6.1, 1991.

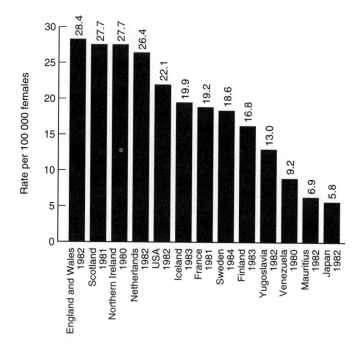

Figure 4.2 International mortality rates for breast cancer. Reproduced from Cancer Research Campaign Factsheet 6.3, 1991.

30%. Non-randomized case–control studies have been carried out in The Netherlands and Florence, results of which have also demonstrated a benefit from screening.

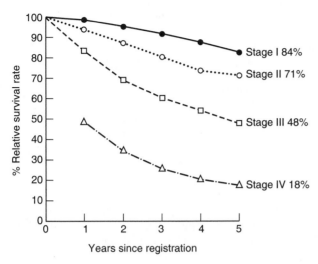

Figure 4.3 Five-year survival for breast cancer patients in the UK, 1975–1980. Reproduced from Cancer Research Campaign Factsheet 6.2, 1991.

Following the consideration by the Forrest Committee in 1986 of available information from overseas studies, a report was presented to the Government stating that: 'screening by mammography can lead to prolongation of life for women aged 50 and over with breast cancer'. The national programme implemented in March 1988 aims to achieve a reduction in mortality from breast cancer in women aged 50–64 years. After about 10 years some 1250 breast cancer deaths are expected to be prevented each year in the UK, provided 70% of the targeted population accept the invitation to be screened.

Guidelines for the National Breast Screening Programme

- Target population: women aged 50–64 years
  - Women aged 65 and over will be screened on request.
  - Women under 50 will not be offered routine screening.
- Screening technique: single, oblique-view mammography
- Interval: three years

There is still debate about the use of single-view mammography and the interval between screens. However, trials are ongoing in certain centres where, in some, two views are taken and in others the interval between screens is reduced. The situation is thus constantly under review.

Factors influencing the effectiveness of a breast screening programme are detailed in Table 4.5. Some of these factors are related to the screening

Table 4.5   Factors influencing the effectiveness of a breast cancer screening programme

Participation of the target population
Sensitivity of the screening test
Specificity of the screening test
Frequency of routine screening
Adequacy of follow-up of those with 'abnormal' mammograms
Effectiveness of treatment of those with breast cancer

Reproduced from Cancer Research Campaign Factsheet 7.1, 1991.

tests and the treatment and follow-up – however, it must be remembered that without the participation of the target population the screening programme will not be as effective and inevitably the results will be affected.

Identification

The FHSA registers are again necessary for identifying eligible women. The accuracy of this data, i.e. names, addresses and ages, is vital in that women are invited according to their age (i.e. 50–64) and, as with the cervical screening programme, if addresses are inaccurate women will not receive their invitations. Health authorities admit that register inaccuracy is one of the main factors affecting the take-up of invitations.

Invitation

The women are sent their invitations from the screening office, the details of which will have been prepared from lists previously checked by each general practice in the targeted area. Usually the invitation will offer a specific appointment giving instructions on how this may be altered if necessary. Information on what is involved in the screening visit is essential and consideration must be given to ethnic minorities who may have special language needs. In areas with a large population of Asian women, problems have been experienced in the uptake of breast screening. However, a randomized controlled trial in Oldham, north-west England, has shown that a personal approach to Asian women was not an appropriate strategy to improve screening attendance. Link-workers made contact with a group of Asian women from seven general practices and no difference was found between the intervention and control groups (Hoare *et al.*, 1993).

Information supplied by the National Health Service Breast Screening Programme (NHSBSP) indicates that in 1990–1 over 70% of women accepted their screening invitation. Regionally this acceptance ranged from 60.2% to 81.7%. The uptake in inner city areas of London affected the overall acceptance rates; once again inaccuracies in the registers led to invitations not being received. A lack of understanding of the potential benefit of breast screening has also affected the uptake – both these issues are now being addressed. An X-ray (or mammogram) is taken of each breast. The breast is placed on a small platform and compressed by the mammography machine. This may cause discomfort, but is essential to prevent movement so as to obtain a clear image and minimize radiation dosage. The mammograms are taken by a specially trained radiographer and the process takes between five and ten minutes. The mammograms are later examined by a radiologist. This examination will show whether there are changes which require further investigation.

The vast majority of women will have mammograms which show no abnormality. They are informed of the result and will be invited again for screening in three years' time. If they are 65 years of age or older by this time, they will have to ask for a further screening appointment. If the mammograms are not clear enough to be accurately examined by the radiologist, the woman will be invited back for repeat screening.

Less than 10% of women screened will have a mammogram which indicates a breast abnormality. They will then be invited to have further tests to determine the nature of the abnormality.

Quality of the screening service

The Forrest Report recognized that if it was to achieve a reduction in mortality by identifying early-stage breast cancer in women, the programme had to set high standards. These covered the following stages of the screening process:

- taking the mammogram;
- identifying and assessing abnormalities;
- follow-up of women with abnormalities.

Evidence has shown that the standards set have been exceeded, which is a great strength of the breast screening programme, and indeed the standards have been revised (NHSBSP, 1993) and now two standards are set that are either 'acceptable' or 'achievable'.

Mammography does not reach an absolute conclusion about the presence or absence of disease, but can only sort the screened population into those with positive and those with negative results.

Notification of results

Usually a woman will receive her results from the screening office within a fortnight, as will her GP. The results of mammograms can be categorized as follows:

- **Normal** – leading to routine recall after the selected interval.
- **'Technical' recall** – because the breast detail is not clearly seen on the film.
- **Abnormal** – the woman will be invited to attend the assessment centre for further investigations. The majority of women with an 'abnormal' result do not have breast cancer but an abnormal result will create anxiety. False reassurance by the GP is neither kind nor justified. A frank discussion of the complexity and limitations of mammography is necessary and an explanation as to why some women are recalled and subsequently found to be normal is essential. These tests take place at an assessment clinic. Further mammograms will be taken and fine needle aspiration may be used to extract a sample of cells from the abnormal area. Most women recalled will not have cancer, although they may have an inflammation, a cyst or a lump, which may be treated, drained or removed. Women with these conditions will be given the results of assessment and invited for screening again in three years' time.

One or two of each ten women attending an assessment clinic may need to have a biopsy to determine whether the abnormality is harmless or cancerous. This should be carried out shortly after the assessment appointment. In a biopsy some of the breast tissue is removed under anaesthetic and is examined under a microscope. If cancer is detected it may be removed at the time of biopsy or the woman may be referred for further treatment and surgery.

If, following investigations, breast cancer is diagnosed, treatment options will be discussed with the woman. She should receive support not only from her GP and the primary health care team but also from the breast nurse counsellor working within the NHSBSP.

If everyone accepted the invitation to be screened up to 3000 lives could be saved annually (ICRF, 1992b). At present the programme attracts just over 70% and it is estimated that 1250 women's lives will be saved per year by the year 2000. However, the take-up rate shows wide variations in different areas – as high as 80% in some and under 50% in others. The ICRF Health Behaviour Unit in London is aiming to identify the reasons why some women attend and others do not. Age, education, social class, attitudes, etc. are being looked at to see whether a pattern can be established. The GP ICRF Research Group in Oxford is examining factors which influence a woman's reattendance for breast screening. Discomfort and embarrassment are high on the list of factors influencing attendance.

Some women choose not to be screened for personal reasons, for example embarrassment, fear of cancer or of the screening test, dislike of medical intervention or because the invitation appears inappropriate in some way. Various factors can influence a woman's decision to accept an invitation to be screened and this issue is discussed in *Breast Cancer Screening* (Austoker, 1990).

The role of the primary care team

The success of the Breast Screening Programme is very dependent on the active involvement of the primary care team. Austoker (1990) suggests that they can help to achieve high levels of uptake by:

1. ensuring the FHSA registers are accurate
2. understanding the organization of the programme and informing women about it
3. being aware of women's anxieties about breast cancer and breast cancer screening
4. being positive and knowledgeable about the breast screening programme
5. following up non-attenders
6. discussing the implications of recall for further investigations
7. discussing the implications of a biopsy
8. discussing treatment options.

PRIVATE SCREENING

Private health screening facilities are available throughout the UK. Many of the organizations involved are well-known and well-respected companies that offer a wide-ranging screening service, often available on a self-referral basis.

Services offered include a range of tests, including basic measurement of height, weight and blood pressure and in addition blood tests, cardiovascular assessment and specific screening tests for bowel cancer and prostate cancer. Cervical smears and mammography are performed when necessary. One company introduces its services by acknowledging the part lifestyle plays in an individual's health status and based on the results of the screening tests will make 'positive recommendations to maintain good health' and emphasizes the need to find 'a suitable balance to fit your own lifestyle'. The more reputable companies will ensure that action is taken regarding appropriate treatment if a serious problem is discovered. Health screening is useful but it is essential that those partaking of such services do not rely on the outcome to the exclusion of visiting their own doctor should a problem arise in the period between screenings. There is also a risk that some clients would view a negative test result as a means of confirming to themselves that no damage had resulted from lifestyle excesses, for example smoking or drinking heavily, and not take advice regarding lifestyle changes. A negative screening test is not a guarantee of continuing good health but an indicator of the state of health at the time of the screening.

It is essential when screening that 'there should be adequate facilities available for the diagnosis and treatment of any abnormalities detected' (as discussed on page 51). It is possible that a client attending for private screening on a self-referral basis may not receive the support and back-up necessary should the test prove positive and further investigations be deemed necessary. This is an important aspect of any screening programme and should be carefully considered by those receiving private screening.

PSYCHOLOGICAL ASPECTS OF SCREENING

Screening is becoming a growing part of the health care system but it has been suggested that screening can 'do more harm than good' in some instances (Marteau, 1990). Many people undergo screening without understanding precisely what the test is for, the accuracy of the test or the implications of any possible test results.

The psychological costs of screening are constantly being assessed, particularly as it appears that high levels of anxiety have been reported in patients participating in many screening programmes, including cervical screening, breast cancer screening and general health screening. Letters sent to people inviting them to attend for screening should clearly state why they are being invited, i.e. a routine screening visit, and also briefly explain the advantages of such a screening test to the individual concerned, how the results will be obtained and possible interpretation of the result. The more knowledge people have about the benefits of undergoing a screening test, the more likely they are to attend (Marteau, 1990). Simply receiving an invitation to a screening exercise can provoke anxiety in some individuals (Nathoo, 1988).

When communicating results to patients it should be remembered that a positive result is usually received with negative feelings (Posner and Vessey, 1988; Quilliam, 1992). Support given at the right time may be helpful, as would explanations with regard to the meaning of a positive screening result. It must be remembered that screening sorts people into 'screen negative' and 'screen positive' and does not produce a definitive diagnosis, particularly in the case of breast screening. Further investigations will be necessary to determine the nature of the screening abnormalities.

In the case of cervical screening all patients should be told the results of smear tests. Some general practices still do not inform patients of a negative result, relying on the suggestion that 'no news is good news'. Clear recommendations that women should receive their test results are still being overlooked by some, with potentially serious physical and psychological consequences. Research has shown that women receiving their smear results, accompanied by an explanatory leaflet including a message that 'most smears showing dyskariosis do not indicate cervical cancer', were less anxious than the women who just received a letter informing them their smear was abnormal and investigations were needed. Good education and counselling from the outset may prevent future psychiatric and psychological morbidity and improve compliance with treatment (Wilkinson *et al.*, 1990).

The Breast Screening Programme has clear guidelines regarding results and all women must receive their results within two to three weeks of the mammogram. A positive result is likely to cause anxiety and thus patients must be given clear information about the implications of such a result and subsequent treatment.

Screening does represent a precarious balance between benefit and harm, but in the absence of any other means of reducing deaths from cancer screening is the only method currently available for tackling certain cancers (Austoker, 1989). However, all screening programmes should include evaluation of the psychological impact of invitation and participation.

EDUCATION AND TRAINING

In 1987 the white paper 'Promoting Better Health' which set out a range of proposals for changing GPs' terms of service and remuneration was introduced. In 1990 it was implemented following a great deal of discussion and controversy. The contract was designed to promote and reinforce the shift from the individual doctor–patient relationship to a broader practice–population focus and from a pre-occupation with treating illness to a concern for preventing illness and promoting health. Following the introduction of the white paper the number of practice nurses almost doubled in one year, and in 1993 the figure stood at about 18 000 part-time practice nurses in the UK. The major implication of the 1990 contractual changes was that practice nurses were being asked to undertake tasks for which they were not always fully trained or prepared. This applied particularly to the taking of cervical smears. Despite the changes implemented in April 1993 when health promotion clinics were phased out and a concept of 'banding' and target setting was introduced, nurses are still expected to undertake 'well woman' screening which involves taking smear tests, teaching breast awareness and performing bi-manual pelvic examinations.

The white paper 'Health of the Nation' (July 1992) aims to secure improvements in the general health of the population of England by increasing life expectancy and reducing premature death. Five key areas are selected for action.

One of these areas covers cancers, with the aim of reducing deaths from lung, breast, cervical and skin cancer, by the year 2000. Nurses will be involved in this area and it is therefore essential they are sufficiently knowledgeable not just in the areas in which they work but also, at the primary care level, in being able to empower clients and patients to make decisions which, in altering lifestyle, will reduce the risk of suffering from ill-health or greatly improve the quality of life.

Nurses must therefore have the knowledge, skill, responsibility and accountability identified in the UKCC 'Code of Professional Conduct' (1992) and 'The Scope of Professional Practice' (1992), which sets out the council's principles on which any adjustment to practice should be based.

Clause 3 of the UKCC 'Code of Professional Conduct' refers to maintaining and improving professional knowledge and competence. Clause 4 stresses the importance of acknowledging any limitation in knowledge and competence and of declining duties or responsibilities unless able to perform them in a safe and skilled manner.

In order for a practice nurse to be fully prepared to undertake well woman screening, she should receive adequate, appropriate and assessed training. There are few courses in the country that fulfil these criteria and thus many practice nurses rely upon their employing GP to teach them how to take a smear. Some of these GPs may be excellent teachers and thus prepare the nurses well for the task; however, some practice nurses receive little or no training, which puts not only the patient but also the nurse at risk.

Taking a cervical smear is not just a matter of sampling the cervix but involves a combination of good communication skills, empathy and a sound knowledge base to ensure the nurse can advise, support and counsel if ever the need arises.

WHAT TRAINING IS AVAILABLE?

Marie Curie cancer screening course for practice nurses

In 1986 the Marie Curie Foundation was awarded a grant of £10 000 per year for three years towards the cost of providing short-course education for practice nurses to increase their skills in taking cervical smears and undertaking bi-manual pelvic examination.

The course was broadened to include information for the practice nurse on breast cancer and breast cancer screening and in particular detailed reference to the NHSBSP, which was being set up on a national basis at that time. The course, which is administered from a central point, has developed and is highly respected as one of the foremost training courses for practice nurses in well woman and cancer screening work.

The courses are constantly assessed and evaluated by a steering committee of practice nurses who are active in the field of nursing and education. Each year approximately 50 courses are held in the UK. Each course lasts five days and is attended by 15–20 students. Days one and two comprise a breast screening module and days three and four a cervical screening module. Each module has a practical component, where the nurses are taught breast examination (with the aim of teaching breast awareness), pelvic examination and taking cervical smears with the aid of teaching models. The two modules are usually taken in consecutive weeks and are followed by a six-month period when the participants are required to prepare a written case study and undertake 15 sessions of supervised practice in each of the areas, i.e. cervical smears, breast examination (including teaching breast awareness) and bi-manual pelvic examination. During this period of supervised practice, the nurses are encouraged to visit a breast screening centre and a colposcopy clinic to give them insight into the complex issues, both physical and psychological, that are inherent in such situations. At the end of the six-month period the practice nurses attend day five of the course, where they have an opportunity to discuss their supervised practice and any practical, theoretical or ethical issues which have arisen in the intervening period.

Each course is led by an experienced and trained practice nurse facilitator who not only organizes the courses and books the speakers, but also coordinates the modules. Marking case studies and assisting if necessary with supervised practice is a major part of the facilitator's role, but giving practical and emotional support during the six-month supervised practice period is often necessary. It has to be remembered that the nurses are employed either part-time or full-time in busy general practices. They encompass many roles within a working day and well woman work is often only a minor part of this work in terms of time, but in emotional and practical terms requires a great deal of commitment. The time required for preparing the case study is both onerous and for many anxiety provoking. Kindly support and encouragement are essential components of the facilitator's role.

Course evaluation

All the courses are evaluated by the participants, the facilitators and the course administrator after the modules and again after the follow-up day has been completed. The steering committee will make modifications as necessary to future courses based on these course evaluations. The constantly changing areas of cervical and breast screening require careful attention to current health policy, and the course notes introduced in 1991 to support the courses have recently been revised and updated to ensure the information is still apposite and accurate.

Women's screening and health promotion course: ENB No. 13

The aim of this course is to educate and train nurses for an advanced professional and specialist role in providing advice, care and support to women of all ages in healthy lifestyles and to perform specialist and appropriate screening procedures safely. This course includes sessions on the practical and theoretical aspects of cervical and breast screening, along with information on sexually transmitted disease, the menopause and general health screening.

BSCC booklet and video

Taking Cervical Smears (BSCC, 1989) is a useful training resource describing clearly how to take reliable cervical smears. It can be used alone but is more valuable as part of an organized training course, for example the Marie Curie cancer screening course.

REFERENCES

Austoker, J. (1989) The pros and cons of screening for cancer. *Cancer Care*. Medicine Group (UK) Ltd, London.

Austoker, J. (1990) *Breast Cancer Screening: Practical Guide for Primary Care Teams*. Cancer Research Campaign, Oxford.

Austoker, J. and McPherson, A. (1992) *Cervical Screening*. Practical Guides for General Practice, no. 14. Oxford University Press, Oxford.

Ayre, J.E. (1944) A simple office test for uterine cancer diagnosis. *Canadian Medical Association Journal*, **51**, 17–22.

Bourn, J. (1992) *Cervical and Breast Screening in England*. Report by the Comptroller and Auditor General, HMSO, London.

Bourne, T., Campbell, S., Steer, C. *et al.* (1989) Transvaginal colour flow imaging: a possible new screening technique for ovarian cancer. *British Medical Journal*, **299**, 1367–79.

Campbell, S., Bhan, V., Royton, P. *et al.* (1989) Transabdominal ultrasound screening for early ovarian cancer. *British Medical Journal*, **299**, 1363–7.

Cancer Research Campaign (1989) Factsheet 3: *UK (females)*.

Cancer Research Campaign (1991a) Factsheet 7: *Breast Cancer Screening*.

Cancer Research Campaign (1991b) Factsheet 17: *Ovarian Cancer – UK*.

Chamberlain, J. (1991) Practical policies for screening for early detection of cancers, in *Reducing the Risk of Cancers* (eds T. Heller, B. Davey and L. Bailey), Hodder & Stoughton, London.

Cuckle, H. and Wald, N. (1991) Screening for ovarian cancer, in *Cancer Screening* (eds A.B. Miller *et al.*), Cambridge University Press and UICC, Cambridge, pp. 228–39.

Department of Health and Social Security (1988) *Cervical Cancer Screening*. Department of Health, London, HC(88)1.

Farmer, R.D.T. and Miller, D.L. (1983) *Lectures Notes on Epidemiology and Community Medicine*. Blackwell Scientific Publications, Oxford.

Forrest, P. (Chair) (1986) *Breast Cancer Screening: Report to the Health Ministers of England, Wales, Scotland and Northern Ireland*. HMSO, London.

Hoare, T. and Thomas, C. (1993) A randomised controlled trial of a linkworker intervention to increase uptake of breast screening by Asian women. Manchester. Poster presented at International Breast Cancer Screening Conference, Cambridge, March 1993.

Imperial Cancer Research Fund (1992a) *Leeds and the North*. ICRF, London.

Imperial Cancer Research Fund (1992b) *Breast Cancer: Saving more Lives*. ICRF, London.

Imperial Cancer Research Fund (1992c) *Cervical Cancer Research Factsheet*. ICRF, London.

Jacobs, I. and Oram, D. (1990) Potential screening tests for ovarian cancer, in *Ovarian Cancer: Biological and Therapeutic Challenges* (ed. F. Sharp *et al.*), Chapman & Hall, London.

Knight, D. and Taylor, V. (1992) *Health Education Breast Screening Training Resource*. NHS Breast Screening Programme/SW Thames Regional Health Authority/Yorkshire Health.

Marteau, T.M. (1990) Screening in practice: reducing the psychological costs. *British Medical Journal*, **301**, 26–8.

Miller, A.B., Chamberlain, J., Day, N.E. *et al.* (eds) (1990) *Cancer Screening*. Report on the workshop to update conclusions on screening for cancer of sites previously considered, and to evaluate some new sites, held at Selwyn College Cambridge, UK, 2–5 April 1990. Cambridge University Press on behalf of UICC.

Nathoo, V. (1988) Investigation of non-responders at a cervical cancer screening clinic. *British Medical Journal*, **296**, 1041–2.

National Health Service Breast Screening Programme (1993) *Standards for the NHS Breast Screening Programme*. Department of Health, London.

Posner, T. and Vessey, M. (1988) *Prevention of Cervical Cancer: The Patient's View*. King Edward's Hospital Fund, London.

Quilliam, S. (1992) *The Positive Smear*. Letts, London.

Wilkinson, C., Jones, J.M. and McBride, J. (1990) Anxiety caused by abnormal result of cervical smear test: a controlled trial. *British Medical Journal*, **300**, 440.

Wilson, J.M.G. and Jungner, R.G. (1968) *Principles and Practice of Screening for Disease*. Public health paper 34, WHO, Geneva.

Wolfendale, M.R., Howe-Guest, R., Usherwood, M. McD. and Draper, G.J. (1987) Controlled trial of a new cervical spatula. *British Medical Journal*, **294**, 33–5.

Young, R.C., Walton, L.A., Ellenberg, S.S. *et al.* (1990) Adjuvant therapy in stage 1 and stage 2 epithelial ovarian cancer. *New England Journal of Medicine*, **322**, 1021–7.

FURTHER READING

Forrest, P. (1990) *Breast Cancer: The Decision to Screen*. Nuffield Provincial Hospitals Trust, London.

Cancer Research Campaign Factsheets on Breast Cancer Screening and Cervical Cancer Screening (and other titles).

Miller, A.B., Chamberlain, J., Day, N.E. *et al.* (eds) (1991) *Cancer Screening.* Cambridge University Press, Cambridge.

Imperial Cancer Research Fund Factsheets (on all forms of cancer, screening and up-to-date information).

Stoll, B. (ed.) (1989) *Social Dilemmas in Cancer Prevention.* McMillan Press, London.

USEFUL ADDRESSES

Health Education Authority, Hamilton House, Mabledon Place, London WC1H 9TX (Tel. 071 383 3833). Provides resources and is a source of health education expertise.

Women's Nationwide Cancer Control Campaign (WNCCC), Suma House, 128/130 Curtain Road, London EC2A 3AR (Tel. 071 729 4688; Helpline: 071 729 2229). Provides information and advice on the early detection and screening of breast and cervical cancer.

Imperial Cancer Research Fund, PO Box 123, Lincoln's Inn Fields, London WC2A 3PX (Tel. 071 242 0200). Research into causes, prevention and treatment of cancer. Useful source of information.

Cancer Research Campaign, 10 Cambridge Terrace, Regent's Park, London NW1 4JL (Tel. 071 224 1333). Information on causes and cures of cancer and education and psychological support for patients.

United Kingdom Coordinating Committee on Cancer Research (UKCCCR), PO Box 123, Lincoln's Inn Fields, London WC2A 3PX (Tel. 071 269 3548/071 269 3249). Provides a forum for the coordination of the activities of bodies funding cancer research and for collaboration in joint projects.

RESOURCES

BSCC booklet and video: *Taking Cervical Smears* (BSCC, 1989).

For further information, contact: Dr Keith Randall, Red Tree House, Pine Glade, Keston Park, Orpington, Kent BR6 8NT.

For breast and pelvic models and further information contact: Philip Harris Ltd, Weston-super-Mare, BS24 9BJ (Tel. 0934 413606).

Chemotherapy and the administration of cytotoxic drugs into established lines

5

Julia Luken and Janice Middleton

INTRODUCTION

The increased use of cytotoxic drug therapy in the treatment of cancer particularly in the out-patient setting has resulted in the need for properly trained nurses to deliver the treatment safely and provide continuity of care. The nurse administering cytotoxic drugs needs to be technically skilled and knowledgeable about the preparation and administration of drugs by the intravenous (i.v.) route. Particular knowledge of the administration, side-effects and regimes used in cytotoxic chemotherapy will prepare the nurse for this role. Awareness of each drug's side-effects will enable the nurse to take action to minimize or prevent these developing. Good communication skills are essential as patient education and information form an integral part of the role. This will encourage patient and family to be active participants in the treatment.

This chapter aims to provide background information for nurses administering cytotoxic drugs and caring for the patients receiving them, including:

- the historical development of cytotoxic chemotherapy;
- outline of a course for nurses;
- cytotoxic drugs and how they work;
- the safe handling of cytotoxic drugs;
- drug-related problems and side-effects.

THE DEVELOPMENT OF CYTOTOXIC CHEMOTHERAPY

The first drug to be used for its cytotoxic effects in the treatment of cancer was nitrogen mustard. During the First World War (1914–18) when mustard gas was used in chemical warfare, soldiers who died were found to have no bone marrow and those who survived had a reduced white cell count (Calvert and McElwain, 1988). Logical appraisal of these facts and research led to the use of nitrogen mustard in the treatment of leukaemia in 1941. Increased understanding of the biology of the cancer cell, drug action and alertness to the properties of plant extracts and synthetically developed chemicals led to the development of a whole range of new anticancer drugs.

Cytotoxic drugs, as their name implies, are poisonous to cells. Most produce their effect by damaging cells which are in the process of division, either killing them or preventing their division. They are therefore particularly damaging to rapidly growing cancers and cause side-effects in active tissues of the host such as the bone marrow, gonads and gut.

Cytotoxic drugs are used in a number of ways. Most commonly they are used:

- to effect a cure in some cancers, e.g. choriocarcenoma, Burkitt's lymphoma and metastatic teratoma;
- prior to radiotherapy or surgery to reduce tumour size;
- after radiotherapy or surgery to eliminate the remaining disease;
- to treat the patient following a relapse;
- for the palliation of advanced disease;
- in research, to develop new treatments.

Several devices are used to make chemotherapy more effective. Drug administration is timed to be damaging to the cancer cells while allowing the body to recover. The latest developments with growth factors suggest that the host's recovery can be stimulated. Combinations of several drugs are used to prevent the cancer cells developing resistance. Anticancer chemotherapy – the use of cytotoxic drugs – is a developing specialty where nurses can extend their traditional role; to do this they have to combine skills training with understanding and experience and keep up to date with developments.

A COURSE IN INTRAVENOUS THERAPY

Nurses who administer drugs through established i.v. lines should be professionally trained to the standard required by their employing authority and consider themselves competent to carry out the actions required. This is their professional responsibility.

Courses to teach nurses the skills needed to administer drugs through established lines are available locally through health authorities and for the administration of cytotoxic drugs at specialist centres. An established

Table 5.1   Specific objectives for the nurse attending the course

Asepsis	Understand the principles of asepsis with reference to the immunosuppressed patient and the methods of management and daily care of intravenous pathways
Equipment	Be aware of the equipment available to safely control the administration of cytotoxic drugs
	Be able to select the right equipment for the job and know how to adapt equipment to the specific needs of the patient
Policies and procedures	The nurse should be able to demonstrate an awareness of district policies related to intravenous management and cytotoxic drug handling
Patient care	Be able to discuss the principles for safe administration of cytotoxic drugs and be aware of the hazards and complications of their use
	Be able to inform the patient on all aspects of their treatment with cytotoxic drugs
	Be aware of short- and long-term side-effects and advise the patient on minimizing them
	Demonstrate communication skills appropriate for patients undergoing cytotoxic therapy

national course, 'administration of cytotoxic drugs into established lines', is available through the Marie Curie Cancer Care Education Department. This course, which is run several times a year at different localities, lasts for three days and aims to prepare a nurse in the skills needed to administer cytotoxic drugs. Following a period of formal teaching, demonstration and practical sessions the nurse will understand the principles of the:

- management of i.v. pathways;
- addition of cytotoxic drugs to i.v. infusions;
- administration of cytotoxic drugs via an established i.v. line;
- care of the patient receiving cytotoxic drugs.

The objectives of the course are specific to the administration of cytotoxic drugs but are applicable to the administration of all drugs in this way (Table 5.1)

EQUIPMENT

Cannulae

The cannula through which cytotoxic drugs are to be administered should have been recently sited. The longer a cannula is in situ the greater the risk of leakage and phlebitis (Plumer, 1982). The position and patency of the cannula must be confirmed using normal saline and careful observation prior to the administration of the drugs. The problems of venous access in patients having cytotoxic drugs require the use of small-gauge cannulae.

Dressings

The insertion site must be considered a breach of the body's first line of defence against infection – the skin. This site should be covered by a sterile dressing (Oldman, 1991). There are several methods of achieving this. The unsterile adhesive tape should not contaminate the insertion site. The insertion site may be covered by sterile gauze dressing (Goodinson, 1990) which can be removed for observation without disturbing the cannula. Observation of the site for signs of infiltration, phlebitis or infection is necessary prior to use. The alternative to tape plus a sterile dressing is a clear, sterile, semi-occlusive dressing, which allows passage of water vapour and gases but is impermeable to bacteria (Oldman, 1991). These must be applied carefully to ensure correct placement.

Administration sets

These must be suitable for the circumstances. The majority of administration sets used in relation to cytotoxic drugs have a very short life. This is due to the way the drugs are administered – through the side arm of a fast-running infusion or as a short infusion under four hours. Therefore cost is important and the cheapest set fulfilling the requirements, e.g. double Y-site, availability of secondary sets, is appropriate. Dedicated sets should only be used with the designated infusion device.

The frequency of administration set changes may vary but research by Maki *et al.* (1987) suggests that every 72 hours is appropriate. The patients receiving cytotoxic drugs are immunosuppressed and more frequent changes may be necessary.

Some drugs are light-sensitive, e.g. dacarbazine. Amber-coloured administration sets are available which protect the drug from light but allow the infusion to be seen and monitored. These sets are marketed by several different manufacturers.

PRACTICES

Asepsis

Strict aseptic technique is of prime importance as the patient is having immunosuppressive therapy.

Frequent handwashing is essential as many nurses have been found to carry antibiotic-resistant Gram-negative organisms on their hands (Goodinson, 1990). As far as is possible a 'no touch technique' should be used. The local policy on the use of gloves when caring for an i.v. site should be followed.

The cannula should be inserted using an aseptic technique. Skin should be cleaned with either a rapidly acting iodine solution in 70% alcohol or a 70% alcohol solution applied with friction for one minute (Goodinson, 1990).

The cannula must be fixed securely in position. Movement of the cannula will not only irritate the vein but may introduce bacteria.

Injection sites are a potential source of contamination and meticulous care must be observed. The latex injection port (Y-site of an administration set) or latex bung should be cleaned with 70% alcohol, which is allowed to dry prior to use. This point of access is preferable to an injection port integral to a cannula. The use of three-way taps increases the number of potential sites for contamination to occur and are not recommended for use with immunocompromised patients.

The use of 0.22 μm in-line filters is much debated, particularly in relation to drug administration. Manufacturers recommend that drug doses below a specific milligram amount per 24 hours should not be administered through the filter. The addition of the filter creates another connection to the system, increasing the potential sites for contamination. Local policy should be followed.

Care of the intravenous site

The i.v. site should be inspected for inflammation and swelling:

- daily;
- prior to drug administration;
- if the patient complains of pain;
- prior to bag changes.

Pain may indicate either extravasation or phlebitis or infection. Any complaints of pain must be thoroughly investigated. If there is any doubt the cannula should be resited.

Intermittent use of a cannula occurs frequently. The cannula should be left between uses with a flush in the lumen to prevent clotting. There is debate over the use of heparinized saline or normal saline. The use of heparinized saline is associated with problems:

- heparin-induced thrombocytopenia;
- incompatibility between heparin and drug administered;
- over-heparinization due to frequent flushing.

Johnstone (1991) reviewed the literature and concluded that:

- there is no good evidence for the use of heparinized saline;

- heparinized saline can cause adverse effects;
- normal saline has a cost advantage.

There are two important points when a cannula is to be left in situ but not in use:

- the final flush should be administered via the rubber bung;
- the needle should be withdrawn under positive pressure.

When removing the cannula a dry dressing should be used and pressure applied for five minutes. An alcohol-impregnated swab will inhibit clotting.

CENTRAL LINES

These are used in patients:

- requiring a lot of venous access, e.g. leukaemic patients;
- with poor or no venous access.

The patients in the first group will have central lines placed as a routine at the start of treatment.

The lines are inserted usually into the subclavian vein and then tunnelled beneath the skin for several inches. This ensures the exit site is well away from the insertion site – an important factor for prevention of infection. The technique for insertion varies with the different lines available but will require either a local anaesthetic or a general anaesthetic. This is a sterile procedure. The position of the line must be checked prior to use, either by insertion under X-ray control or by chest X-ray on completion of the procedure.

There are many systems in use:

- silicone (Hickman/Broviac) lines;
- polyurethane lines;
- implantable systems.

All these lines may stay in situ for long periods of time. They can be used for all venous access requirements:

- taking blood samples;
- administration of fluids;
- administration of blood and blood products;
- parenteral nutrition;
- drug administration.

The care of these lines is very important and a strict aseptic technique must be maintained at all times.

Lines with external access may be cuffed or uncuffed. The cuffed line has a Dacron cuff which is sited in the skin tunnel. This fibroses into the tissue. A stitch is required to hold the line in place until fibrosis occurs – approximately 10 days – at which time it may be removed. This ensures there is no focus for infection. Uncuffed lines must retain the stitch to hold the line in place.

Each unit should have a policy on the dressing of these lines: what dressing is used, frequency of changes and, for cuffed lines, whether a dressing is necessary when the patient is at home. The patient should be taught how to care for the line at home:

- flushing if required;
- hygiene;
- how to change the dressing;
- contact number for help.

The implantable systems use similar lines but an access port is implanted beneath the skin. There is therefore no exit site on the surface of the skin. Some patients find this cosmetically more acceptable and the risk of infection is reduced. The access port requires dedicated needles to access it – Huber needles with a long, shallow bevel to prevent coring of the port material. The disadvantage of this system is that the patient still requires a needle to be inserted through the skin although it is reported that the area of skin over the port becomes numb.

Hickman/Broviac lines should be flushed with heparinized saline. This is usually required either on a daily basis or the minimum of weekly flushing. The polyurethane lines can be flushed with normal saline and experience suggests this should be weekly. The implantable systems should be flushed with heparinized saline at four- to six-week intervals.

Complications

These central lines are susceptible to all the complications of any centrally placed line whether for long-term use or not, e.g. air embolism, bleeding. The length of time these lines are left in situ coupled with the immunosuppression of the patients involved make them susceptible to additional complications.

The major complication of long-term use of central lines is infection. This may be of the tunnel and is usually easily treated. Systemic infections may also occur either with the line as the source – the line being colonized with the infecting organism – or from an alternative source with the line being colonized as a secondary event. These infections must be treated with appropriate drug therapy administered via the line to sterilize it. Persistent infective colonization of the line may necessitate removal of the line.

Clotting of the line may occur. This may be due to poor flushing technique or poor/faulty connections. The line should be gently aspirated using a 2 ml syringe, then saline gently flushed down the line. Undue pressure should not be used as this may damage the line or result in a thrombus being dislodged. If these measures do not free the line it may be filled with urokinase to dissolve the clot (Barrus and Danek, 1987).

PATIENT INFORMATION

Information must be offered using language the patient can understand and may need repeating on several occasions. The information should be given verbally to allow questions and be reinforced with written material.

Information for patients is essential for many reasons. Knowledge facilitates coping. Lack of knowledge in advance of a possibly threatening event can impede coping (Leventhal and Johnson, 1983). The patient can develop a 'schema' – a picture – of the event (Dodd, 1984). This is believed to be a positive effect but may be negative. Negative effects may be the result of information gleaned from friends or relatives. Therefore specific information relating to what will happen when this patient comes to this unit for treatment is important.

Initial information about the treatment should be given prior to the patient's decision to accept cytotoxic drug therapy. This will include the number of treatments required, when the treatment will be administered, how the treatment will be administered, where the treatment will be administered and the expected side-effects of treatment. The information is necessary to allow the patient to make an informed decision to commence this treatment. The inclusion of a friend or relative, at the patient's discretion, in the discussions may be helpful.

Detailed information about the side-effects of treatment should be given at the time of treatment. This must be specific. The information must relate to the specific drugs and protocol with which the patient is being treated. Locally produced written information, to reinforce the verbal presentation, designed for each individual regimen used in that unit is the ideal. The ideal is not always realistic! There are many booklets written for patients about cytotoxic drugs available which can be used. These of necessity contain information about all the side-effects produced by cytotoxic drugs. All of these side-effects will not be applicable to an individual patient. The booklets should be carefully marked for each patient to indicate the side-effects relevant to him/her and his/her treatment. This should prevent a patient worrying about a side-effect not associated with the treatment.

It is relevant to augment the side-effect information with advice and help available locally. The inclusion of advice will aid the patient to develop coping strategies to control the situation. These strategies may well minimize or prevent a side-effect from occurring (Dodd, 1984). Local information, e.g. wig-fitting arrangements, is essential and must be added to a general booklet to complete the information provided.

COMMUNICATION SKILLS

The nurse who is actively involved in the administration of cytotoxic drugs needs to be technically skilled to deliver the drugs safely and equally skilled in communication methods. Communication skills used appropriately will provide essential support for the patient and family during long periods of cytotoxic drug treatment. Information-giving is an essential element of care (Coughlan, 1993).

Basic communication skills consist of listening and attending (Morrison and Burnard, 1992). Attending is the act of fully focusing on the other person – to give them your whole attention. Close and sustained attention leads to effective listening.

Listening is more than hearing what the other person says – it can be identified at three different levels (Morrison and Burnard, 1992):

1. Language
   - what is said
   - how it is said
   - the use of metaphors
   - special phrases.
2. Para-language
   - volume
   - pitch
   - fluency
   - silences/pauses.
3. Non-verbal
   - facial expression
   - gestures
   - touch
   - body movement
   - body position
   - eye contact.

The first level of listening is the act of hearing what is being said. The second level is to listen to the 'whole' conversation including non-verbal and para-linguistic behaviour. At the third level the listener becomes self-aware and empathy can develop. In this stage:

> the client feels listened to, the counsellor feels she is understanding the client and a level of mutuality is achieved in which both people are communicating, both rationally and intuitively. (Morrison and Burnard, 1992)

There are aids to effective listening:

- close attention
- non-judgemental approach

- appropriate environment
- physical comfort
- avoidance of interruption.

There are blocks to effective listening:

- lack of attention
- nurses attitude, e.g. to cancer
- unsuitable environment
- physical discomfort
- interruptions
- lack of privacy.

The basic communication skills of listening and attending are appropriate skills to be used by cancer nurses. In most hospital situations patients feel that nurses and doctors are too busy to stop and listen. The patient feels guilty about taking up valuable time.

When the nurse is administering cytotoxic drugs the time it takes to do this safely is time that can be used to give close and sustained attention to the patient. This is a rare opportunity to take time to listen and develop a relationship. Over months of treatment this relationship can allow trust to build, enabling the patient to confide problems. This cooperation can promote a more positive approach to treatment and provide the emotional and physical support that is essential to the patient and family. Tschudin (1988) observes that to communicate with another person effectively is to help that person. (See also Chapter 9 on communication.)

CYTOTOXIC DRUGS

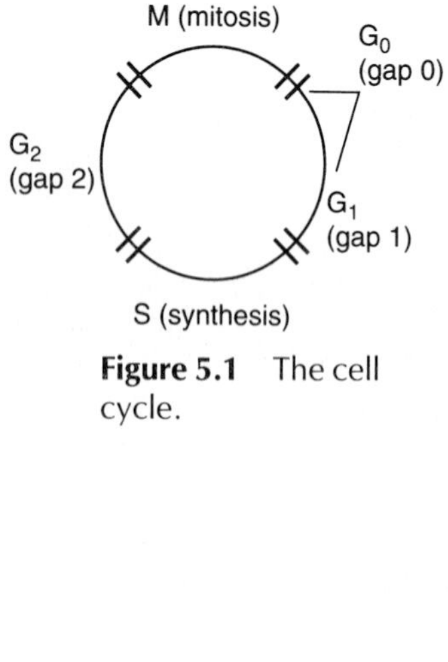

Figure 5.1 The cell cycle.

Cytotoxic drugs are toxic to all dividing cells. This means that they act against the cells of the host as well as those of the cancer.

The dividing cell passes through four phases of activity: G_1, S, G_2 and M (Figure 5.1). G_0 (gap 0) denotes the resting phase, where cells remain until stimulated to divide.

When a cell is stimulated to divide it enters the cycle at G_1 (gap 1) and is triggered into the S (synthesis) phase. During this phase the nucleic acids RNA (ribonucleic acid) and DNA (deoxyribonucleic acid) are replicated for the two daughter cells and the cell enters a second resting phase, G_2 (Robinson, 1993).

The final phase in cell division is mitosis (M); during this phase the spindle is formed and the DNA is divided for the two daughter cells as they are formed and finally separate. These cells then enter the resting phase G_0 or continue in the cycle to produce more cells.

The time taken for a cell to complete all phases of the cycle depends on the type of cell and is related to the time spent in G_1 (Groenwald *et al.*,

1992). Normal cells only divide to replace cells lost through death or damage and during body growth (Tortora and Anagnostakos, 1987). Cancer cells do not necessarily divide at a faster rate than normal cells but they do not recognize the controlling mechanisms. Cancer cells therefore divide continuously and erratically.

Cytotoxic drugs interfere with cell division and do not affect cells in the G_0 phase. Cytotoxic drugs act on all dividing cells, therefore normal tissues are also affected. Treatment has to be planned with these facts in mind.

PRINCIPLES OF TREATMENT

PULSING TREATMENT

Pulsing is the usual routine for the administration of cytotoxic drugs. The drugs are given, followed by a rest period. This allows:

- normal cell recovery;
- non-dividing (G_0) cells to be recruited into the dividing cycle;
- reduced toxicity.

Pulsing drug administration exploits a difference between normal and cancer cells. Cancer cells do not have the same capacity for recovery as normal cells. The cancer cell population is reduced by a percentage with each pulse of cytotoxic drugs. The resting period must be long enough to permit normal cell recovery but not long enough to allow cancer cell recovery. This is monitored by the full blood count (FBC). The length of time varies with the drugs used, the protocol used and individual patient response, e.g. treatment may be administered:

- once a week;
- on day 1 and day 8 of a 14-day cycle;
- on day 1 of a 21-day cycle;
- on day 1 and day 8 of a 28-day cycle;
- on days 1–5 of a 21-day cycle.

There are many variations.

DRUG COMBINATIONS

Many drug regimens use several different drugs. The number of drugs in a combination may be as few as two or as many as six or more. The reasons for drug combinations are to:

- increase cell kill due to synergistic action of the drugs;

- increase cell kill by using drugs which act at different phases of the cell division cycle;
- reduce development of drug resistance.

DURATION OF TREATMENT

The number of pulses of cytotoxic drugs required to complete treatment varies according to the protocol used. Assessment of the patient and disease response to treatment may be required at specific stages in the protocol. Many regimens give six pulses of treatment. There is evidence to show that some patients are under-treated (i.e. disease returns rapidly at the end of treatment) and others may be over-treated. New protocols, especially for treatment of teratoma, are attempting to select the patients with good prognostic disease features for less treatment and those with poor prognostic disease features for more intensive treatment.

DRUG CLASSIFICATION

There are two methods of classifying cytotoxic drugs:

1. according to activity on the cell cycle;
2. chemical group.

The first method divides the drugs into:

- phase-specific drugs – known to act at a specific stage in the cell dividing cycle;
- cycle-specific drugs – includes drugs known to act at more than one stage and those where stage of activity is unknown.

This classification is complex. The knowledge of the specific stage of activity within the cell dividing cycle is necessary when drug regimens are devised.

The second method is more frequently used and classifies cytotoxic drugs by their chemical action. There are five groups:

1. alkylating agents
2. antimetabolites
3. vinca alkaloids
4. antimitotic antibiotics
5. miscellaneous.

Alkylating agents

Drugs of this group in common use include **chlorambucil, cyclophosphamide, ifosfamide, melphalan, mustine,** and the nitrosureas **carmustine** and **lomustine.** This group of cytotoxic drugs developed from the observed effects of mustard gas. Agranulocytosis was noted in people exposed to mustard gas during the First World War.

The activity consists of the formation of a cross-link between the two strands of DNA which prevents separation necessary for cell division (Burgen and Mitchell, 1985).

The nitrosureas have a similar action and may therefore be placed in this group. They are lipid soluble, which allows crossing of the blood–brain barrier (Groenwald *et al.*, 1992).

Antimetabolites

Drugs in this group in common use include **cytarabine, 5-fluorouracil mercaptopurine, methoterxate** and **thioguanine**. The development of these drugs began in the 1940s.

The antimetabolites act by affecting either the synthesis or the introduction of purines and pyrimidines into nucleic acid (Burgen and Mitchell, 1985). They are similar to natural metabolites essential for cell function and compete with the natural metabolite. Where used they alter the molecule and thereby the function (Groenwald *et al.*, 1992). This prevents the formation of new DNA or RNA.

Vinca alkaloids

Drugs in this group include **vinblastine, vincristine** and **vindesine**. Vinblastine and vincristine are plant alkaloids derived from the South American periwinkle *Vinca rosae*.

The action of these drugs is to interfere with the protein tubulin. This protein is essential for spindle formation (Burgen and Mitchell, 1985).

Antimitotic antibiotics

Drugs in this group in common use include **actinomycin, bleomycin, daunorubicin, doxorubicin, epirubicin** and **mitomycin**. These drugs are fungal in origin.

The activity of the antimitotic antibiotics is to insert a ring between adjacent turns of DNA helix. This distorts the helix, inhibiting replication (Burgen and Mitchell, 1985).

Miscellaneous

Drugs in this group in common use include **asparaginase, carboplatin, cisplatin, mitozantrone,** procarbazine and the podophyllotoxins, e.g. **etoposide**. This group covers all drugs which cannot be categorized into the other four groups. This may be due to lack of knowledge of their mode of activity or to the drugs having more than one action.

Drugs other than cytotoxic drugs are also used to treat cancers.

Glucocorticoids

The drugs from this group commonly used to treat patients with cancer are **dexamethasone** and **prednisolone**. These drugs are used for their inhibition of lymphocyte production, depression of the anti-inflammatory response and production of a euphoric state. The desired action will vary with the context in which they are used.

HORMONE THERAPY

Hormones including oestrogens, progesterones, androgens and anti-adrenal drugs are used to treat tumours which are hormone-dependent and therefore sensitive to this mode of treatment (see Chapter 8).

BIOTHERAPIES

Biotherapy makes use of naturally occurring proteins which are cell regulators. They control the proliferation and maturation of cells. These proteins are called cytokines. Several of these proteins associated with the immune system have been identified and a few are available for clinical use. Others are the subject of research and development. Cytokines are used as supportive therapy to stimulate white blood cells (other than lymphocytes) to cover neutropenic episodes in susceptible patients and as active therapy in hairy cell leukaemia, renal cell carcinoma and advanced melanoma.

- Supportive therapy:
  - colony-stimulating factors (CSFs)
  - interleukin 3 (IL-3).
- Active therapy:
  - interferon (IFN)
  - interleukin 2 (IL-2).

Full details of these drugs, their actions and side-effects are discussed in Chapter 8.

SAFE HANDLING OF CYTOTOXIC DRUGS

Cytotoxic drugs are known to be carcinogenic (cause cancer), mutagenic (cause gene mutations) and teratogenic (affect embryonal tissue). The effects of long-term, low-dose exposure are not known but the properties of the drugs already stated suggest they may be hazardous. The short-term effects of exposure to the drugs can result in irritation of the skin, eyes and mucous membranes. Exposure to cytotoxic drugs should therefore be avoided by all concerned with their use.

The principles for handling the drugs are:

- protect the patient;
- protect yourself;
- protect the environment.

PROTECT THE PATIENT

The patient is equally susceptible to the problems of exposure as the nurse administering the drugs. Care should be taken to protect the skin. All connections between drug (syringe or container) and the patient should occur away from the patient's skin where possible. If this is not possible the skin should be protected.

PROTECT YOURSELF

The most hazardous part of handling cytotoxic drugs is the preparation of the drugs. The safest method of preparing these drugs is in a laminar flow cabinet conforming to Australian standard, ref. AS2567 or modified LAF class 2 BS5726 and BS5295 (Royal College of Nursing (RCN), 1989). An aseptic technique is essential and therefore drug preparation by pharmacy staff using such a cabinet, preferably situated in the clean preparation area, is the best environment for handler and drug. Bench-mounted cabinets are available conforming to the same standards and offering the same protection for the person preparing the drug: however, the drug itself is not prepared to the same high standard and should be used as soon as possible after preparation. The drug can only be stored for a maximum of 24 hours or less, dependent upon drug stability.

Pharmacy-based facilities are becoming more widely available. The drugs are prepared on an individual patient basis, arriving in the clinic or ward clearly labelled with the patient's name, the drug, dose and expiry time. This system offers safety for those preparing the drug and for patients receiving the drug.

However, where this facility is not available or out of pharmacy hours it may be necessary for drugs to be prepared by other members of staff. Any member of staff preparing these drugs should have received appropriate training (RCN, 1989).

The area and practices used should comply with the Control of

Substances Hazardous to Health (COSHH) Regulations 1988. Protective clothing should be worn **but** protective clothing is **no** substitute for good technique:

- gloves – should be of adequate thickness; either PVC (polyvinyl chloride) or latex rubber are appropriate (Laidlaw *et al.*, 1984; Thomas and Fenton-May, 1987);
- goggles – to conform to BS2092 (RCN, 1989);
- plastic apron or water-resistant gown;
- plastic or water-repellent armlets (not necessary with water-repellent gown);
- respirator face mask – when reconstituting dry powder in a glass ampoule – to BS 2091;
- ampoule necks should be wrapped in gauze prior to being broken.

The administration of cytotoxic drugs is less hazardous to the handler, therefore gloves of the appropriate thickness are sufficient.

PROTECT THE ENVIRONMENT

Care should be taken to prevent contamination of the area in which the drugs are being prepared.

Luer lock connections should be used on all equipment, particularly syringes. This is to prevent accidental disconnection which may endanger patients, staff preparing the drugs and those administering the drugs.

Air inlet devices should be used when preparing drugs supplied in rubber-stoppered vials. This will equalize the pressure in the vial with the atmosphere, preventing aerosol spray from the drug contaminating the air. There are numerous devices available: some are integral to the drawing-up needle and others are inserted separately.

Addition of diluent to dry powder preparations should be done slowly and carefully down one side of the vial.

Drug preparation should occur over a tray. This may be plastic or metal to prevent accidental spillage contaminating a large surface area.

Air bubbles from a drug-filled syringe should be expelled back into the vial or into a clean needle sheath.

A good technique in conjunction with the precautions discussed should offer adequate protection but must be inferior to that of the laminar flow cabinet situated in a clean area of pharmacy.

DISPOSAL OF WASTE

All waste contaminated with cytotoxic drugs should be disposed of according to local policy. **Disposable equipment should be incinerated.**

- **Needles, vials and ampoules** should be discarded into a suitable container which should conform to the British Standard Specification for Sharps Containers 1990 (Holloway, 1992).

- **Syringes** may be discarded as above or classed as dry waste and placed in a bag for incineration (yellow bag).
- All other disposable equipment should be classed as dry waste and placed in a bag for incineration.

Non-disposable equipment should be washed in warm, soapy water and dried.

- **Unused cytotoxic drugs** should also be incinerated at a temperature of 1000°C. This may be done by returning unused drugs to the pharmacy.
- **Body fluids** – includes body fluids and linen or clothing contaminated either by the drugs themselves or by excreta from a patient receiving cytotoxic drug therapy (Harris and Dodds, 1985). Local infection control policies should cover this (RCN, 1989).

SPILLAGE

- **Skin** should be washed with copious amounts of water. Soap may be necessary to remove colour from a drug left on the skin. This must be reported as an accident; appropriate forms should be completed and managers informed.
- **Eyes** should be washed with a sterile eyewash solution but if not available water may be used. As some cytotoxic drugs may cause corneal ulceration the eye should be seen by a medical practitioner – an ophthalmologist if possible. This must also be reported as an accident, appropriate forms completed and managers informed.
- **Clothing** should be changed immediately and treated as contaminated linen according to local policy.
- **Hard surface**
  – Wet spillage: protective clothing (plastic apron and suitable gloves) should be worn. Disposable cloths or paper towels should be used and discarded for incineration as previously. Surfaces should be washed thoroughly using warm, soapy water and dried (RCN, 1989).
  – Dry spillage: protective clothing including a face mask should be worn. Wet paper towels should be carefully laid over the powder until it may be wiped as for wet spillage (RCN, 1989).

ADMINISTRATION

GOOD PRACTICE

All cytotoxic drugs should be administered through an indwelling i.v. needle. This is to ensure the needle can be fixed in place, reducing the risk of drug entering the tissues (extravasation). Cannulation with a hypodermic needle should never be used for cytotoxic drug administration. Therefore following the placement of an indwelling needle good practice should incorporate the following:

- Flush with normal saline to check needle position and patency.
- Administer drug using appropriate method.
- Flush between each drug with normal saline.
- Flush following last drug with normal saline.

INTRAVENOUS ADMINISTRATION OF CYTOTOXIC DRUGS

This is the most common route of administration. There are four methods of administering intravenous cytotoxic drugs:

1. bolus injection;
2. bolus injection into a fast running infusion;
3. continuous infusion;
4. intermittent infusion.

Bolus injection

This may be done by direct attachment of a syringe to an indwelling needle/cannula, by a syringe and hypodermic needle via an injection port of an administration set or by a syringe and hypodermic needle through a rubber bung attached to an indwelling needle/cannula.

Bolus injection into a fast running infusion

This method is recommended for most vesicant agents (cause tissue necrosis if extravasated). It requires the indwelling needle/cannula to be connected to an infusion of a compatible fluid. The drug is administered via the injection port at the same time as the fluid infusion is running, diluting the drug as it is administered.

Continuous infusion

This may require the infusion of either a large volume of fluid or a small volume.

Large-volume administration dilutes the drug to be infused in a bag of compatible fluid: 250 ml, 500 ml or 1 l. Each bag is administered over a prescribed period of time. Therefore several bags of diluted drugs may be required to complete treatment. A peripheral or a central line may be used for this method. The patient remains in hospital for the period of treatment.

Small-volume administration can be done using a syringe driver or an ambulatory infusion system. The drug is diluted in a syringe or dedicated container. The length of time taken to administer each syringe/container depends on the stability of the drug and the system being used. These parameters also determine how many syringes/containers are required to complete a treatment. These systems must use a central line. The patient is not required to remain in hospital for the duration of the treatment and arrangements will need to be made to change bags/containers as necessary. A contact number accessing help 24 hours a day seven days a week during the treatment period is essential.

Intermittent infusion

This method is used for drugs which require dilution and administration over periods of half an hour to four hours. The volume is dependent upon the drug being used and the dose. The time required for the infusion varies with the drug and with the protocol being used. Patients may either be in-patients or out-patients.

OTHER METHODS OF ADMINISTRATION OF CYTOTOXIC DRUGS

Although the majority of cytotoxic drugs are administered i.v. there are alternative methods: **intracavity**, **intramuscular**, **intrathecal**, **oral** and **subcutaneous**.

PROBLEMS ASSOCIATED WITH INTRAVENOUS ADMINISTRATION

Extravasation

This is the leakage of intravenously administered fluid or drugs into the surrounding tissues. There are some solutions – hypertonic, acid, alkaline – and drugs which cause tissue necrosis when extravasated. The cytotoxic drugs which have this ability – vesicant agents – are **actinomycin, dacarbazine, daunorubicin, doxorubicin, mithramycin, mitomycin, mustine**, the **vinca alkaloids – vinblastine, vincristine** and **vindesine** – and **etoposide** – the latter is highly irritant and should be treated as a vesicant.

Everyone administering these drugs should be aware of which drugs are vesicant and their potential for tissue damage. Each unit involved in administration of cytotoxic drugs should have a policy for treating the problem when it occurs (RCN, 1989). Whatever the policy decided upon in a unit it must be commenced immediately an extravasation has occurred. The person administering the cytotoxic drugs must have the authority to do this without reference to others. Once the policy has been put into action then senior medical and nursing staff must be informed. The patient should be seen by the medical staff as soon as possible and definitely prior to leaving the hospital. The details of the occurrence and the subsequent treatment must be fully documented in the patient's records.

Research in this area is limited, therefore there is no one definitive method of treatment (Larson, 1985). The use of heat or ice packs is common. Heat is thought to increase the blood supply and aid dispersion of the drug. It may increase the metabolic rate and lead to a rise in cellular damage (Plumer, 1982). Ice decreases the blood supply, reducing absorption of the drug into the tissues (Plumer, 1982). The use of plastic surgery particularly with reference to delayed healing of doxorubicin extravasation is widely advocated (Larson, 1985; Rudolf and Larson, 1987; Cox *et al.*, 1988).

Venous access

The problems of cannulation are outside the scope of this chapter. The nurse administering cytotoxic drugs should be aware which sites of venous access are suitable for each situation.

Continuous infusions of cytotoxic drugs through a peripheral line should, in order of preference, use:

* forearm, non-dominant arm;
* forearm, dominant arm;
* back of hand, non-dominant arm;
* back of hand, dominant arm.

These sites allow maximum use for the patient, necessary over a prolonged period of time.

Bolus injection sites include:

* back of either hand;
* forearms;
* antecubital fossa;
* inside of wrist (site of desperation!).

Short infusions may use the same sites other than the antecubital fossa. It is very painful and therefore difficult to keep the elbow straight for even a short period of time. The risk of movement increases the chance of extravasation.

If more than one attempt at cannulation is necessary second sites should for preference be on the other arm. If the same arm must be used the second site must be distal (further up the arm) to the first.

The lower limbs are not suitable for administration of cytotoxic drugs.

Patients who have had a mastectomy or dissection of axillary lymph nodes should receive their i.v. cytotoxic drug therapy using the opposite arm.

The use of a pre-existing cannula for cytotoxic drug administration is not recommended. There is an increased risk of venous damage.

The nurse must ensure the cannula is sited satisfactorily and suitably prior to administering any cytotoxic drugs.

DRUG-RELATED PROBLEMS

Anaphylaxis

This is a problem to be alert for when administering any drug, but is more common when using **asparaginase** intravenously. A test dose should be administered and the patient observed closely. Medical help should be immediately available during administration.

Acute local allergic reactions

This is most frequently seen when small, fragile veins are used to administer **doxorubicin, daunorubicin** and **epirubicin**. First there is redness (erythema) along the venous pathway. This is followed by the patient complaining of itchiness around the cannulation site. A blotchy urticarial rash with raised pale-coloured welts may then appear. An increase in the dilution of the drug may resolve the situation. Resiting of the cannula is dependent upon many variables. The fact that a small, fragile vein is being used indicates venous access is difficult and the patient's preference should be considered. The site should be flushed well prior to removing the cannula and frequently at this stage the rash and erythema will begin to resolve (Plumer, 1982).

Phlebitis

Vinblastine, mustine and **5-fluorouracil** are irritants and can cause phlebitis.

Mustine should be administered via a fast running infusion and flushed well with saline. The irritant nature of this drug frequently results in phlebitis, even with the use of all precautions.

Vinblastine may cause phlebitis in some patients. The dilution of the drug in twice the volume of diluent can resolve the problem. It may be helpful to use a diluent free of preservative as this could be an irritant.

Venous discoloration

5-fluorouracil and **mustine** cause a brown discoloration along the venous pathway used for administration. The discoloration following mustine administration may be associated with phlebitis. The effect is long lasting and may cause distress to patients.

Muscle pain

This may be due to venous spasm. The patient will complain of pain in the upper arm on the side of drug infusion. Slowing the infusion reduces the pain but care must be taken to ensure that **carmustine** and **dacarbazine** are infused within the time of drug stability.

SIDE-EFFECTS OF CYTOTOXIC DRUGS

Knowledge of the function of cytotoxic drugs at a cellular level forms the basis of an understanding of treatment regimens, their side-effects and patient management.

Cancer cells and normal cells have similar cell cycle times, but normal cells have a zero growth rate, i.e. replace one for one to repair and repopulate after death or damage. Side-effects are more acute in those tissues that divide for repair and replacement most frequently (Robinson, 1993).

BONE MARROW DEPRESSION

Myelosuppression is a life-threatening side-effect. There are a few exceptions but almost all cytotoxic drugs exhibit this side-effect to a greater or lesser degree. Stem cells in the bone marrow replicate continually. Stem cells are affected by cytotoxic drugs, therefore the number of new cells produced is diminished. The cells produced (Priestman, 1989) are:

- red blood cells   approx. lifespan   120 days
- white blood cells   approx. lifespan   4–5 days
- platelets   approx. lifespan   9–10 days

A full blood count taken before the next treatment will show whether the bone marrow has recovered. Interim blood counts may be ordered to monitor progress.

It is obvious that the cells with the shortest lifespan are the most vulnerable. The granulocyte is in fact the most susceptible. The first effect to be seen is a fall in white blood cell count in the peripheral blood approximately seven days after the cytotoxic drug is administered, with a return to normal levels approximately three weeks after treatment. The majority of cytotoxic drugs commonly produce a moderate effect but there are variations in severity. Mild or occasional effects are seen with bleomycin and **vincristine**; severe or dose-limiting effects are seen with **amsacrine, carboplatin, cisplatin, daunorubicin, doxorubicin, etoposide, melphalan, mustine** and the **nitrosureas** (Priestman, 1989).

There are also some variations in the duration of myelosuppression. The effect of mustine is seen in approximately two to three days. Mitomycin C, carmustine and lomustine have a late effect, requiring a four- to six-week delay between treatments.

Nursing actions for white blood cell depression

1. Provide written and verbal information to the patient and relatives about the serious nature of this side-effect and the subsequent risk of infection.
2. Practise and teach aseptic and good hygiene techniques (Priestman, 1989).
3. Educate the patient and relatives in prevention of exposure to known infections.
4. Teach the patient and relatives how to recognize and report early signs of infection.
5. Provide a 24-hour contact telephone number to report such signs and symptoms.

Nursing actions for platelet depression

1. Provide written and verbal information to the patient and relatives about this side-effect.
2. Avoid trauma to the patient, e.g. intramuscular injections.
3. Educate the patient and relatives to avoid trauma.
4. Teach the patient and relatives about early signs of haemorrhage, e.g. headache, nosebleeds, blurred vision, bruises, petechiae, blood in urine or other blood loss. Any of these signs must be reported.
5. Educate about the avoidance of certain drugs that would aggravate blood loss, e.g. aspirin.

Nursing actions for red blood cell depression

1. Provide written and verbal information to the patient and relatives about this side-effect.
2. Teach the patient and relatives about the symptoms of anaemia, e.g. tiredness, dizziness.
3. Observe for signs of anaemia, e.g. pallor, shortness of breath.
4. Suggest that the patient allows more time for rest.
5. Explain the procedure of blood transfusion if appropriate.

NAUSEA AND VOMITING

Many cytotoxic drugs cause nausea and vomiting, with the dose and number of emetic drugs in a regimen being significant. There are some drugs which are highly emetic: **actinomycin D, cisplatin, dacarbazine** and **mustine.**

Epithelial cells lining the gastrointestinal tract are extremely sensitive to cytotoxic drugs. The rate of cell division in this part of the body is only slightly lower than in bone marrow cells. All parts of the gut can be affected from the mouth to the large bowel, but the small intestine has a highly rapid cell turnover (24–48 hours), making it particularly sensitive. A short time after treatment with cytotoxic drugs villi mitosis ceases, therefore there is a loss of mucosa cells, which results in nausea and vomiting. This usually starts within 24 hours of treatment and may persist for a few days to one week.

Specific receptors ($5-HT_3$ receptors) in the gut are stimulated, which leads to the stimulation of the vagus nerve. This in turn stimulates the vomiting centre in the medulla, resulting in vomiting (Roberts, 1992).

Receptors in the chemoreceptor trigger zone in the brain are also responsible for chemotherapy-induced nausea and vomiting, stimulated by changing chemical levels in the brain and cerebrospinal fluid. Grunberg *et al.* (1992) discussed these mechanisms and their aetiology in a review of chemotherapy-induced emesis.

There is also a psychological component of nausea and vomiting, known as anticipatory vomiting. This occurs before actual drug administration and may be stimulated by particular smells, sights or sounds associated with treatment.

Nursing actions for nausea and vomiting

1. Provide information to the patient regarding his or her particular drug regime. Not all cytotoxic drugs cause vomiting, and if they do so the effect is variable.
2. Provide an appropriate antiemetic regime based on the drugs being given and the patient's previous experience. Assess the effectiveness of the chosen antiemetic at future treatment visits. Change if necessary.
3. Give instructions regarding antiemetic administration. Prophylactic and regular use has proved the most effective. The use of antiemetic suppositories may be more appropriate than tablets.
4. Give psychological support to prevent and reduce the stress of anticipatory nausea and vomiting. Reassure patients that they are not 'mad' and explain that this behaviour is a conditioned response. The use of a drug such as lorazepam, which has an amnesic effect, can be very helpful. A relaxed, friendly environment and the use of

distraction such as music or relaxation tapes may be used (Contanch, 1983).

5. Offer dietary advice; this is best in written as well as verbal form, to be used by the patient and their family throughout treatment. For example: eat little and often instead of three large meals a day; eat cold, ready-prepared food to avoid cooking smells; try fizzy drinks; eat what you fancy; try 'snack' foods. If there is persistent anorexia or weight loss provide nutritional counselling regarding methods of increasing calorie and protein intake without adding to food volume (Stollery, 1991).

6. Encourage self-care and independence (Richardson, 1991).

STOMATITIS

The drugs most likely to cause a sore mouth include **actinomycin D, bleomycin, cytosine arabinoside, daunorubicin, doxorubicin** and **methotrexate.**

Oral mucosa cells are damaged by cytotoxic drugs and their regrowth is inhibited. The effect occurs between five and seven days after treatment. The result is a painful, red, often ulcerated mouth. The pain may result in eating, drinking and speaking becoming a miserable struggle.

Infection can also occur due to immunosuppression and tissue damage. The infection may be bacterial, e.g. staphylococcus; fungal, e.g. candida; or viral, e.g. herpes simplex.

Nursing actions for stomatitis

1. Provide information about this side-effect so that good oral hygiene habits can begin.

2. Give instructions about keeping the mouth clean. A mild non-astringent antiseptic mouthwash, e.g. saline solution (one teaspoon of salt to one pint of water) may be used after meals and at bedtime (Pritchard and Mallett, 1992).

3. Give advice about teeth. Use a soft brush, to prevent unnecesary abrasions to the gums and oral mucosa. If dental care is required during chemotherapy treatment the dentist must be made aware of the cytotoxic drug therapy. Dentures are to be removed and cleaned as thoroughly as possible.

4. Remind the patient to include care to the lips. Lips kept soft and supple with a lip salve or Vaseline will be less likely to crack and become infected or sore.

5. Provide information about diet; suggest the avoidance of hot, spicy foods.

6. Stress the benefits of increasing oral fluids.

7. Educate the nursing staff, patient and family to inspect and assess the mouth. Teach the signs of early fungal infection. This must be reported and treatment started to avoid further spread, e.g. oesophagitis.
8. Provide written instructions to follow if mouth soreness develops. Use the saline mouthwashes every two hours. Use a mouthwash with local anaesthetic properties, e.g. Difflam, before meals to reduce the pain. Failure to improve with these measures requires medical intervention and the patient must be instructed to use the contact telephone number to report the situation.

ALOPECIA

The drugs most likely to cause alopecia are **cyclophosphamide, daunorubicin, doxorubicin, etoposide** and **epirubicin.**

Hair loss is not the inevitable result of cytotoxic drug therapy. Some drugs may cause mild alopecia – thinning of the hair rather than total baldness, e.g. vindesine. Others have no effect on hair growth.

There is a suppression of growth in hair follicle cells. The hair loss is reversible.

Loss begins three to six weeks after treatment starts and is usually limited to head hair, but body hair can also be lost. The growth of facial hair in men is greatly reduced; shaving may only be necessary every two to three days. This news is often well received! Eyebrows and eyelashes are affected in some patients.

Hair loss is a devastating side-effect for the patient and family. It is often seen as an outward sign of cancer in an otherwise fit and well-looking person. It presents an altered body image which can be difficult to deal with for both men and women. To help deal with hair loss nurses can provide practical advice and psychological support.

Nursing actions for alopecia

1. Provide information about the extent and nature of hair loss, stressing that hair will regrow.
2. Provide practical help for dealing with hair loss before it occurs, e.g. obtaining a wig, giving ideas for hats, scarves and use of jewellery. A photograph album showing patients happily managing and living with their hair loss can be useful, as can self-help support from other chemotherapy patients.
3. Advise about gentle care of the hair and scalp to minimize loss, e.g. avoid perms, bleaching agents, hot brushes and tight rollers, but use mild shampoos and gentle washing.
4. Allow time to discuss the psychological impact of hair loss. Even with adequate preparation the sight of baldness can be distressing.

5. Suggest the use of a towelling turban to wear at night so that hair lost in bed can be easily and less distressingly dealt with.
6. There are several booklets available (*How To Cope With Hair Loss*, from Wessex Cancer Trust; *Coping With Hair Loss*, from BACUP).

Scalp cooling

Some patients may have heard that scalp cooling can prevent hair loss. It has only been shown to be effective in the case of doxorubicin and this depends on precise timing and normal liver function (Satterwhite and Zimm, 1984). Scalp cooling should not be performed when there is any possibility of cancer cells circulating in the scalp vessels, and the patient's consultant should give permission for the procedure (Pritchard and Mallett, 1992).

TASTE CHANGES

Commonly accompanying the side-effect of nausea are changes in taste. This manifests as a loss of taste acuity and an over-emphasis on the sense of smell or food aversions, i.e. 'fads or fancies'. Along with other side-effects this may contribute to loss of appetite and weight loss. Also some chemotherapy drugs give a strange taste during administration, for example:

- cyclophosphamide – metallic taste/hot sensation;
- bleomycin – unpleasant taste and/or smell;
- mustine – unpleasant taste and/or smell.

Nursing actions for taste changes

1. Inform the patient and family about this possibility and explain the impact it may have on appetite.
2. Reassure that it is temporary, therefore 'fads and fancies' can be indulged.
3. Give advice to the family about reducing cooking smells.
4. Offer further nutritional counselling if it becomes necessary; monitor appetite during course of treatment.
5. Provide mints, boiled sweets, drinks, etc. to detract from the unpleasant taste during chemotherapy administration. Sucking half a lemon has been known to be preferable to the taste of bleomycin!
6. Suggest the use of alternative seasonings, e.g. herbs and spices.

See Stollery (1991) under 'References' and Hunter and Janes (1988) in the 'Further reading' section.

HAEMORRHAGIC CYSTITIS

The drugs responsible for this side-effect are **cyclophosphamide** and **ifosfamide**.

Symptoms can range from dysuria to acute haematuria. The metabolites of these drugs irritate the bladder. It can be prevented by an increase in fluids. Mesna is an agent that can prevent bladder irritation by being given at the time of treatment with ifosfamide and high doses of cyclophosphamide. It converts the damaging metabolites to harmless compounds (Priestman, 1989).

Nursing actions for haemorrhagic cystitis

1. Inform the patient about the possibility of this side-effect and educate about the signs and symptoms of cystitis.
2. Give specific instructions to patients receiving cyclophosphamide about increasing daily fluids, e.g. 6–8 pints of fluid daily for three days following i.v. administration; 3–4 pints of fluids daily during the course of oral administration.
3. Educate the patient to empty their bladder often to minimize the contact time in the bladder.

URINE DISCOLORATION

Some of the highly coloured drugs are noticeably excreted in the urine:

- daunorubicin – red urine;
- doxorubicin – red urine;
- mitozantrone – blue/green urine;
- mitomycin – blue/green urine;
- epirubicin – red urine.

Nursing actions for urine discoloration

Inform the patient of this possibility and reassure that it is harmless.

RENAL TOXICITY

This can be caused by **cisplatin, methotrexate** and **carboplatin**.

Acute renal tubule damage can be caused by cisplatin. It should always be used with pre- and post-treatment hydration to force adequate diuresis in order to minimize nephrotoxicity. (Lawson, 1993).

Methotrexate given in high doses can also produce tubular necrosis, much of the drug being excreted unchanged in the urine. Precipitation can occur in the tubules, causing severe damage. To avoid this the urine must be rendered alkaline, by using sodium bicarbonate, i.v. or orally, before, during and for 24 hours after treatment with an increase in hydration.

If there is poor renal function resulting in inadequate renal clearance other cytotoxic side-effects can be enhanced or prolonged.

Nursing actions for renal toxicity

1. These drugs should always be given in specialist centres with experienced supervision. Reasons for monitoring renal function need to be well understood.
2. Monitor and record the pre- and post-treatment hydration accurately.
3. Supervise the use of sodium bicarbonate by testing and monitoring the urine pH.
4. Give an explanation to the patient about the process to maintain their cooperation with the hydration regime.

NEUROPATHIES

Peripheral neuropathies

All the **vinca alkaloids** are neurotoxic, affecting sensory, motor or mixed nerves. The symptoms are tingling of the hands or feet, numbness, and weakness leading to loss of deep reflexes, becoming irreversible with cumulative doses.

Cisplatin occasionally has similar neurotoxic effects (Holden and Felde, 1987). This side-effect produces dose-limiting affects; the drug is withdrawn or doses reduced when symptoms appear, to avoid irreversible neuropathies.

Nursing actions for peripheral neuropathy

1. Inform the patient and encourage him or her to report the early symptoms of sensory disturbance.
2. Reassure about the generally reversible nature of the neuropathy but that it may take many weeks.
3. Question and monitor the patient for early symptoms.
4. Educate the patient and family about safety related to sensorimotor impairment, e.g. touching hot objects, dropping cups of hot drinks, kettles, etc.

Gastrointestinal neuropathy

The **vinca alkaloids** can cause similar neurotoxic effects on the nerve plexuses in the bowel wall, resulting in constipation and pain, occasionally leading to obstruction. Patients who have undergone abdominal surgery are more vulnerable.

Nursing actions for gastrointestinal neuropathy

1. Inform the patient of this possible side-effect.
2. Give dietary advice to minimize constipation.

Audio neuropathy

Hearing loss can be a side-effect of **cisplatin** treatment. Damage can be caused to the eighth cranial nerve causing tinnitus, high-frequency sound loss and deafness. Doses may need to be limited to avoid permanent damage. Baseline audiography may be prescribed before treatment begins.

Nursing actions for audio neuropathy

1. Inform the patient of the side-effect and encourage him or her to report any changes in hearing.
2. Make observations of any changes and report.
3. Educate the family to report any changes.

FOOD INTERACTIONS

Procarbazine is a mild monoamine oxidase inhibitor used for its cytotoxic effect in some regimens. The manufacturers suggest that food restrictions associated with these drugs are unnecessary but food containing tyramine should not be eaten in excess (Marmite, cheese). The Pharmaceutical Society has produced a patient leaflet, which is available.

Nursing actions for food interaction

Inform the patient and discuss foods not to be eaten in excess.

ALLERGIC REACTIONS

Allergic or hypersensitivity reactions can occur with any of the cytotoxic drugs. The process is the production of antibodies after exposure to the antigen (the drug); subsequent doses will then result in the allergic response. This response can range from mild (rashes and rhinitis) to severe (pulmonary distress and full anaphylactic shock). The drug most likely to cause an allergic reaction is **asparaginase**. Test doses are often recommended and adrenaline given if an emergency situation develops.

Mild allergic reaction to **bleomycin** is not uncommon, appearing about six hours post treatment with fever, chills and shaking. It is usually given in conjunction with hydrocortisone to reduce the symptoms.

Nursing actions for allergic reactions

1. Be aware of possible allergic reactions and know the early signs and symptoms of anaphylaxis. Be prepared to administer emergency care, and at all times be able to summon medical help.
2. Inform the patient if delayed reaction is a possibility, e.g. bleomycin, and provide instructions for treatment, e.g. paracetamol.

SKIN CHANGES

Hyperpigmentation

The drugs commonly responsible are **actinomycin D, bleomycin, busulphan** and **cyclophosphamide**.

This results in brown discoloration of the skin in exposed areas, skin creases and pressure areas, e.g. knees, elbows, knuckles.

Nail discoloration

Caused by **bleomycin, cyclophosphamide** or **doxorubicin**, this may be seen as discoloration or ridging of the nails.

Finger-tip ulceration/blisters or hardening of the skin

This can be caused by **bleomycin**.

Radiation skin reactions

Drugs responsible include **actinomycin, daunorubicin** and **doxorubicin**. A 'recall' reaction can happen at previously irradiated sites.

Sun skin reaction

Hypersensitivity to sunshine can occur during or immediately after treatment with **doxorubicin**.

Nursing actions for skin changes

Be aware of these specific reactions in order to give explanations, reassurance and advice to the patient.

CARDIOTOXICITY

The drugs responsible are **daunorubicin** and **doxorubicin**.

Cardiomyopathy is due to direct damage to cardiac muscle. It has a cumulative effect and is irreversible. Clinical symptoms can include pericarditis, left-ventricular dysfunction, arrhythmias and cardiac failure. It is usually suggested that a total dose does not exceed $550 \, mg/m^2$ of doxorubicin and $500–600 \, mg/m^2$ of daunorubicin (Priestman, 1989). Patients over 70 are likely to be more susceptible and those patients with a history of heart failure should probably have an alternative drug. Baseline electrocardiograph prior to **anthracycline** treatment is recommended.

Nursing actions for cardiotoxicity

1. Give a brief explanation regarding tests ordered and subsequent monitoring that may be required.
2. Check for total cumulative dose being reached.
3. Observe for signs of cardiac dysfunction.

PULMONARY TOXICITY

Bleomycin is the drug most likely to cause problems in as many as 40% of patients, causing severe pneumonitis and fibrosis of the lung tissue (Groenwald *et al.*, 1992). The effects are usually dose related and limit the total lifetime dose of bleomycin to 300 iu (Priestman, 1989). The toxicity is compounded by chest irradiation, other pulmonary conditions and age (over 70 years). Clinical symptoms may appear slowly over several months, with a dry cough, shortness of breath and changes on chest X-ray. If these symptoms occur the drug must be discontinued. The damage is usually irreversible and can be fatal.

Busulphan-induced lung toxicity manifests over several years (up to 10 years) and is related to duration of treatment rather than total dose. The incidence is less than that for bleomycin, being 2–10% (Groenwald *et al.*, 1992).

Carmustine-induced lung toxicity is associated with a cumulative total dose and occurs in 20–30% of patients (Groenwald *et al.*, 1992).

Nursing action for pulmonary toxicity

1. Provide a brief explanation and educate about the signs and symptoms of early pulmonary toxicity.
2. Observe for signs and symptoms of pulmonary toxicity.
3. Be aware that these patients may pose an anaesthetic risk.
4. Check for total cumulative dose being reached.

FERTILITY

Male

Spermatozoa are formed by stem cells and are therefore vulnerable to the effect of cytotoxic drugs. The result is a reduced sperm count (Averette *et al.*, 1990). The extent of the infertility depends on the type of drugs used. Alkylating agents have an especially high risk of causing permanent sterility (Priestman, 1989). There may also be decreased libido due to the general effects of chemotherapy, e.g. fatigue, anxiety, nausea and altered body image.

Female

Ova are formed before birth and therefore there is not the same effect as in men. Oestrogen levels fall, frequently causing women to have irregular menstruation or amenorrhoea during treatment; depending on age, this may lead to an early menopause.

Pregnancy during or soon after a course of cytotoxic treatment can result in serious fetal damage with gross abnormalities (Priestman, 1989). There is also concern about long-term genetic defects. Alkylating agents and methotrexate have a particularly high teratogenic and mutagenic risk.

Nursing actions for infertility

1. Information about sterility should be provided when treatment options are being discussed with the patient.
2. Counselling can be offered and is often helpful when dealing with this possible life-long effect (Averette *et al.*, 1990).
3. Provide reassurance about temporary impotence and/or loss of libido.
4. Sperm banking should be offered in appropriate cases.
5. Provide contraceptive advice to both sexes.

CONCLUSION

Nurses working in the oncology specialty need to continue to update their knowledge. New cytotoxic drugs and refinements to treatment regimens occur frequently.

The administration of cytotoxic drugs must be seen in the context of the whole care of the patient. The outcome of the nursing interventions should always be to encourage the patient and their family to live as normal a life as possible.

REFERENCES

Averette, H.E., Boike, G.M. and Jarrell, M.A. (1990) Effects of cancer chemotherapy on gonadal function and reproductive capacity. *Ca-A Cancer Journal for Clinicians*, 40(4), 199–209.

BACUP (undated) *Coping With Hair Loss*. BACUP, London.

Barrus, D.H. and Danek, G. (1987) Should you irrigate an occluded IV line? *Nursing*, 17(3), 63–4.

Burgen, A.S.V. and Mitchell, J.F. (1985) *Gaddum's Pharmacology*. Oxford University Press, Oxford.

Calvert, H. and McElwain, T. (1988) Principles of chemotherapy, in *Oncology for Nurses and Health Care Professionals*. Vol. 1: *Pathology, Diagnosis and Treatment* (eds R. Tiffany and P. Pritchard), Harper & Row, Beaconsfield.

Contanch, P. (1983) Relaxation techniques as an anti-emetic therapy, in *Anti-Emetics and Cancer Chemotherapy* (ed. J. Laszlo), Wilson & Wilkins, Baltimore.

Coughlan, M.C. (1993) Knowledge of diagnosis, treatment and its side-effects in patients receiving chemotherapy for cancer. *European Journal of Cancer Care*, 2, 66–71.

Cox, K., Stuart-Harris, R., Abdini, G. *et al.* (1988) The management of cytotoxic-drug extravasation: guide lines drawn up by a working party for the Clinical Oncology Society of Australia. *Medical Journal of Australia*, 148, 185–9.

Dodd, M.J. (1984) Measuring informational intervention for chemotherapy knowledge and self-care behaviour. *Research in Nursing and Health*, 7, 43–50.

Goodinson, S.M. (1990) Keeping the flora out: reducing risk of infection in IV therapy. *Professional Nurse*, 5(11), 572–5.

Groenwald, S.L., Frogge, M.H., Goodman, M. and Yarbro, C.H. (1992) *Treatment Modalities*. Jones & Bartlett, Boston.

Grunberg, S., Leonard, R.F.C., Smyth, J. *et al.*, (eds) (1992) Chemotherapy induced emesis: a review of aetiology, mechanisms, methodology and prospects for clinical management. *British Journal of Cancer*, 66 (Suppl.), S1–76.

Harris, J. and Dodds, L.J. (1985) Handling waste from patients receiving cytotoxic drugs. *Pharmaceutical Journal*, 235(6345), 289–91.

Holden, S. and Felde, G. (1987) Nursing care of patients experiencing cisplatin-related peripheral neuropathy. *Oncology Nursing Forum*, 14(1), 13–19.

Holloway, J. (1992) Safety from sharps. *British Journal of Nursing*, **1**(8), 389–90.

Johnstone, J.M. (1991) Heparinised saline: is the heparin really necessary? *Australian Nurses Journal*, **20**(8), 31–3.

Laidlaw, D.L., Connor, T.H., Theiss, J.C. *et al.* (1984) Permeability of latex and polyvinyl chloride gloves to 20 anti-neoplastic drugs. *American Journal of Hospital Pharmacy*, **41**, 2618–23.

Larson, D.L. (1985) What is the appropriate management of tissue extravasation by anti-tumour agents? *Plastic and Reconstructive Surgery*, **75**(3), 397–405.

Lawson, N. (1993) Cisplatin and carboplatin: a guide to administration. *European Journal of Cancer Care*, **2**(1), 16–20.

Leventhal, H. and Johnson, J.E. (1983) Laboratory and field experimentation: development of a theory of self-regulation, in *Behavioral Science and Nursing Theory* (eds P.J. Woolridge, M.H. Schmitt, J.K. Skipper Jr and R.C. Leonard), Mosby, St Louis.

Maki, D.G., Botticelli, J.T., LeRoy, M.L. and Thielke, T.S. (1987) Prospective study of replacing administration sets for intravenous therapy at 48 vs 72 hour intervals. *Journal of the American Medical Association*, **258**(13), 1777–81.

Morrison, P. and Burnard, P. (1992) *Caring and Communicating*. MacMillan Press, London.

Oldman, P. (1991) A sticky situation? Microbiological study of adhesive tape to secure cannulae. *Professional Nurse*, **6**(5), 265–9.

Plumer, A.L. (1982) *Principles and Practice of Intravenous Therapy*. Little, Brown & Co., Boston.

Priestman, T.J. (1989) *Cancer Chemotherapy: An Introduction*. Springer-Verlag, London.

Pritchard, A.P. and Mallett, J. (1992) *Manual of Clinical Nursing Procedures*, 3rd edn. Blackwell Scientific Publications, Oxford.

Richardson, A. (1991) Theories of self-care: their relevance to chemotherapy-induced nausea and vomiting. *Journal of Advanced Nursing*, **16**(6), 671–6.

Roberts, T. (1992) *Nausea and Vomiting in Cancer Patients*. Managing Cancer 1(3), Synergy Medical Education, London.

Robinson, S. (1993) Principles of chemotherapy. *European Journal of Cancer Care*, **2**, 55–65.

Royal College of Nursing (1989) *Safe Practice with Cytotoxics*. Scutari Projects, Harrow.

Rudolf, R. and Larson, D.L. (1987) Etiology and treatment of chemotherapeutic agent extravasation injuries: a review. *Journal of Clinical Oncology*, **5**(7), 1116–26.

Satterwhite, B. and Zimm, S. (1984) The use of scalp hypothermia in the prevention of doxorubicin-induced hair loss. *Cancer*, **54**, 34–7.

Stollery, R. (1991) *Eating Well During Your Treatment*. Bristol-Myers Squibb, Hounslow.

Thomas, P.H. and Fenton-May, V. (1987) Protection offered by various gloves to carmustine exposure. *Pharmaceutical Journal*, June 20th, 775–7.

Tortora, G.J. and Anagnostakos, N.P. (1987) *Principles of Anatomy and Physiology*. Harper & Row, New York.

Tschudin, V. (ed.) (1988) Counselling, in *Nursing the Patient with Cancer*, Prentice Hall, London.

Wessex Cancer Trust (undated) *How To Cope With Hair Loss*. Wessex Cancer Trust, Southampton.

FURTHER READING

Allwood, M. (1990) *Cytotoxics Handbook*. Radcliffe Medical Press, Oxford.

Calvert, H. (1988) The role of chemotherapy, in *Oncology for Nurses and Health Care Professionals*. Vol. 1: *Pathology, Diagnosis and Treatment* (eds R. Tiffany and P. Pritchard), Harper & Row, Beaconsfield.

Eli Lilly & Co. Ltd (undated) *Cytotoxic Chemotherapy*. Eli Lilly, Basingstoke.

Health and Safety Executive (1988) *Control of Substances Hazardous to Health (COSHH) Regulations*. HMSO, London.

Holmes, S. (1990) *Cancer Chemotherapy*. Austin Cornish, London.

Hunter, M. and Janes, E.M.H. (1988) Nutrition in cancer care, in *Oncology for Nurses and Health Care Professionals*. Vol. 2: *Care and Support* (eds R. Tiffany and P. Webb), Harper & Row, Beaconsfield.

Illier, H.J., Bornmann, L. and Herdrich, K. (undated) *Safe Handling of Cytotoxic Agents*. Astra Pharma AG, Frankfurt.

Speechley, V. (1991) Nursing patients having chemotherapy, in *Oncology for Nurses and Health Care Professionals*. Vol. 3: *Cancer Nursing* (eds R. Tiffany and D. Borley), Harper & Row, Beaconsfield.

An education package produced by the International Society of Nurses in Cancer Care in collaboration with Glaxo is described by:

Hawthorn, J. (1991) The management of nausea and vomiting induced by chemotherapy and radiotherapy: a comprehensive guide. *European Journal of Cancer Care*, **1**(1), 23–6.

Radiotherapy: its nature and scope 6

Philippa Green and Shaun Kinghorn

INTRODUCTION

Radiotherapy has emerged as a major treatment intervention in the local management of cancer. Recent developments have focused on trying to minimize the side-effects and to increase its potency in achieving cure and effective palliation. Such progress has been accompanied by a body of research, which has helped caring professionals become more adequately versed in the unique needs of the patient requiring radiotherapy.

The aims of this chapter are to provide an overview of:

- the historical development of radiotherapy;
- the nature and scope of radiotherapy;
- the role of the nurse and other health care professionals in caring for the patient receiving radiotherapy;
- the psychological and social consequences associated with radio-therapy;
- strategies which may help the patient and family come to terms with this daunting form of treatment.

HISTORICAL VIEW

It is just under 100 years since the discovery of radiation, in both its natural, and man-made forms. Radiation in its natural form has been present since the formation of the earth, yet despite this it was radiation in its artificial form that was discovered first. It was a German physicist, Wilhelm Konrad Röntgen, who in 1895 discovered X-rays; he had been carrying out experiments using cathode rays and barium platino-cyanide and was studying the fluorescence produced by these (Deeley, 1976). This was recognized as an exciting discovery in the field of medicine when it was realized that this method could be used to display the bones in the tissues of the body. This was the beginning of diagnostic radiology and Röntgen is now regarded as the 'father of radiation physics and diagnostic radiation', which now play a large part in cancer treatment.

If we now look at the discovery of naturally occurring radiation we find the first discovery being made by a physicist called Henri Becquerel in 1897. He had been looking at the magnetic and phosphorescent properties of some of the rare earths – uranium in particular – as it was thought that uranium had the power to hold light and to give this out as phosphorescence in the dark. Becquerel thought that this may be a similar phenomenon as that reported by Röntgen or alternatively that this was a property of uranium itself.

It was through his experiments that he was able to establish that uranium was a naturally radioactive substance. His work did not stop there. He continued to work with a couple of scientists called Marie and Pierre Curie. It was in 1898 that two more naturally occurring radioactive materials were discovered by the Curies; the first they called polonium, while the second and more widely known substance was radium, which was contained in pitchblende. Following the discovery of the therapeutic values of X-rays and radium they were hailed as a cure for many diseases which had previously been described as incurable. Other ailments such as tuberculosis, kidney stones, asthma, arthritis, acne and many other non-malignant conditions were also treated with radium. In addition to these it was used to treat nearly every malignancy known (Deeley, 1976).

The use of both X-rays, as discovered by Röntgen, and radioactive substances, as discovered by Becquerel and the Curies, have developed simultaneously since the turn of the century. The first successful treatment of a malignancy was recorded in 1899 in the USA and was for a malignant tumour of the nose; the patient was reported as being disease free in 1920 (Raven, 1990).

When radiation was first being used the patient would have been exposed to either repeated X-rays over a number of hours or the radioactive material for long periods of time, as described by Deeley (1976) and Raven (1990).

As a result of this patients experienced severe side-effects and long-term damage to the skin and other healthy tissues, and some even died. It was in the period 1920–35 that research was done to find a way of administering the maximum amount of radiotherapy to the tumour but minimizing the amount of damage done to the healthy tissues of the body. The research led to a technique, now known as fractionation, being used; this involves radiation being delivered in smaller doses every day over several weeks, so giving the same overall dose but allowing the healthy tissue time to repair as described by Regaud, Coutard and Hautant in 1922 (Holmes, 1988; Hall and Cox, 1989; Nias, 1990).

As well as the use of fractionation to help minimize the damage to healthy tissue a technique was introduced in 1925 whereby the radiation was delivered to the patient from more than one direction. It was initially used in the treatment of breast cancer because it had been noted that when using a single direct dose of radiation to the breast, damage was caused to the lungs.

The use of two directed beams of radiation meant that the tumour received a greater dose of radiation and only a small part of the lung was exposed to radiation (Deeley, 1976).

The last major development during the 1920s was that of brachytherapy, which involved low-activity radioactive substances being implanted either through tumour-bearing tissue or into a body cavity in close proximity to the tumour. The radioactive substance would be left in place for several days. The first malignancy this treatment was used for was uterine cancer. The treatment was initially developed in Paris and became known as the 'Paris technique' (Hall and Cox, 1989; Raven, 1990).

Following this period the advances that have been made in radiotherapy are of a technical nature, with improvements in the machines. A greater understanding has been reached as to how radiation actually works.

HOW RADIOTHERAPY WORKS

When discussing how radiotherapy works it is important to have a basic understanding of the physics involved. When we talk about radiotherapy we are referring to ionizing radiation, which is radiation that has the ability to penetrate the tissues of the body as well as being able to destroy cells within the tissue.

Ionizing radiation comes in the form of rays of which there are four types: alpha, beta or gamma rays from radioactive isotopes, and X-rays produced using electricity. These have different strengths and absorption depths.

Radioactive substances or isotopes are classed as such because of their atomic structure. All matter is composed of atoms, the structure of which is shown in Figure 6.1. Within the nucleus of an atom are the neutrons and the positively charged protons. Surrounding the nucleus in orbit are negatively charged electrons; the atom is normally neutral, with equal numbers of protons and electrons. Changes in the number of neutrons in the nucleus leads to instability of the atom and the emission of radioactivity.

In an attempt to attain stability the radioactive isotope emits rays of charged particles (Souhami and Tobias, 1986). Isotopes are referred to by the element's name followed by a number. This number identifies the atomic weight, which is the total number of both the neutrons and protons within the nucleus of the atom (Souhami and Tobias, 1986;

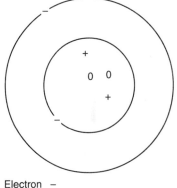

Electron −
Proton +
Neutron 0

Figure 6.1 Structure of a stable atom.

Table 6.1 Half-life of more commonly used radioactive isotopes

Element	Symbol (radioactive form)	Half-life
Radium	^{226}Ra	1620 years
Caesium	^{137}Cs	30 years
Cobalt	^{60}Co	5.3 years
Iridium	^{182}Ir	74 days
Iodine	^{131}I	8 days
Gold	^{198}Au	2.7 days
Yttrium	^{90}Y	2.5 days

Holmes, 1988). Any element which has an atomic weight greater than 209 is a naturally occurring radioactive isotope, for example radium-226 and uranium-238 (Holmes, 1988).

Electrons are emitted from the destabilized atom of the isotope; these in turn link up with another formerly stable atom, causing it in turn to become unstable. The process whereby an electron is lost by one atom and links up to another atom is called ionization. When the process of ionization occurs within living tissue the chemical change which results is damaging, leading to a biological change within the cell and eventually to cell death.

As the radioactive isotope emits ionizing radiation its radioactivity is reduced; this process is referred to as decay. The activity of an isotope can be measured and the length of time it takes for the radioactivity to be reduced by half is known as the half-life. The half-lives of the more commonly used radioactive isotopes are shown in Table 6.1. As you will see, the table includes some substances which are not normally considered to be radioactive. These artificial radioactive isotopes are produced by bombarding the non-radioactive elements with neutrons inside a nuclear reactor (Walter, 1977; Copp, 1991).

Biological effects of radiation

The target of radiation damage is the genetic structure of the cells: the deoxyribonucleic acid (DNA) which is present in the cell nucleus. During cell division the DNA is copied so that the genetic information can be passed on to the daughter cells. There are four phases in the division process or cell cycle:

1. G_1 = pre-synthetic phase – enzymes are produced to aid the synthesis of DNA;
2. S = synthesis – DNA synthesis occurs in readiness for cell division;

3. G_2 = pre-mitotic phase – proteins and RNA are synthesized prior to cell division;
4. M = Mitotic phase – the cell divides to produce two identical daughter cells.

When the cell leaves the cell cycle it enters the phase called G_0, the resting phase, and will only re-enter the cell cycle when stimulated to do so. Because the DNA is the target, the greatest damage radiation causes occurs to cells when they are in the S and G_2 phases just before mitosis and during mitotis itself (Holmes, 1988).

The damage caused by ionizing radiation can be used therapeutically to treat patients who have cancer by inflicting damage on cancer cells, particularly those which reproduce rapidly. Unfortunately the ionizing radiation also causes damage to the healthy cells. Some cells and tissues in the body are more sensitive to the effects of ionizing radiation than others. As was identified earlier, the target of the damage is the DNA within the cells and because the most damage is done just before or during mitosis, cells which have a high mitotic rate are more susceptible to damage from radiation. These tissues are termed radiosensitive and show early acute reactions to radiation. They include the bone marrow, skin, hair follicles and gastrointestinal tract epithelium; fortunately these tissues are generally able to repair themselves quickly because of their high mitotic rate. On the other hand, tissues that have a slow or non-existent mitotic rate tend to show late effects of damage and take longer to repair themselves. Some may not be capable of repair (Copp, 1991).

These are important points to remember when caring for patients receiving radiotherapy and observing for potential side-effects from the radiotherapy treatment.

Measurement of radiation

Measurement of the radiation dose given to a patient is very important because treatment has to be planned and is prescribed in the same way as drug therapy. When radiotherapy was first used there was no means of measuring the amount of radiation being given to the patient and often it was only the extent of skin damage which could be used as an indicator of dose to the radiotherapist. This was known as the 'erythema dose base'. Another method of dose assessment used early on was called 'the pastille dose'; this was based on the change in colour of a tablet exposed to radiation. It was not until 1928 that a measured unit of dose was defined and was called the roentgen (Deeley, 1976). This was the measure of one unit of radiation in the air (Crown, 1978).

During the 1950s it became apparent that the roentgen was not an accurate enough measure and what was needed was a measure of the amount of radiation being given to the patient. The first measure developed was called the rad (radiation absorbed dose). This traditional dose has now been replaced by an internationally recognized unit called the gray, equivalent to 100 rads. Another measure used is called the sievert, previously called the rem, which is used to describe the dose equivalent: the dose equivalent is the absorbed dose multiplied by a reactive effectiveness of the type of radiation involved (Holmes, 1988). These measurements are used when prescribing the dose of treatment and when measuring the amount of radiation to which someone has been exposed.

Radiation protection

Important as it is to measure the dose of radiation being given to the patient, it is equally important to be aware of the amount of radiation to which staff are exposed. Radiation protection guidelines were brought into being in 1928 when the International Commission on Radiological Protection was formed (Harris and Jackson, 1987).

The dangers associated with radioactivity had not been fully understood by the early radiation workers, many of whom went on to develop radiation-induced tumours (Oliver, 1988; Walter, 1977). Now that the dangers have been recognized there are strict guidelines in force in each department and in 1985 statutory regulations were updated in the UK (see HMSO Guidelines).

For staff working with radioactive substances the tissues at risk are the bone marrow and the gonads; they are susceptible to the same damage as that of a patient receiving radiotherapy. All staff working with radiation are monitored strictly by wearing a 'film badge', which is checked every four weeks and can indicate the amount and type of radiation the wearer has been exposed to. This ensures that the maximum permissible dose is not exceeded in any way. There are three fundamental methods of reducing radiation hazards which staff are exposed to: they are distance, shielding and time.

The first is **distance**: the further away from the radioactive source you are the less radiation dose you receive – an example of the inverse square law (Figure 6.2).

The second is that of having a **barrier**: usually a thick lead shield between the radioactive source and the member of staff.

Third, is that of **speed**: the less time spent with the patient who has a radioactive implant, then the less the staff are exposed to radiation. However, this can cause difficulty and distress for the patient, who may already feel a sense of isolation because of the disease; this is discussed later in the chapter.

Anderson (1980) stated that it has to be appreciated that the principles underlying the methods of radiation protection are generally restrictive in nature and in consequence are often in direct conflict with the principles

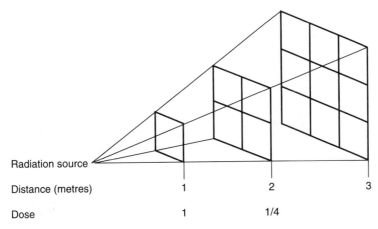

Radiation source

Distance (metres)   1   2   3

Dose   1   1/4

Figure 6.2   Illustration of the inverse square law.

that determine high standards of patient care. Relatives and other visitors also have to be protected and it is usually done by the use of clear signs indicating that a patient is being treated using a radioactive isotope.

Patients receiving brachytherapy (pp. 128–33) are usually nursed in side wards wherever possible and the length of time visitors can stay is restricted. Anyone who thinks they may be pregnant, and children under the age of 18, are not allowed to visit a patient with a radioactive source in situ.

The use and scope of radiotherapy

The aim of radiotherapy is to destroy as many of the tumour cells as possible whilst only damaging a small amount of the healthy tissue. To do this radiotherapy can be given in two different ways, each of which produces its own unique problems and potential side-effects, which are discussed below. Radiotherapy is not always given with the express purpose of curing the patient of cancer. Sometimes the disease may have been at an advanced stage when the diagnosis was made or the cancer may have progressed despite treatment. For these patients radiotherapy may be used to alleviate or ameliorate some of the symptoms of the cancer. This is known as palliative radiotherapy.

Radiotherapy is only one of the modes of treatment used to fight cancer, the others being surgery and chemotherapy. Frequently patients now receive more than one type of treatment (radiotherapy, surgery, chemotherapy) in an attempt to cure their cancer. It is beneficial from a medical perspective to have more than one means of attacking the cancer, but as you can imagine from the patient's point of view it all adds to the

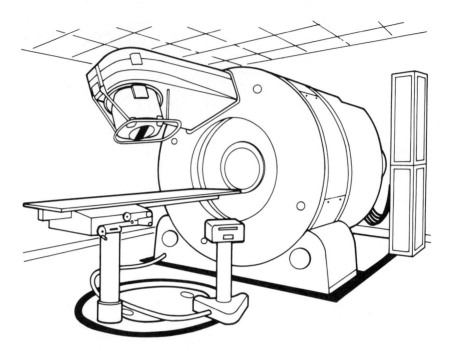

Figure 6.3 Diagram of linear accelerator. (Redrawn with permission from Walter, J. (1977) *Cancer and Radiotherapy*, 2nd edn, Churchill Livingstone, Edinburgh.)

trauma experienced, not only from the disease itself but also from the treatments.

It is also important to remember that radiotherapy is still used in the treatment of some non-malignant conditions, such as keloid scars, menorrhagia, thyrotoxicosis and benign pituitary tumours. As a consequence patients and their relatives may have had previous encounters with radiotherapy which are not necessarily as treatments for cancer. These experiences may affect how they accept the proposed treatment using radiotherapy.

EXTERNAL BEAM RADIOTHERAPY

External beam radiotherapy, or teletherapy as it is also known, is the treatment of cancer by directing rays of ionizing radiation towards the tumour site from a distance. These rays are produced either electrically by a machine called a linear accelerator (Figure 6.3) or from a piece of radioactive material, usually cobalt, which is housed in the head of a machine.

The linear accelerators operate at different voltages, so one machine may be better to use in the treatment of a deep-seated tumour than another, for example. The linear accelerators offer greater accuracy than the cobalt machines and because a higher percentage of the dose is aimed at the tumour site the skin receives less radiation. Skin reactions when using the linear accelerator are generally less aggressive than were seen in the past, so they are referred to as 'skin sparing'. Skin sparing also occurs as a result of the use of multiple fields when treating the cancer as well as dose fractionation – dividing the total dose to be given and administering that over 5–40 treatment sessions, as mentioned earlier in the chapter.

PLANNING

Unlike treatments in the past a great deal of planning goes into the administration of radiotherapy nowadays. Planning is usually carried out on a machine called a simulator, which is an X-ray machine that incorporates an image intensifier which actually mimics the movements of the treatment machine (Oliver, 1988; Holmes, 1986b). This enables the radiotherapist to see the patient on the treatment couch and also see an X-ray of the proposed treatment site at the same time. The radiotherapist will then mark the area to be treated on the X-ray and the radiographers will then apply the marks onto the patient's skin, using gentian violet or a special marker ink which does not easily come off. These marks on the skin enable the radiographers to set up the treatment machine and direct the radiation accurately each time the patient receives radiotherapy.

Accuracy is very important because the beams are aimed in a manner which administers a high dose of radiation to the tumour whilst trying to reduce the exposure of healthy tissue to the damaging rays. The planning process is lengthy in some instances, possibly taking several days; this is essential to maximize the effects of the radiotherapy. Computers now play a large role in the radiotherapy departments and, in particular, they are of benefit in the planning process, producing 'map-like' diagrams of the tumour in relation to the vital organs in the vicinity and showing the percentage dose of radiation each will receive. This is an area where research and development is taking place, with the latest simulators able to produce three-dimensional pictures of the tumour within the body. The aim in using computerized planning machines is to improve accuracy in the direction of the radiation beams and to show how effective treatment is at intervals during a course of radiotherapy.

HEADSHELLS

With all external beam radiation treatment it is essential that the patient lies still during the treatment. For patients with tumours of the head and

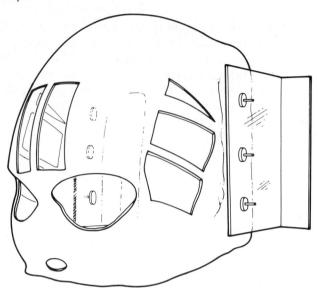

Figure 6.4 Perspex headshell. Redrawn with permission from Souhami, R. and Tobias, J. (1986) *Cancer and its Management*, Blackwell Scientific Publications, London.

neck the use of a perspex headshell is one of the best ways of achieving immobilization, consistency of treatment and greater accuracy (Figure 6.4). These shells are made by the technicians who work in the 'mould room', which should be located in close proximity to the radiotherapy department. The perspex shells are made individually from a plaster impression (Souhami and Tobias, 1986).

SHIELDING

If vital organs are in the treatment field then lead blocks of different sizes can be used to shield these organs. The shields can also be used to try to get uniformity of dose within the body. If on the other hand a higher dose of radiation was required nearer the surface or on the skin, then blocks of wax can be placed between the machine and the patient; this will absorb some of the radiation dose, but the higher dose will be given to the skin.

SIDE-EFFECTS AND NURSING CARE

Because of the accuracy of the planning of the treatment, the use of fractionation and multiple treatment fields, the side-effects which can be experienced by the patients are substantially reduced, but they still remain as potential problems. It is important to inform the patient of these, because if a side-effect occurs this may be perceived by the patient as a deterioration in the condition. As stated by Holmes (1986b) and Oliver (1988), the role of the nurse when caring for the patients receiving radiotherapy is to try to minimize, control and possibly prevent some of the side-effects of this treatment, as well as intervening in problems associated with the disease itself. It is important to remember and to reinforce with the patient that the potential side-effects will only relate to the area of the body being treated with radiotherapy. The extent of the radiation reactions will vary depending upon the dose of treatment being given, the volume and type of normal tissue included in the treatment field, the frequency with which it is being given and also on whether the patient has had, or is having, chemotherapy (Holmes, 1988).

As indicated by Holmes (1986a, 1986b) there are three categories of side-effects, which depend upon the tissues involved:

1. Acute side-effects which occur during or shortly after treatment. These are seen in tissues that have a high reproduction rate, such as skin, bone marrow or gastrointestinal tract lining. These are also the tissues that are able to recover rapidly, as previously mentioned, so nursing care is focused on helping the patient to cope with the side-effects and trying, if possible, to minimize these effects.
2. Subacute side-effects can occur weeks to months following the completion of a course of radiotherapy. Prompt recognition of these is important as it is difficult to differentiate between progression of the disease and side-effects.
3. Lastly, there are late chronic side-effects, which can occur from between one and five years after treatment. These are seen in tissues which have a slow reproduction rate and can sometimes be difficult to treat. Effects can include fistulae formation, severe fibrosis and tissue necrosis.

   Possibly one of the worst late side-effects is that of carcinogenesis, which is not usually seen until many years following the therapeutic treatment.

The most common side-effects of radiotherapy are described below.

Skin reactions

Any beam of radiation directed at the human body must pass through the skin and will exert some effect on the very sensitive germinal layer (Oliver, 1988). More accurate planning of treatment, improved treatment machines and techniques such as fractionation and the use of multiple fields theoretically will reduce the occurrence of skin reactions.

There are three grades of skin reaction – erythema, dry desquamation and moist desquamation – and these can occur as acute or subacute reactions. There appears to be no consensus on an agreed protocol for caring for the patient's skin during treatment; if a skin reaction occurs the care tends to vary very much from one radiotherapy centre to another. It is now generally accepted by most radiographers and oncology nurses that the skin within a treatment site can be washed without increasing the incidence of skin reactions; this was also shown in a randomized trial by Campbell and Illingworth (1992). The myth that water caused the skin to burn is slowly petering out.

Care does have to be taken not to wash the treatment marks off and some centres offer tattooing as an alternative. This involves having a small subcutaneous injection of a dye, similar in size to a freckle; this mark will be permanent. The radiographer's marks are points of reference needed to ensure the accurate setting up of the treatment machine. If the area is washed it should be treated gently; perfumed soaps should be avoided at all costs and the areas should be patted dry. The application of purified talcum powder is still encouraged, as this has a cooling effect on the skin.

Exposing the area being treated to air, but not the sun, is beneficial as it reduces friction on the skin, which exacerbates skin reactions.

Erythema is reddening of the skin with irritation, similar to mild sunburn, and is treated by encouraging more 'exposing', the use of talcum powder and wearing loose cotton clothing where possible.

Treatment of skin reactions

Dry desquamation follows on from erythema; the skin becomes darker red and feels tight and painful. Skin emulsion analogue creams are safe to use in treated areas, such as Natuderm or even Baby Oil. No creams containing metals should be used as this could exacerbate a potential skin reaction.

Moist desquamation follows on from dry desquamation. The skin blisters and splits, resulting in production of serous exudate following loss of the surface epithelium. Again treatment of this type of reaction varies from centre to centre. Some centres dress the area with Flamazine, although this has to be removed before further radiotherapy is given. Antibiotic sprays offer useful prophylaxis against infections developing.

Late skin reactions can also occur, which can include hyperpigmentation, necrosis and telangiectasia. These late effects on the skin are difficult to treat and can leave the patient with a long-term problem.

Radiotherapy may be used to treat fungating wounds, which should be dressed in the normal way; a topical antibiotic such as metronidazole is useful as it can also reduce odours produced by these wounds.

Hair loss

Hair loss causes concern for patients embarking on a course of radiotherapy. Often the patient will have heard many myths about the effects of radiotherapy and it is important to deal with these and give the patient correct information regarding hair loss. Hair will be lost if it is within the area of the body being irradiated, for example axillary hair will be lost during radiotherapy to axillary nodes, or alopecia may occur if the brain is being treated.

Hair loss will occur two to three weeks into treatment and the hair will grow back following completion of the radiotherapy.

People accept these facts in different ways and time must be spent with them helping them to adjust. Hair-pieces and wigs can be provided now, but often patients prefer to use alternatives such as head scarves, turbans or hats.

Nausea and vomiting

The amount and severity of the nausea and vomiting will depend upon which area of the body is being treated, the dose and frequency of treatment. If the gastrointestinal tract is included in the treatment field nausea and vomiting are definitely potential problems. Prior to commencing treatment the patient should be informed of this and asked to inform the nurse or radiographer if he or she is experiencing problems so that prompt action can be taken. Antiemetic therapy may be helpful in the management of nausea and vomiting. Other therapies have much to offer the patient at this time: relaxation, visualization, reflexology, aromatherapy and acupressure are all beneficial, as are all forms of diversionary technique. Hypnotherapy can also be useful for patients who have severe problems. It is important to encourage a good fluid intake in an effort to prevent electrolyte imbalance and/or dehydration.

Bone marrow depression

Bone marrow depression is the only systemic side-effect caused by radiotherapy and occurs if the treatment field contains large areas of cell-producing bone marrow (Holmes, 1986b). The presentation and treatment of this side-effect are similar to those of bone marrow depression caused by chemotherapy. Close observation for signs of marrow depression should be made and blood samples taken weekly so that prompt action can be taken if necessary.

Nutritional requirements

It is important that patients are encouraged to maintain a good fluid intake and have a well-balanced diet, as this can help the patient to complete their treatment with fewer problems.

A high fluid intake helps the body to excrete the breakdown products from cell destruction which are toxic to the body. A high-protein, high-calorie diet helps the body to repair and regenerate the damaged healthy tissues (Holmes, 1986a). The maintenance of weight and dietary intake may be affected either by the disease or by the radiotherapy. If any part of the gastrointestinal tract is involved in the treatment field then this can have an effect on the nutritional intake of the patient (Holmes, 1987).

Dietary supplements such as Complan or Ensure are of great value and should be encouraged, as should patients' and families' involvement in care. Early referral to the dietitian before problems become established is beneficial, the dietitian being a valuable resource for both the patient and health care professionals.

Oral hygiene

Oral hygiene is important as the mouth can be the entry site of infection when the white cell count is low. If the patient is having treatment for cancer of the mouth or tongue, oral problems may be exacerbated. Assessment of the mouth prior to and during treatment is of great value (Eilers *et al.*, 1988). Meticulous oral hygiene needs to be taught to the patient, along with the signs which alert to infection developing. Patients may experience taste alterations as a result of their radiotherapy and can be assured that these should revert to normal once treatment is over.

Bowel problems

When radiotherapy is being given to treat pelvic tumours, altered bowel habits can present a problem in the management of the patient. Diarrhoea is usually the first acute reaction experienced by the patient; the treatment for this is the encouragement of fluids to prevent dehydration, a low-fibre diet because high-fibre intake can exacerbate the diarrhoea, and the administration of antidiarrhoeal medication. If the diarrhoea persists and becomes severe the patient may be rested from their treatment until the diarrhoea subsides.

Tenesmus can present as a subacute side-effect which is usually treated with topical application of steroids.

A late side-effect of pelvic irradiation may be radiation proctitis, which can develop into haemorrhagic proctisis. The treatment of this, in some severe cases, is the removal of the damaged bowel and possible formation of a colostomy.

Thankfully these side-effects are greatly reduced as a result of improved machinery and techniques.

Urinary problems

The problems occur initially as a result of inflammation caused by the radiation. The acute reaction produces symptoms of cystitis. Urinary tract infection must be ruled out and if infection is not the cause then a high fluid intake is encouraged and a mixture of potassium citrate may be given, but this is not always effective. This side-effect can be very distressing, particularly if it causes interruption in sleep patterns. Incontinence may also become a problem during treatment and then nursing care is aimed at maintaining good levels of hygiene as well as skin integrity.

Haemorrhagic cystitis can present as a late side-effect which requires prompt accurate diagnosis and treatment.

The kidneys may be damaged if they are in the field of treatment, so great care has to be taken to reduce damage. The patient may be prescribed steroids to reduce the inflammation caused by the treatment.

Sterility

Sterility and/or reduced fertility is a side-effect which can be experienced by both men and women receiving irradiation. This is because the gonads, ovaries and testes are particularly sensitive to radiation. As pointed out by Oliver (1988), sympathetic counselling should be given along with full explanation of this prior to commencing treatment.

Eyes

The eyes will be affected by radiotherapy if they are within the treatment field. Conjunctivitis may be an early reaction to the radiotherapy. Lead shields may be used; this involves having a thin lead cover inserted under the eyelids to shield the eyes during treatment. The procedure itself can be very uncomfortable and care has to be taken not to damage the eye during insertion of the shield.

Late effects of radiation on the eyes may be 'dry eyes' or cataract formation.

WHOLE BODY IRRADIATION

Whole body irradiation is used in the treatment of leukaemic patients in preparation for bone marrow transplantation. The patient will have radiotherapy to the whole body, no shielding, twice a day at a high dose. The patient will also be receiving high-dose chemotherapy. The aim of this treatment is to ablate any malignant cells in the bone marrow as well as ablating the bone marrow totally, in the hope that the subsequent bone marrow transplant will not be rejected.

As a result of the intensity of this treatment the side-effects tend to be acute. Severe nausea and vomiting can present as problems and are treated by use of regular antiemetics. A pre-medication of an antiemetic and a steroid is given prior to each dose of radiotherapy in an effort to lessen the side-effect. Neutropenia is a desired side-effect initially, but can last for weeks following the treatment. Septicaemia, bacterial or fungal infection, pneumonitis and marrow failure are a few of the acute problems which may be experienced.

Some of the long-term side-effects are cataract formation, arthritis and sterility (Bareford, 1988). It is important that the patients are aware of these side-effects prior to giving informed consent to undergo the procedure.

RECENT DEVELOPMENTS

There have been few new innovations in the field of radiotherapy since the 1930s. The machinery has improved but the techniques remain the same. Research has been done to find out if drugs can make tumours more sensitive to the effects of radiotherapy, but without much success.

More recently some radiotherapy centres have been undertaking a trial using hyperfractionation of the radiotherapy. Continuous hyperfractionated accelerated radiotherapy treatment (CHART) involves the radiotherapy being given at eight-hourly intervals on 12 consecutive days. The aim is to produce a better tumour response. As a result of this intense treatment the acute side-effects can be increased in severity. The patients are admitted to hospital for the duration of their treatment, allowing for early detection and prompt treatment of any of the side-effects.

The main focus of attention at the moment seems to be on increasing the accuracy with which the treatment is delivered; the advent of three-dimensional planning, described above, will assist in this.

BRACHYTHERAPY

Brachytherapy is treatment using ionizing radiation at a short distance from the tumour site. To achieve this, radioactive isotopes can either be implanted into tumour-bearing tissue, known as interstitial treatment, placed inside body cavities which are in close proximity to the tumour, known as intracavity treatment, or placed directly onto the tumour. The radioactive isotopes used for these treatments are known as sealed sources because the radioactive isotope is encased in plastic or steel. As mentioned above, this form of administering radiotherapy treatment has been used since the 1920s.

Radium was the only radioactive isotope available for use in this way until after the Second World War and the advent of nuclear reactors, which enabled the production of artificial radioactive isotopes such as cobalt-60, caesium-137, iridium-192 and gold-198 (Baker, 1979).

It is important to remember that with all radioactive implants the duration of the treatment is calculated very precisely, taking into account the dose of radiation prescribed and the radioactivity of the actual source being used.

Because the half-life of the radioisotopes changes as they decay, the length of time treatment takes (even delivering the same dose) will vary from patient to patient. It is therefore difficult to tell the patient the exact duration of their treatment; this can sometimes present problems for patients who may need to make arrangements (such as for child care, or to notify their employer) while they are in hospital.

The most commonly used radioisotopes in brachytherapy are caesium-137, iridium-192 and gold-198.

EXTERNAL APPLICATORS

For the application of a radioactive source to a tumour the radioactive source can be encased in a perspex mould or shell, which can then be placed over the lesion, for example on the skin. The shell is placed onto the affected area and left there continuously or intermittently until the prescribed dose of radiotherapy has been administered.

The nursing care of these patients depends very much on the site of the skin lesion and whether the radioactive mould is left on continuously or not. A skin reaction may develop whilst the treatment is in progress or shortly after the patient has been discharged from hospital. The advice for treating the skin reaction is similar to that for a skin reaction caused by external beam radiotherapy. Patients can continue to be self-caring during their treatment. Radiation protection should not be a problem if the guidelines are adhered to.

INTERSTITIAL TREATMENT

Radium was used in the past in the form of needles but more frequently now iridium-192 is used in the form of needles or wires. The iridium wires can be inserted through the tumour-bearing tissue or the bed of the tumour, following surgical removal and radiotherapy. Gold-198 can also be used in the form of grains.

When the radioactive wires are inserted into the mouth or tongue (Figure 6.5), oral hygiene and nutrition may present as problems; both should be fully discussed with the patient prior to the treatment commencing.

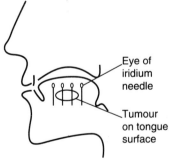

Figure 6.5 Iridium needle implant to the tongue.

Mouth care given is similar to that for patients having external beam radiotherapy, with two- to four-hourly mouthwashes being encouraged, both during treatment and on discharge home. Nutritional intake may be affected during treatment and a soft or liquid diet may be required; advice from the dietitian should be sought. For the patient, the main concerns may be the isolation that must be endured during the treatment, the discomfort of the treatment and the problems he or she may have with communication. Again these concerns should be discussed prior to the patient undergoing the treatment and plans of care made to try to minimize these problems, should they occur.

When the wires are implanted into the breast (Figure 6.6) the problems are quite different. The implant is less uncomfortable, and the patient can be self-caring and ambulant within the cubicle in which she is nursed. Prior preparation of the patient is very important and has a great bearing on how well the treatment will be tolerated. This treatment is generally given following a course of radiotherapy, so skin reactions can present a problem if the patient has had previous radiotherapy. The skin should be assessed prior to the wires being inserted.

The first stage of treatment is the insertion of nylon tubes to the site; this is done under general anaesthetic. When the nylon tubes are in place an X-ray will be taken to enable accurate measurement of the length of radioactive wire required. When the wire has been cut and the duration of the treatment calculated, the radioactive wire can be inserted into the nylon tube; this is done by the medical staff using long-handled forceps. Once the radioactive wires are in situ the patient will be restricted to the cubicle. The site of the insertion of the wires will be checked regularly during the treatment for signs of a skin reaction, haemorrhage or infection. If the skin shows signs of a reaction developing, the patient should be encouraged to 'expose' the area to the air, reducing the friction which is so often the cause of a treatment reaction. The wires will be removed at the designated time by the medical staff, and after removal of the wires the patient can go home within one hour.

The care of the skin will be explained to the patient prior to discharge, as will the signs to look for if a skin reaction was to develop. One important point to stress to the patient is that she is no longer radioactive once the wires have been removed.

Gold-198 is used in the form of grains which can be implanted into mucous membranes such as the mouth or vagina, and because its radioactivity reduces so quickly it can be left in place following insertion. The patients will generally be admitted for the insertion of the gold grains under a general anaesthetic and will not be discharged home until the radioactivity is at a safe level, which happens fairly quickly because of its short half-life. If the gold grains become dislodged over time they do not present a danger to anyone and can either be kept for posterity or disposed of!

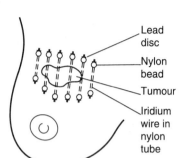

Figure 6.6 Iridium wire implant to the breast.

Lead disc

Nylon bead

Tumour

Iridium wire in nylon tube

Intracavity treatment

This was the first brachytherapy treatment to be used in the 1920s when uterine cancers were treated by inserting radium into the uterus and vagina.

This treatment can be given before or after both surgery or external beam radiotherapy. As mentioned previously, radium was the only isotope used until the development of caesium; this has taken the place of radium in the treatment of gynaecological cancers because it causes less damage to healthy tissue than radium.

The applicators are inserted in theatre with the patient under an anaesthetic. Following insertion of the applicator an X-ray is taken to ensure its correct positioning. On return to the ward the patient is given analgesia as required and the applicator is loaded manually by medical staff. The applicators used vary in composition from centre to centre.

While the applicator is in place the patient will have to lie as flat as possible so as not to dislodge the applicator. She will have a urinary catheter in situ to keep the bladder empty, and an enema or suppositories are given to clear the bowel prior to the patient going to theatre, because bowel movement can also cause the applicator to be dislodged. During the time the applicator is in place regular checks for signs of haemorrhage or development of infection have to be made.

Because the patient has to lie flat in bed for the duration of treatment, she will be prone to the complications of bedrest, so preparation and patient education prior to the procedure are again vitally important.

One of the major drawbacks from the medical and nursing aspect of this treatment is that when caring for the patient the staff will be exposed to radiation, so presenting a problem with regard to radiation protection.

Remote afterloading

One area where advances have been made in brachytherapy is with the development of remote afterloading machines. This machine was designed to resolve some of the problems of radiation protection. The patient will undergo the same preparation and procedure in theatre, whether that be insertion of vaginal applicator or tubes into the breast; the difference and benefits are seen on return to the ward. The applicator or tubes are attached to tubes coming from a remote afterloading machine: the selectron unit. The machine has stored safely within it some radioactive pellets, usually caesium. Once the machine is linked to the applicator the radioactive pellets can then be quickly transferred from the shielded container into the applicator to deliver the treatment.

The major advantage is that when the patient needs any nursing attention, at the press of a button the machine withdraws the radioactive pellets from the applicator. This means that staff involved in giving direct care are no longer being exposed to radiation. The one negative aspect from the patients' point of view is the fact that they still have to be isolated for the duration of the treatment and again prior information is important in helping them to accept this.

There are now two types of remote afterloading machines: a low-dose-rate machine which contains caesium pellets, and a high-dose-rate machine which contains iridium.

The low-dose machine can be used to treat gynaecological cancers and also oesophageal cancers using a specially designed applicator. This treatment offers good palliation for patients with cancer of the oesophagus who are having dysphagia. The high-dose machine, known as a Microselectron, has the potential for more applications. It can be used to treat the same conditions as the low-dose-rate machine, but the duration of the treatment is shorter. It can also be used to treat bronchial tumours, and some centres are using the machine to apply radiation to the tumour site during an operation – intra-operative radiation – but this technique is fairly new.

UNSEALED SOURCES

Unsealed radioactive isotopes can be used to actually target some malignant tumours. These isotopes may be either injected into the bloodstream or ingested, thereby gaining access into the bloodstream and allowing them to get straight to the tumour-bearing tissue. Radioactive iodine (^{131}I) is used in the treatment of cancer of the thyroid. The thyroid normally takes up iodine; therefore by making iodine radioactive you can target thyroid tissue in the body even if metastases have developed. The patient is admitted to have the treatment and, because of the radioactive iodine being taken up into the bloodstream following its ingestion, everything about that patient becomes radioactive – sweat, saliva and, in particular, urine.

The patient should be nursed in a side ward or a purpose-built suite where he or she has access to a toilet and possibly a bathroom. During the stay in hospital the patient will be monitored daily by the medical physics staff and will be discharged home only when the radiation levels are safe. The reduction in radioactivity occurs as a result of the body excreting the radioiodine in the urine and the decay of radioactive iodine. Prior to being given treatment the patients have to stop taking any thyroid replacement tablets and during treatment diet should be iodine-free to enable a good take-up of the radioactive iodine.

Not all cancers of the thyroid respond to this treatment; it is mainly those cancers which are well differentiated that respond well, rather than the poorly differentiated or anaplastic thyroid cancers. Radioactive iodine is also used to treat thyrotoxicosis and for diagnostic purposes but in these cases much smaller doses are used, given on an out-patient basis.

Radioactive colloids, such as yttrium, can also be used in the treatment of malignant effusions such as pleural effusions or ascites by being injected into either the pleural or peritoneal cavity. Again the radioisotope will have a relatively short half-life, so that the patient can be discharged home shortly after the procedure has been carried out. Radioactive phosphorus is used in the treatment of polycythaemia and can be used in the treatment of bone metastases, as the phosphorus is readily taken up by the bone.

PALLIATIVE RADIOTHERAPY

Radiotherapy can be used effectively to alleviate some of the symptoms produced by advanced cancers when curing the disease may not be possible. The aim of this treatment is to relieve symptoms, thereby giving some quality of life without experiencing the side-effects of radiotherapy to the extent to which they would cancel out the beneficial effect of the treatment. Bone metastases are often very responsive to radiotherapy and it can be used to effect pain relief for many patients.

Radiotherapy for bone metastases can be given in one of two ways, depending upon the extent of the spread of the disease. If a patient presents with a pathological fracture of a bone, for example the femur or a rib, then the radiotherapy can be directed straight towards those areas and the treatment given over one to two weeks.

If the patient presents with widespread bone metastases these can be treated by giving half-body irradiation as a single exposure (Copp, 1991). The patient may experience severe nausea or vomiting as a result of this treatment and will usually have a pre-medication prior to receiving the radiotherapy; they will also need good antiemetic cover following the treatment.

The patient receiving half-body irradiation will need support prior to and following this treatment, which is often given on an out-patient basis.

Bleeding can become a problem for patients with advanced gynaecological cancers. For these patients a short course of external beam radiotherapy or intracavity treatment can help to reduce or stop the bleeding and hopefully improve the quality of life at that time.

RADIATION IN COMBINATION

Radiotherapy is not the only means to treat a tumour. It is often used in conjunction with other forms of treatment, mainly surgery and/or chemotherapy. In some diseases radiotherapy may be used prior to surgery to effect a reduction in tumour bulk or, as is more likely the case, the radiotherapy is given following surgery if it is felt some cells may still be present.

In some diseases, such as cancer of the breast, radiotherapy and chemotherapy are used in combination; this is referred to as adjuvant chemotherapy, the benefit being that the chemotherapy will hopefully attack any micro-metastases in the body whilst the radiotherapy is being given to the breast area and possibly the axilla. As a result of this the side-effects may well be compounded by the fact that the patient is receiving both chemotherapy and radiotherapy.

RADIOTHERAPY AND CHILDREN

For some paediatric cancers the treatment regimes include a course of radiotherapy and often in these instances the course of radiotherapy is a long one.

Often the children will have to undergo a (short-acting) general anaesthetic to ensure they lie still during the treatment. Because the radiotherapy regime is long the problems associated with frequent anaesthetics, together with the side-effects from the treatment itself, will certainly take its toll on the child. A great deal of psychological support is needed not only for the child but also for the parents and family. Copp (1991) points out that the side-effects from the radiotherapy will present earlier in children than they would in adults and, depending upon where the treatment is directed, the child's growth may be affected in the long term.

The topic of children's tumours and their treatment is covered in more depth by Arnfield (1988).

RADIOTHERAPEUTIC EMERGENCIES

There are some conditions which are classed as emergencies in the field of oncology, although the diagnosis itself dictates urgency in obtaining treatment. There are conditions which can develop secondary to the primary disease, such as superior vena cava obstruction which can be potentially life threatening, but in which quick treatment with radiotherapy, in some cases, can offer to alleviate the distressing symptoms by decreasing the bulk of the tumour (Copp, 1991).

Spinal cord compression is another condition where radiotherapy, if given in the early stages of development, can offer to alleviate the distressing symptoms and possibly halt the progress of the disease.

Steroids are also used at this time and can often give some relief from the distressing symptoms.

Having covered the ways in which radiotherapy is administered and the physical manifestations of the side-effects resulting from this treatment, we now focus on the psychological problems which may be experienced by those patients receiving radiotherapy for treatment of cancer.

RADIOTHERAPY: PSYCHOSOCIAL PERSPECTIVES

An extensive outline of the nature, scope and biological effects of radiotherapy, as well as the implications for nursing care, have been presented. This knowledge in isolation is not sufficient to meet the holistic needs of patients and their families. Card and Fielding (1986) mention that there is clearly growing interest in accommodating the psychological needs of those with cancer. This interest has provided the impetus for research into the psychological sequelae associated with the adminis- tration of radiotherapy. These enquiries over the last decade have highlighted that receiving radiotherapy can be detrimental to the psychological and social well-being of an individual (Hughson *et al.*, 1987; Christman, 1990; Peck and Boland, 1977).

RADIOTHERAPY AND SOCIETY: FRIEND OR FOE?

An appreciation of society's perceptions of radiotherapy is fundamental in identifying the patient and family's potential and actual fears regarding this mode of treatment. Decker *et al.* (1992) mention that cancer treatments often cause stress, anxiety and depression. These experiences may be exacerbated by myths that the patient may hold with regard to radiotherapy. Gilmore and Fairclough (1992) mention that radiation remains a taboo subject, shrouded in mystery yet paradoxically sen- sationalized by the media. Society's relationship with radiation is one of conflict. Issues such as Sellafield, Hiroshoma and the Christmas Island experiments implicate radiation in the aetiology of cancer. In contrast, radiation is used as a therapeutic source in the management of cancer. On this theme Cull (1991) notes that society is often confused between the carcinogenic and therapeutic properties of radiation. Locked up in these images are common fears of being burned and society's unease with the technology used in the administration of radiotherapy. This uncertainty on the issue of safety and radiation extends to health care professionals as well as members of the general population.

Few treatment modalities possess this 'Jekyll and Hyde' image. Such a scenario has implications for the management of the patient receiving radiotherapy.

Any pre-treatment preparation must accomodate an in-depth assessment of the patient's and family's beliefs regarding radiotherapy. This assessment would need to address the following issues:

1. Explore the patient's/family's knowledge of radiotherapy.
2. Explore the patient's/family's emotional response at the prospect of receiving radiotherapy.
3. Ascertain if any family or friends have had radiotherapy and explore the effects this has on the patient's attitude towards radiotherapy.

Ironically, the emergence of nursing models has expanded our vision of the nature of the assessment process, but at the same time may ignore the patient's and family's unique psychological construct of radiotherapy. An assessment of the patient's perception of radiotherapy may associate this treatment with pain, hair loss, or impending death. Bond (1982) mentions that the social and psychological aspects of cancer are not adequately addressed by health professionals. Research into society's knowledge of cancer suggests that images of this disease are dominated by visions of pain and eventual death. Although the majority of misconceptions surround the process of receiving radiotherapy, uncertainty often also surrounds its purpose. Watson (1991) states that some patients believe that radiotherapy is only used for palliation. For others radiotherapy is tantamount to a death sentence. It is evident that more empirical scrutiny is essential if a clearer picture of society's image of radiotherapy is to be achieved.

An attempt to clarify this situation is made by Eardley (1986), who examined patients' knowledge of, and attitude towards, radiotherapy. This study involved interviewing 39 patients receiving radical radiotherapy to head and neck tumours in a regional radiotherapy unit.

Each patient was interviewed three times; interviews coincided with admission, shortly before discharge and finally when the patient was at home. Eardley acknowledges that the study did not examine the patients' knowledge of 'X-ray treatment' prior to admission. One finding from the study was that it was evident that a wide range of understanding and knowledge of radiotherapy existed among those involved in the research. According to Eardley 43% of the patients noted that they were surprised that the treatment was completely painless: 'I expected to feel something . . . the X-ray going through', 'I was wondering what it would be like . . . whether it would be hot, with X-rays going through'. Patients in this study also found the treatment surprisingly simple (29%). The study also reinforced the assertion that patients felt unprepared for treatment with radiotherapy and many were left feeling unclear as to what side-effects they might expect. Despite not addressing patients' preconceptions of radiotherapy, the study is useful in acknowledging the existence of misconceptions concerning treatment with radiotherapy.

RADIOTHERAPY AND THE FAMILY

Although the principal focus of radiotherapy is to cure or relieve symptoms, its effects also extend to those who are not receiving the treatment. Cassileth and Hamilton (quoted by Bond, 1982) describe how cancer affects the family in three ways:

1. It may upset the future plans and orientations of the family.
2. It threatens or disrupts existing patterns of family interactions.
3. It alters the constellations of family contacts/reference groups.

When relating these principles to the patient receiving radiotherapy it becomes apparent that radiotherapy is potentially disruptive in all the aforementioned areas. Radiotherapy treatment centres may be a considerable distance from the patient's home, therefore a large portion of the patient's and family's day may be disrupted by travelling to and from the centre by ambulance or public transport.

It was noted earlier in the chapter that treatment using unsealed or interstitial sources imposes limitations on the time and distance patients and families may share together for safety reasons. At this crucial and uncertain time for the patient and family neither party may be able to offer the physical contact which may be crucial to a climate of mutual support. Such a scenario may also inhibit meaningful conversation amongst family members.

Oberst *et al.* (1991) note, in research which centred on examining the self-care demands of patients receiving ambulatory radiotherapy for the treatment of cancer and its associated distresses, that patients experienced a marked disruption in lifestyle. It also emerged that a strong family system was significant in coping with radiotherapy and that when such support is not available additional nursing support may be necessary. The diagnosis of cancer and its attending treatment may be sufficient to discourage close contact between the extended and nuclear family.

PSYCHOLOGICAL REACTIONS TO RADIOTHERAPY

Most patients receiving radiotherapy seem to cope effectively. For others the process of receiving treatment for cancer appears to be stressful (Oberst *et al.*, 1991). As early as the late 1970s Peck and Boland (1977) discovered that receiving radiotherapy is associated with emotional distress and anxiety. This assertion is supported by Graydon (1988), who conducted a study involving 79 patients who were receiving radiotherapy for lung cancer (21 patients) or breast cancer (58 patients). None of the patients in the study had previously had radiotherapy. Each patient was interviewed twice, initially during the first week of radiotherapy and finally following the course of radiotherapy. The interviews focused on symptoms experienced, the patient's emotions, individual concerns and the nature of the patient's social support network. It was discovered that high emotional distress in the initial stages of radiotherapy was associated with poorer resumption of their usual activities following treatment. The implications of this research are that receiving radiotherapy is stressful and that this emotion may have a detrimental effect on the quality of life for the patient beyond the completion of treatment. In the battle against cancer, multiple modes of treatment may be instigated to offer cure or effective palliation.

Hughson *et al.* (1987) examined the psychosocial effects of radiotherapy following mastectomy. The purpose of the study was to elicit if post-operative radiotherapy induced more psychological and social morbidity than that seen in a control group who had mastectomy with no further treatment. Forty-seven patients who received post-operative radiotherapy and 38 patients who received no further treatment were involved in the study. It was noted that three months after mastectomy those patients who had completed radiotherapy had significantly more somatic symptoms and social dysfunction than those not treated with radiotherapy. The social dysfunction took the form of the patient feeling indecisive or uncommunicative. The evidence that radiotherapy did not induce excessive depression or anxiety was a surprise to the researchers in this study. Hughson and his colleagues concluded that those who received radiotherapy may be upset by their treatment but the study failed to confirm that depression and anxiety were more common than in those given no further radiotherapy.

It is also suggested that any psychological morbidity associated with radiotherapy tends to be short lived. Despite the findings of the above study it is premature to suggest that radiotherapy imposes minimal disruption to the psychological welfare of the individual. Depression and anxiety are just two of a plethora of experiences which can emerge from treatment of this nature. Earlier in the chapter it was noted that radiotherapy can be administered using unsealed sources, by external beam and via the interstitial route.

The scanty research to date has focused on patients receiving radiotherapy by external beam who could be classified as self-caring. Treatment using unsealed sources such as iodine-131 for thyroid tumours and interstitial treatment such as iridium wire implants for breast cancer offer scenarios in which the patient receives treatment for a longer period of time. This may last for several days in both of these examples. The need to follow radiation safety protocols means the cancer patient has minimal contact with both relatives and carers. This may be the first time the patient is alone to ponder his or her plight of having a cancer. Receiving radiotherapy via selectron for a gynaecological malignancy using uterine afterloading devices leads to long periods of isolation. These periods of isolation may be therapeutic, allowing the patient to come to terms with the present and the future, but they might also exacerbate fears and anxieties. One thing is for certain: research into the patient's experience of 'isolating' forms of radiotherapy is needed.

Radiotherapy can also bring about structural alteration in the genitalia which may require psychological and physical rehabilitation. The psychological sequelae of radiotherapy are therefore implicated in body image disturbance.

The emotional toll of radiotherapy seems to be linked to the site in which the radiotherapy is targeted. This becomes evident in Eardley's (1986) extensive research which was referred to earlier; this examined patients' experiences of receiving radiotherapy for head and neck tumours. It is evident that a number of the patients experienced distressing symptoms as a result of radiotherapy. One patient is quoted as saying 'I did feel depressed – it was my mouth, I was frightened of going to sleep because of what I expected to find in the morning [i.e. bleeding from the mouth]. I got a bit worried, thinking has the treatment done the trick, or do I have to go through that again?' This study revealed that 47% had felt depressed following discharge from hospital. Another patient is quoted as saying 'I was very frightened when my neck broke out, we all wondered what it was – we didn't know about it. It really did look dreadful . . . you wonder all sorts'. In contrast is Hughson's assertion that psychological disruption as a result of radiotherapy is minimal and transient in nature. Eardley's study infers that radiotherapy for head and neck tumours is very much more traumatic. Words such as 'frightened', 'depression', 'irritable' and 'fed-up' seemed to characterize the experience of the patient receiving radiotherapy.

Why are patients so worried about receiving radiotherapy? It appears that a number of reasons underpin such anxiety:

1. fear of the technology involved in administering radiotherapy;
2. fear of being separated from sources of support for the duration of the treatment;
3. having radiotherapy may symbolize the person's fear that the tumour is still present and has not been clearly excised;
4. fear of the distressing symptoms which may emerge as a result of the radiotherapy.

In conclusion, it can be elicited from available research that radiotherapy is benign in its impact on psychological welfare, but can in certain instances be distressing and an ingredient in the development of long-term psychological problems.

IMPROVING THE PSYCHOLOGICAL WELL-BEING OF THE
PATIENT RECEIVING RADIOTHERAPY

A great deal of emphasis is now being placed on meeting the holistic needs
of the patient. In the light of the research already cited, nurses and other
caring professions have a responsibility to inaugurate and sustain
initiatives which can enhance the psychological well-being of the patient
receiving radiotherapy. Since cancer care is very much multidisciplinary
in nature, collaboration between radiotherapists, radiographers and
nurses would appear essential irrespective of whatever strategy is
employed. Cull (1991) outlines three supportive interventions that offer a
useful framework, which if used in an integrated manner may enhance
psychological adjustment to radiotherapy:

1. educational
2. interpretive
3. cathartic.

Educational

Close (1992) mentions that over the last two decades health care
professionals have become increasingly aware of the need to educate
patients. Frith (1991) mentions that the rationale for providing patients
with information prior to and during diagnostic and therapeutic procedures is well established. This information is not only necessary to
minimize the side-effects of radiotherapy, but also to help clear up
misconceptions about this mode of treatment.

Understanding a treatment modality and its effects can facilitate a
feeling of control. The need for control would appear essential if the
patient is to develop a 'fighting spirit' as described by Greer and Moorey
(1989). Without this information the existence of inaccurate beliefs
regarding radiotherapy will persist and an air of pessimism dominate the
patient's view of the future. Cassileth (quoted by Bond, 1982) discovered
that 98% of patients desired information on possible side-effects and that
disappointment and anger may follow if this information is not forthcoming (Frith, 1991). It is overwhelmingly clear that patients receiving
radiotherapy are in need of extensive patient education prior to and
during the treatment phase. Frith (1991) outlines six areas in which
patients require information relating to radiotherapy:

1. correction of misconceptions relating to previous knowledge;
2. information on the nature of radiotherapy;
3. a description of the radiotherapy room, using photographs of the
   machinery, or a visit, if at all practical;

4. procedural, sensory and behavioural information relating to the actual administration of radiotherapy;
5. information on the side-effects to be expected and behaviour information on their management;
6. the knowledge that individuals react in different ways to treatment.

These six areas offer a comprehensive framework of the patients' anticipated informational needs. Patient education is of course not as easy as simply a nurse or other health care professional providing the appropriate information. Nichols (1984), in his work with renal patients, offers a useful model of informational care which fits in well with the informational needs of the patient receiving radiotherapy. Nichols suggests that informational care consists of the following stages:

1. **Informational exchange.** This stage would be characterized by the patient sharing with the health care professional fears and expectations relating to radiotherapy.
2. **Giving information.** At this point information about radiotherapy could be delivered using a variety of methods, e.g. video, booklets, visits to treatment areas.
3. **Final accuracy check.** This is perhaps the most important stage as it is the role of the health care professional to ascertain the patient's degree of understanding and level of retention of information.

A great deal of emphasis is currently placed on the nurse/health care professional giving information. Successful patient education seems to be the successful integration of interpersonal skills, approachability, giving information and of course follow-up.

Currently, there is a wide selection of booklets available to help the patient and family understand the nature of radiotherapy, e.g. BACUP, *Which? Consumer Guide to Understanding Cancer* and more recently Speechley and Rosenfield's *Cancer Information at your Fingertips* (1992). It is beyond the scope of this chapter to expand further on these sources, but questions dealt with include 'What is radiotherapy?', 'Will I be radioactive after treatment?' and 'Are there any side-effects?' and offer some insight into the role of these sources. To date very little evidence exists on the effectiveness of this mode of delivering information to patients. Hagopian (1991) investigated the effects of sending out structured patient information to patients receiving radiotherapy in the form of a weekly newsletter. The patients in the study who read the booklet scored higher in the post-knowledge test in comparison to the control group. It was hypothesized that this difference would also emerge in a reduction in side-effects in those who studied the booklets. The results of this issue suggest that no significant difference existed between the control group and the group who had studied the booklet.

One must be cautious in proclaiming that information booklets are a panacea for all patients' informational needs. In a study which has had an influence on the construction of patient information material, Byrne and Edeani (1984), looking at the knowledge of medical terminology amongst 125 hospital patients, noted that just over 9% had no knowledge of radiation. Just over 50% did not provide a clear understanding of what radiation is and only 36% understood what radiation is. This study implies that patients prescribed radiation treatment are likely to have scanty knowledge of the therapy they are going to receive. Perhaps health care professionals involved in caring for the patient receiving radiotherapy should have a cohesive plan for educating the local community on the nature of radiotherapy. Radiotherapy patient education is, at the moment, a reactive entity rather than being proactive in nature. Open days in radiotherapy units for the public and health care staff could do much to enhance society's understanding of radiotherapy. More openness and public education regarding radiotherapy are much needed. Booklets are of course not the only medium by which the patient and family can become acquainted with the nature of radiotherapy. North *et al.* (1992), describing research on the use of tape-recorded consultations, suggest that this can help cancer patients retain information, and illustrate the need to further explore the value of using audiotapes as a means of educating patients about treatment interventions. Similarly short videos focusing on the nature of radiotherapy played in out-patient waiting areas may help dispel myths held by the patient and the family. Irrespective of whether or not patient education influences the outcome of treatment, Eardley (1986) suggests that on humanitarian grounds attempts should be made to inform patients about the nature of radiotherapy.

INTERPRETIVE

Patients' interpretation of radiotherapy being painful and the cause of much pain and discomfort seems to be locked up in the technical face of the treatment. Having cancer means entering a very different universe, in which the carers use a new and peculiar language. Card and Fielding (1986) advocate the idea of staff spending time to elicit patients' specific fears. Part of the time must be used to unravel technical jargon which the patient may have been exposed to.

   The nurse or radiotherapist has a key role in interpreting the patient's emotional journey through this anxiety-provoking experience. Such a strategy may seem unrealistic in a treatment centre where hundreds of patients may be treated on a daily basis. The sheer volume of patients may be one reason why the psychosocial needs of the patient receiving radiotherapy are overlooked. Another reason is provided by Oberst *et al.* (1991), who examined the self-care burdens of patients receiving radiotherapy. Because patients may be classed as ambulatory, hidden fears may be overlooked by the caring team. As well as helping patients identify strategies for coping with the total experience of cancer treatment, the emergence of complementary therapies has opened up new horizons in terms of stress induced by fear of cancer treatments. Decker *et al.* (1992) carried out research in which a total of 82 patients of mixed gender received relaxation training in adjunct to radiotherapy. The authors of this study noted reductions in tension, depression, anger and fatigue in the group receiving relaxation training.

CATHARTIC

The onset of cancer marks a period of crisis (Pinell, 1988). Throughout this experience the need to release pent-up emotions comes to a head immediately before, after or during treatment. During the cancer experience, irrespective of whether the treatment is palliative or curative, support in the form of counselling may be necessary. Young and Mayer (1992) mention that in some centres radiographer counsellors have been employed. Perhaps it would be more beneficial to the patients if all staff involved in the care of the patient receiving radiotherapy were competent in supporting patients psychologically.

PSYCHOLOGICAL CARE: SETTING STANDARDS TOGETHER

No one discipline has a monopoly in meeting the psychological needs of the patient receiving radiotherapy.

The advent of standard setting via a variety of methods has provided an avenue where members of the multidisciplinary team can work together in enhancing the quality of life for patients receiving radiotherapy. Standard setting may facilitate interdisciplinary collaboration and a shared understanding of the patient's holistic needs for the duration of a course of radiotherapy.

CONCLUSION

It becomes evident that caring for the patient with cancer requiring radiotherapy is a demanding task. Radiotherapy paradoxically can alleviate physical distress but at the same time can be the cause of debilitating emotional and physical discomfort. Quality care for the patient receiving radiotherapy seems increasingly dependent on good interdisciplinary collaboration and an expanding knowledge base founded on research.

REFERENCES

Anderson, W. (1980) Radiotherapy: radiation protection methods. *Nursing Times*, **76**(2), 45–8.

Arnfield, A. (1988) Children's tumours, in *Nursing the Patient with Cancer* (ed. V. Tschudin). Prentice Hall, London.

Baker, J. (1979) Radiotherapy: implants and applicators. *Nursing Mirror*, **148** (Suppl. 10), 37–40.

Bareford, C. (1988) Leukaemias, in *Nursing the Patient with Cancer* (ed. V. Tschudin), Prentice Hall, London.

Bond, S. (1982) Communication in cancer nursing, in *Cancer Nursing: Recent Advances in Nursing*, Vol. 3 (ed. M.C. Cahoon), Churchill Livingstone, Edinburgh, pp. 3–30.

Byrne, T.J. and Edeani, D. (1984) Knowledge of medical terminology among hospital patients. *Nursing Research*, **33**(3), 178–81.

Campbell, I.R. and Illingworth, M.H. (1992) Can patients wash during radiotherapy to the breast or chest wall? A randomised control trial. *Clinical Oncology*, **4**(2), 78–82.

Card, I. and Fielding, R. (1986) Caring for the cancer sufferer: a survey of therapy radiographers' problems. *Radiography*, **52**(602), 57–9.

Christman, N. (1990) Uncertainty and adjustment during radiotherapy. *Nursing Research*, **39**(1), 17–20.

Close, A. (1992) Patient power: strategic planning in patient education. *Nursing Standard*, **6**(43), 32–5.

Copp, K. (1991) Nursing patients having radiotherapy, in *Oncology for Nurses and Health Care Professionals*, Vol. 3 (ed. D. Borely), Harper & Row, London.

Crown, V. (1978) Principles of radiotherapy, in *Cancer Nursing* (ed. R. Tiffany), Faber & Faber, London.

Cull, A. (1991) Lung cancer, in *Cancer Patient Care: Psychosocial Treatment Methods* (ed. M. Watson), BPS Books/Cambridge University Press, Cambridge.

Decker, T., Cline Elsen, J. and Gallagher, M. (1992) Relaxation as an adjunct in radiation oncology. *Journal of Clinical Psychology*, **48**(3), 388–93.

Deeley, T.J. (1976) *Principles of Radiation Therapy*. Butterworth, London.

Eardley, A. (1986) Patients and radiotherapy: 3. Patients' experiences after discharge. *Radiography*, **52**(601), 17–19.

Eilers, J., Berger, A.M. and Peterson, M.C. (1988) Development, testing and application of oral assessment guide. *Oncology Nursing Forum*, **15**(3), 325–30.

Frith, B. (1991) Giving information to radiotherapy patients. *Nursing Standard*, **4**(34), 33–5.

Gilmore, M. and Fairclough, C. (1992) Putting radiation in perspective. *Journal of Cancer Care*, **1**(3), 183–6.

Graydon, J. (1988) Factors that predict patients' functioning following treatment for cancer. *International Journal of Nursing Studies*, **25**(2), 117–24.

Greer, S. and Moorey, S. (1989) *Psychological Therapy for Patients with Cancer: A New Approach*. Heinemann Medical Books, London.

Hagopian, G. (1991) The effects of a weekly radiation therapy newsletter on patients. *Oncology Nursing Forum*, **18**(7), 119–203.

Hall, E.J. and Cox, J.D. (1989) Physical and biological basis of radiation therapy, in *Radiation Oncology: Rationale, Technique, Results* (eds W.T. Moss and J.D. Cox), Mosby, St Louis.

Harris, S.J. and Jackson, D.F. (1987) Radiation and the nurse. *Professional Nurse*, 2(12), 385–7.

Holmes, S. (1986a) Radiotherapy: planning nutritional support. *Nursing Times*, 82(16), 26–9.

Holmes, S. (1986b) Radiotherapy: minimising the side-effects. *Professional Nurse*, 1(10), 263–5.

Holmes, S. (1987) *Nutritional Problems in the Cancer Patient*. Nursing Series, Ballière Tindall, London.

Holmes, S. (1988) *Radiotherapy*. Austin Cornish, London.

Hughson, A.V.M., Cooper, A.F., McArdle, C.S. and Smith, D.C. (1987) Psychosocial effects of radiotherapy after mastectomy. *British Medical Journal*, 294, 1515–18.

Nias, A.H.W. (1990) Radiation biology, in *Treatment of Cancer* (eds K. Shikora and K.E. Halnan), Chapman & Hall, London.

Nichols, K. (1984) *Psychological Care in Physical Illness*. Croom Helm, London.

North, N., Cornbleet, M., Knowles, G. and Leonard, R.C.F. (1992) Information giving in oncology: a preliminary study of tape-recorder use. *British Journal of Clinical Psychology*, 31, 357–9.

Oberst, M.T., Hughes, S.H., Chang, A.S. and McCubban, M.A. (1991) Self-care burden, stress appraisal and mood among persons receiving radiotherapy. *Cancer Nursing*, 14(2), 71–8.

Oliver, G. (1988) Radiotherapy, in *Nursing the Patient with Cancer* (ed. V. Tschudin), Prentice Hall, London.

Peck, A. and Boland, J. (1977) Emotional reactions to radiation treatment. *Cancer*, 40, 180–4.

Pinell, P. (1988) How do cancer patients express their points of view? *Sociology of Health and Illness*, 9(1), 25–45.

Raven, R.W. (1990) *The Theory and Practice of Oncology*. Parthenon, Casterton, Carnforth, Lancashire.

Souhami, R. and Tobias, J. (1986) *Cancer and Its Management*. Blackwell Scientific Publications, London.

Speechley, V. and Rosenfield, M. (1992) *Cancer Information at your Fingertips*. Cass, London.

Walter, J. (1977) *Cancer and Radiotherapy*, 2nd edn. Churchill Livingstone, Edinburgh.

Watson, M. (ed.) (1991) *Cancer Patient Care: Psychosocial Treatment Methods*. BSP Books/Cambridge University Press, Cambridge.

Young, J. and Mayer, E. (1992) The role of the radiographer counsellor in a large centre for cancer treatment: a discussion paper based on an audit of the work of a radiographer counsellor. *Clinical Oncology*, 4(4), 232–5.

7 Surgery and the cancer patient

Annie Topping

INTRODUCTION

Surgery is the oldest and probably the most widely used medical approach for the management of cancer and possibly the modality most familiar to nurses. The newer approaches – chemotherapy and radiotherapy – were originally administered in specialist centres, whereas surgery was and continues to be performed along with operations for non-malignant conditions. The individual undergoing surgery for cancer has been nursed in general surgical wards and this, it could be suggested, has delayed the development of surgical oncology as a specialist area for nurses and doctors alike. This may change with increasing consumer demands within a 'market' health service and a specialist multidisciplinary approach to care for the individual with cancer.

This chapter sets out to discuss the range and scope of cancer surgery and issues relating to the management of care for individuals undergoing surgery and their subsequent recovery and rehabilitation. Cancer patients, because of the nature of the disease and the treatments used in its management, do have special needs. Care planning, therefore, should be based upon an understanding of the underlying knowledge concerning the physical and psychological processes which are manifested in malignant disease.

HISTORICAL PERSPECTIVE

In the classical Greek period two different theories relating to the nature of cancer emerged, both based on the concept of humours – blood, phlegm, yellow bile and black bile – which were the physical representations of the four universal elements. These elements – fire, air, wind and earth – had the qualities of hot, cold, dry and moist ascribed to them.

Black bile was associated with cancer, being of the earth and moist. Hippocratic writings suggested that cancer was a systemic disease and cautioned against interfering with hidden cancers within body cavities. Galen advocated removal of tumours or drainage of the 'black bile' which accumulated from cancer and, it could be proposed, took a more locoregional approach (Gallucci, 1985; Havard and Topping, 1991).

The humoral theories were gradually replaced as advances in knowledge provided contrary evidence, particularly Harvey's theories in relation to circulation and the discovery of the lymphatic system — lymphatic fluid being considered significant in the development of cancer. John Hunter, the father of modern surgery, believed that cancer was a locoregional disease and therefore advocated ligation of vessels which supplied the tumour and removal of local lymph nodes. Descriptions of surgical procedures for specific tumours make harrowing reading, particularly prior to anaesthetics and any real understanding of sepsis. Yet surgery was performed, although often at great cost in terms of mortality.

The landmarks in terms of modern cancer surgery, such as Bilroth performing a subtotal gastrectomy in 1881 and Halstead developing his technique for radical mastectomy in 1890, were only made possible by the introduction of general anaesthesia and changed practices in relation to antisepsis. Further developments such as antibiotic therapy, intensive care and nutritional support have allowed extensive and often radical surgical procedures to be performed.

These radical approaches were initially advocated in the absence of effective alternative treatment for solid tumours. Secondly the notion of local control (en bloc resection with lymph node dissection) effecting cure was a widespread belief. It is now suggested that although a degree of improved survival did result, many individuals died from distant metastatic disease or peri-operative complications. The current thinking that the majority of individuals have distant, microscopic, metastatic disease on presentation supports a multimodality approach and obviates the need for radical surgery in a number of cases. This change has been brought about by:

- greater understanding regarding the nature and spread of cancer;
- improved technology to enhance diagnosis and staging of disease;
- chemotherapeutic and radiotherapeutic developments;
- advances in surgical technique and biotechnology;
- consideration of quality of life.

THE SCOPE OF CANCER SURGERY

Although there have been considerable developments, surgery alone cannot effect a cure unless malignant disease is confined to its primary

Table 7.1   The scope of cancer surgery

Type	Example
Cancer prevention	Colectomy (familial polyposis coli)
	Orchidopexy (testicular cancer)
Diagnosis	Orchidectomy (testicular tumours)
	Lumpectomy (breast cancer)
Staging	Staging laparotomy (Hodgkin's disease)
Treatment of primary tumour	Abdominoperineal resection (bowel cancer)
Reconstruction/rehabilitation	Breast reconstruction
Palliative	Oophorectomy (breast cancer)
Adjuvant	Para-aortic node dissection
Iatrogenic	Excision of radionecrotic tissue
Resection of metastases	Partial hepatectomy
To facilitate access	Tunnelled central venous catheters
	Arterial access for limb perfusion
	Insertion of interstitial radioactive needles (cancer of the tongue)
Emergencies	Tracheostomy
Cytoreductive	'Debulking' laparotomy

site. Surgery should be considered as one in a list of approaches which can be advocated as part of an individual's care package. However, surgery should not just be seen as the means by which tumour is removed but as having an important contribution to make in terms of restoring form and function. Increasingly the quality of life achieved following cancer treatment is an important consideration and one of the central tenets of rehabilitation of the cancer patient. Surgery can play an important part in that recovery.

The scope of cancer surgery today is broad and the trend away from single-modality treatment has not reduced the valuable and diverse role of surgery. Table 7.1 outlines the scope of cancer surgery and examples of its application. This diversity is increasing along with technological advances. The use of lasers is an example of the application of new techniques. Originally they were used to reduce tumour mass and relieve symptoms in rectal cancer, particularly where patients were too frail to sustain general anaesthetic (Bown *et al.*, 1986). There is currently a trial in progress monitoring the efficacy of laser therapy in destroying malignant tissue in breast cancer. Early results suggest the use of lasers may be an effective treatment, so in the future management of breast lumps may be very different, with lumpectomy becoming a more infrequent procedure.

The principles underpinning the use of surgery in cancer are as follows:

1. Surgery remains important and is sometimes the only approach suitable for the individual with cancer.
2. Surgical excision generally includes removal of tumour beyond its margins and will include normal tissue.
3. The surgical procedure performed should be carried out with consideration of eventual cosmetic appearance and residual functional abilities.
4. Multimodality approaches are increasingly being used owing to the micrometastasis theory of cancer.

CANCER PREVENTION

In the area of cancer prevention, for some cancers there remains debate; this in effect means surgical management versus surveillance. Surgery is effective in the management of certain familial diseases, although offering prophylactic oophorectomy or bilateral mastectomy to a young women with strong familial tendency to ovarian or breast cancer requires sensitive and supportive information giving and counselling. The decision to advocate surgery should be based upon presence or absence of symptoms, the risk, histological evidence, ease of monitoring, and the eventual outcome in terms of body image, lifestyle effects, and fertility.

DIAGNOSIS

Although suspicion of cancer may be evident from radiological or physical examination, confirmation should be established from actual tissue. This can be achieved by a variety of methods, the choice usually determined by the method which affords the best result, offset by consideration of cost, disturbance to the patient and ease of performance (Ames, 1986).

An incisional biopsy involves removal of a portion of tissue and can be performed under a general or local anaesthetic, e.g. shave or punch biopsy, whereas an excisional biopsy involves excision of the complete tumour with little or no margin of normal tissue, e.g. lump biopsy. A needle biopsy is used to aspirate fluid or tissue from the tumour, whereas an exfoliative technique such as the Papanicolaou (Pap) smear allows examination of cells from a scrape or smear of tissue. Endoscopy may be used to gain access to suspicious tissue from normally inaccessible sites such as the bladder or bronchus. The instrument used can be rigid or flexible.

Whatever approach is used, a two-step process to diagnosis and treatment is increasingly being adopted. This affords the individual and important others the opportunity to assimilate a cancer diagnosis before considering treatment options.

STAGING

This is undertaken to determine the full extent and stage of disease. In some cases a diagnostic laparotomy may be performed to assist the surgeon in planning the extent of resection and monitoring for the presence of hidden metastases. This is becoming increasingly infrequent with the advances in radiological imaging using computed axial tomography (CAT) or nuclear magnetic resonance (NMR) and chemical assay tests to monitor tumour markers. In Hodgkin's disease staging may include laparotomy, splenectomy, liver biopsy, retroperitoneal node biopsy and the placement of clips to denote borders for future radiotherapy treatment (Szopa, 1987).

Another infrequent use of surgery is the 'second-look laparotomy', which was advocated as a follow-up after recovery from original curative surgery to check for absence or presence of disease. It is more commonly used for cancers which recur locally such as ovarian tumours. This also has a place in assessing response to other treatment modalities, such as radiotherapy or chemotherapy.

TREATMENT OF PRIMARY TUMOUR

There is still a major role for surgery as a definitive treatment. Success in terms of cure is dependent on the nature, i.e. tendency to metastasize via the bloodstream, of the particular cancer (Westbury, 1988). Skin cancers, excluding melanoma, early tumours of the rectum and colon, and differentiated thyroid cancer, can be effectively managed by surgical approaches. Surgical approaches may involve:

1. local excision – removal of the tumour with a margin of normal tissue;
2. en bloc dissection or wide excision – removal of the tumour, regional nodes which drain the tumour and tissue containing drainage channels, and any tissue or structure locally infiltrated or contiguous.
3. management of cancer in situ – involves local excision or application of cryo-, laser or electrical probe to ablate tissue; endoscopy is often used initially to visualize the tumour.

Traditional radical surgery is increasingly being abandoned where advances in other treatment modalities may improve or provide similar results in terms of disease control, with less loss of function or body image disturbance.

RECONSTRUCTIVE OR REHABILITATIVE SURGERY

Many major surgical resections for cancer can leave the individual with loss or change of functional ability or body image change. Increasingly it is being recognized that cure without consideration of outcome is not enough. Advances such as the end-to-end anastomosis (EEA) using a stapling device have reduced the numbers of stomas raised. The development of myocutaneous skin flaps and their use in head and neck surgery and breast reconstruction has improved the cosmetic effects of primarily curative surgery. Also techniques originally developed for use in benign conditions are increasingly being used in the management of malignant disease such as the continent urinary reservoir or pouch (Cumming et al., 1987). Greater control over life and freedom are reported as benefits of continent urinary or faecal diversion over traditional stoma surgery.

In the past reconstructive surgery was often delayed to allow a period where the individual could be monitored for recurrence. Early reconstruction is now increasingly being performed and is supported by research which suggests it may assist psychological recovery in breast cancer (d'Angelo and Gorrell, 1989; Stevens et al., 1984).

PALLIATIVE SURGERY

For the individual whose disease makes life difficult and in some cases intolerable palliative surgery may prove beneficial. Cancer can present on or near the skin surface and cause pain, ulcerate, and become infected and odorous. Secondary bone metastases can cause pain. Gastrointestinal, airway, biliary and uretic obstructions can all be managed surgically. Surgical management even when there is evidence of extensive metastatic disease can improve the quality of life of some individuals and therefore can justify the demands of surgery, and in some cases very extensive surgery.

ADJUVANT SURGERY

Increasingly surgery is being used to support management of cancers by other modalities. Tumours which are sensitive to radiotherapy or chemotherapy may be treated initially by that approach followed by surgery to remove residual tissue. Residual para-aortic node enlargement in testicular cancer (teratoma) is often removed surgically after completion of chemotherapy. Similarly in osteosarcoma of the limbs chemotherapy is administered to destroy metastatic tissue and reduce the size of the primary tumour. This is followed by limb-sparing bone resection.

Sometimes surgery is required to mediate the effects of other modalities. Radiotherapy can result in local skin necrosis, development of rectal or colonic fistulae, bladder and vaginal contractions, ureteric strictures, etc., whereas some chemotherapy regimes can cause intestinal inflammation which can lead to perforation. A wide range of chemotherapeutic agents can be toxic if they extravasate and in severe cases grafting may be necessary to provide skin coverage. Iatrogenic complications can for some individuals create greater problems than the original cancer and therefore sensitive and supportive management is important.

Occasionally, in selected cases, there is a place for resection of metastases. This usually means that control of the primary tumour has been achieved and removal of a solitary mass will result in cure of disease. There are reports of successful outcomes in cases with isolated metastases involving bone, liver, lung and brain (Beattie, 1984; Fortner, 1984).

Sometimes surgery is performed to reduce the size of tumours – cytoreductive surgery. This controversial approach is based on the notion that if the amount of tumour cell mass is reduced other therapies such as chemo- or immunotherapy may be rendered more effective.

SURGERY TO FACILITATE ACCESS

With the development of devices to assist in the delivery of treatment surgery is used to implant the devices to improve access, delivery and patient comfort. These devices may be for the delivery of chemotherapy, as in ventricular, inter-arterial and venous access reservoirs and catheters. Advantages include reduction in discomfort, greater compliance with treatment regimes, and ease of access for monitoring, sampling, delivery of drugs to support therapy, e.g. antiemetics, etc. However, some individuals experience body image disturbance and feel restricted by these devices. Also they are not without potential and actual problems related to infection, displacement, blockage and occlusion.

The delivery of brachytherapy often involves the surgical insertion of the actual isotope or a device to contain the isotope. This may be intracavity as in gynaecological cancer or interstitially as in breast, and head and neck cancer.

EMERGENCY SURGERY

The management of oncological emergencies by surgical measures remains highly controversial and often presents a real ethical dilemma, often with decision-making acted out at the bedside. Whatever procedure is involved the outcome should be symptomatic relief with improvement in the quality of life. Some may argue that non-intervention may in some instances be more humane and warrants consideration.

Cancer does unfortunately produce life-threatening conditions such as airway obstruction or carotid artery erosion which require immediate action to prevent death. Other events such as gastrointestinal perforation or obstruction allow consideration of potential outcome and provide time to initiate supportive management prior to surgery.

THE SURGICAL EXPERIENCE

Care of the individual with cancer often requires the employment of innovative strategies. It can prove difficult in some cases to achieve even baseline needs in relation to pain, nutrition and wound care. Pain management in the peri-operative period can be more demanding if the individual has been requiring opiate analgesia pre-operatively. Wound healing can be severely retarded by poor nutritional status, previous radiotherapy, delayed or depressed immunological responses or drug therapy (e.g. steroids). Psychological and social influences may also have an effect on surgical recovery. In the remaining part of this chapter these and other issues such as altered body image will be addressed in greater detail.

WOUND HEALING

The goal of care in relation to wound healing is that individuals receive full assessment and appropriate intervention in order that complications are minimized and comfort and healing are promoted (Luthert and Robinson, 1993, p. 127). Unfortunately for some individuals perfect wound closure and healing is not possible. Torrance (1985) proposes that:

> Wound healing is only one aspect of the body's response to injury and the whole person, not just the visible injury, must be treated.

This holistic approach is particularly pertinent for the individual with cancer. It should be remembered too that people with cancer may also have other underlying conditions which predispose them to difficulties with healing.

Wound healing is said to have four sequential overlapping stages (Westaby, 1985; Messer, 1989). These phases are:

1. the acute inflammatory phase;
2. the destructive phase;
3. the proliferative phase;
4. the maturation phase.

The inflammatory phase

In the first seconds of tissue damage bleeding into the area occurs. This allows the movement of leucocytes into the site and platelets to congregate along vessel walls and edges. Once the bleeding ceases and histamine is released plasma proteins, leucocytes, antibodies and electrolytes exude into the tissues and produce local inflammation and heat.

The process of repair and defence against infection occurs when macrophages and leucocytes migrate to the wound due to a chemotactic response. Individuals with underlying conditions such as diabetes may have reduced numbers of macrophages and this can result in delayed healing. Large clots, necrotic tissue and sometimes sutures can prolong this phase (Wilson-Barnett and Bateup, 1988, p. 204).

The destructive phase

Macrophages and polymorphonuclear leucocytes debride necrotic tissue and ingest bacteria, thereby removing them from the area. This degradation process causes increased osmolarity; therefore there can be local swelling, which in some sites could cause problems, possibly resulting in ischaemia. Also this level of activity exerts greater cellular oxygen demands and therefore individuals with hypoxic wounds (e.g. in peripheral vascular disease) are more susceptible to infection.

Proliferative phase

Endothelial cells and fibroblasts proliferate and collagen is synthesized. This results in an increased supportive quality in the wound produced by the random organization of collagen. This mechanism is dependent on oxygen, vitamin C and iron being present. New granulation tissue, consisting of capillary loops, supporting collagen and glycoprotein, can be formed in a disorderly way. It can grow into dressings such as gauze and can be easily damaged. Clean, moist conditions are said to accelerate granulation.

The maturation phase

Collagen fibres become reorientated and enlarged through a process of lysis and resynthesis. This produces enhanced tensile strength.

THE EFFECTS OF CANCER AND CANCER THERAPIES ON WOUND HEALING

Radiotherapy

Regardless of body site, radiation must penetrate skin to reach its target site. Modern treatment planning is based upon reducing side-effects whilst maximizing accuracy of dose, and therefore skin-sparing strategies are used. Tissue changes, it is suggested, can be directly related to dose increments, frequency and total amount delivered. It is suggested that doses above 40 Gy can produce permanent damage such as scarring, reduced blood supply and fibrosis. The individual undergoing surgery following radiotherapy may experience poor wound healing, assuming the surgery is within the field of the previous treatment. This may manifest as delayed healing or more severe problems such as dehiscence or fistula development. Increased susceptibility to infection may also be problematic (Wilson-Barnett and Bateup, 1988, p. 209).

Chemotherapy

Experimental animal studies examining the effects of cytotoxic therapy on wound healing indicate a variety of problems. These include decreased wound strength, inhibition of contraction, reduced collagen production, inflammatory response and vascularization due to effects on cell proliferation. However, Ferguson (1982) when reviewing clinical studies failed to obtain evidence which supported the experimental work, although other explanations such as lack of comparability of wound assessment measures across studies or administration of agents begun once wound healing was well established could explain paucity of clinical evidence. Work by Westaby (1981) indicated that pre-operative cytotoxic chemotherapy resulted in the absence of healing following suture removal post-operatively in patients undergoing thoracic surgery.

Immunosuppression

The immune system is significant and contributes to the inflammatory response, phagocytosis, and hormonal and cell-mediated immunity. Individuals who can be considered at risk from delays in wound healing are:

- those individuals who have immunological diseases which compromise phagocytosis (leukaemia) or cell-mediated immunity (Hodgkin's disease);
- older people who may have impaired immunological functions and

may be malnourished and experiencing decreased essential organ functioning (Chvapil and Koopman, 1982);

- individuals who have underlying conditions which may delay healing, such as diabetes mellitus or malnutrition;
- individuals taking drugs which may compromise healing. The effects of steroids on healing have been debated but some studies show a decreased tensile strength of closed wounds, slower rates of epithelialization and neovascularization, and inhibition of wound contraction.

Choosing the right dressing

No one dressing is suitable for all wounds (Turner, 1983). The vast array of products available can be confusing and therefore recognition of the performance criteria necessary to promote healing may help in the selection process. For optimum conditions for healing a dressing should:

- remove exudate and toxic elements, and therefore needs to be absorbent;
- maintain a high humidity at the interface between wound and dressing;
- allow gaseous exchange of oxygen, carbon dioxide and water vapour;
- provide thermal insulation;
- be impermeable to microorganisms;
- be free of particulate contaminants;
- not result in trauma when changed.

Other qualities, such as acceptability, safety and sterilizability, are discussed in more specialist texts such as Turner *et al.* (1986), Morgan (1990) and Thomas (1992). As well as the dressing the nurse needs to consider the preparations used for cleansing and their potential effects on the environment and the healing process. Brennan and Leaper (1985) demonstrated that many antiseptic agents exert some effect on the local wound environment and some were detrimental to and retarded healing. Williams *et al.* (1985) showed that frequent dressing changes had an adverse effect on experimental wounds. Therefore as a rule of thumb, unless special circumstances exist, in the unproblematic surgical wound it would seem that:

- disruption and cleansing should be minimized;
- cleansing with a non-toxic agent, e.g. normal saline, should only be performed when exudate and debris have accumulated.

THE PATIENT UNDERGOING FORMATION OF A STOMA

A stoma or ostomy is an opening constructed surgically where an end, or ends, or loop of gut is brought onto the body surface. This can be: to allow access to the stomach or jejunum for feeding purposes – an **input stoma**; or more commonly to provide an exit for faecal or urinary material – an **output stoma**, which can be of a temporary or permanent nature.

Stomas can be fashioned for a variety of reasons but the focus of this section will be the cancer patient who requires ostomy surgery. It is estimated that something like 52 000 people in the UK have stomas. Approximately 30 000 have permanent colostomies, most commonly performed for rectal cancer. About 7500 patients have urinary diversion stomas which are usually performed for bladder cancer (Coloplast Ltd, 1987). From these figures it can be seen that a large proportion of individuals who have ostomy surgery are also coping with the diagnosis of, and a life with, cancer. With advances in technique and developments in early diagnosis the numbers of people facing and living with a stoma are anticipated to fall.

The aim of any care is to promote independence, ideally self-care, and adjustment. Rehabilitation is deemed successful when the ostomist has mastered altered elimination and begins to resume or broaden social activities and interaction (Dudas, 1983), although it should be recognized that adaptation and adjustment are dynamic and ability to cope may change in response to altered status, particularly health status. As many ostomists are elderly, reduced manual dexterity or diminished acuity may create difficulties in someone who was previously independent and self-caring. Similarly a recurrence of cancer can seriously threaten confidence and reopen issues that had been previously successfully managed (Dudas, 1986; Topping, 1987).

Most authors recognize that the provision of structured teaching, and proper physical and psychological care, play a major part in reducing difficulties and promoting rehabilitation (Devlin *et al.*, 1971; Breckman, 1981; Topping, 1987; Wade, 1989). This supportive process should ideally begin pre-operatively and continue for a lengthy period post-operatively (Wilson and Desruisseaux, 1983; Oberst and Scott, 1988).

PRE-OPERATIVE PREPARATION

Client assessment and subsequent care planning will focus predominantly on two dimensions of care, namely physical preparation and psychological care, although there will and should be considerable overlap in order that quality intervention is achieved. Table 7.2 identifies potential problem areas and suggests actions. These nursing activities may be assumed by a ward-based nurse or clinical nurse specialist dependent upon local circumstances. For example, in some centres stoma siting is performed by a clinical nurse specialist, and in others by medical staff.

Table 7.2   Potential problems in relation to stoma formation

Problem	Possible nursing activities
1. Lack of knowledge concerning surgery	Planned verbal information reinforced by written information. Areas which should be addressed: type of stoma planned, effects on elimination, rationale for surgery, how stoma is cared for, anticipated recovery regime
2. Attidues to stoma	Opportunity for the patient (and relatives) to discuss feelings about planned surgery and impact on future. Topics which may emerge are: effects on relationships, body image concerns, cancer diagnosis and prognosis, being different, etc. Concerns should be addressed positively yet realistically
3. Nutritional needs	Provide high calorie/low residue fluids and diet. Ensure patient understands why this is necessary
4. Bowel preparation needs	Inform patient of bowel cleansing procedure. Administer medication or lavage as per local procedure. Ensure privacy and that toilet and hygiene facilities are in close proximity. Monitor for evidence of shock, severe dehydration, distress, etc.
5. Skin preparation	If the patient has a history of allergies or skin problems instigate patch testing with tape, barrier creams, appliances, wafers, etc. Note outcome on medical and nursing notes
6. Siting of stoma	The following factors should be considered: dexterity, physical characteristics (such as skin folds, scars, dressing practices), eyesight, planned incision

IMMEDIATE POST-OPERATIVE CONSIDERATIONS

The goal of independence and ideally self-care is paramount and therefore elements of patient teaching which may help accelerate knowledge development should be included as part of all interventions. For example, when monitoring the stoma for colour, perfusion, swelling, bleeding and output, 'normal' appearance and function can be discussed. Familiarity with changed body, appliances, and gradual participation may encourage confidence and feelings of ownership and control.

POST-OPERATIVE REHABILITATION

In an ideal world all patients who undergo stoma formation would take responsibility for care of their changed elimination. Unfortunately, particularly in the severely debilitated or disorientated individual, it may be more realistic to teach a carer stoma management concurrently. Mastery of stoma care is often perceived as the major milestone in the process of adaptation. This concentration of effort may mask or submerge other concerns such as the underlying disease and its effect on living. Over a period of time the input by health care professionals may change from predominantly educational to more supportive (Hurney and Holland, 1985; Oberst and Scott, 1988).

As mentioned earlier, stoma surgery can result in body image disturbance and severe sexual difficulties. These can include loss of self-esteem, feelings of real disgust in relation to loss of control over elimination patterns, difficulties in love-making and effects on fertility. Honest, open yet non-threatening assessment and discussion of the problems experienced should be the baseline of practice. Many individuals have never talked about their sexual practices or preferences and find it a very difficult area to discuss.

Ostomy surgery, particularly where the rectum has been excised, can result in quite major dysfunction. In men erectile and ejaculatory difficulties may be transiently (up to two years) or permanently experienced. Information regarding prosthetic surgery and referral to an appropriate specialist may prove beneficial to the man with erectile difficulties.

Women may experience pain or discomfort during penetrating sexual intercourse due to weaknesses in the posterior vaginal wall or perineal scarring. Advice and treatment may be helpful in resolving or reducing the impact of these difficulties. Simple advice such as use of lubrication (water-soluble lubricant, e.g. K-Y Jelly, Replens) or saliva, perhaps encouraging greater foreplay before penetration, or offering alternative positions for love-making, are all strategies which may help the woman experiencing dyspareunia.

DISCHARGE PREPARATION

The patient or carer should, on discharge:

- be able to empty, clean, change, prepare and dispose of appliances;
- understand how diet, medication and fluid intake may effect output;
- recognize and maintain clean intact peristomal skin with a healthy stoma;
- appreciate and recognize signs of complications and what action to take;
- understand how to obtain further supplies of appliances and accessories;
- be aware of community resources.

Additionally, written information and instructions should be given for reference purposes, as should appropriate advice regarding social activities, travel, holidays and healthy living prior to discharge.

CHOOSING THE RIGHT EQUIPMENT

Many factors are involved in choosing the right appliance from the selection on the market. The major consideration is type and volume of effluent. The overriding issue should be selection which allows freedom to take on or resume previous activities and provide a sense of security.

From the range available many pouches and pouching systems have design features which may be useful for specific problems. Integral activated charcoal filters are one such feature; these absorb odour and allow flatus to escape. Although modern appliances have effective adhesive, some ostomists prefer to use a belt attached to either an integral or add-on attachment for added security. Some use tape to provide additional adherence to flange or baseplate edges. Advice regarding removal of adhesive debris and type of tape should be given if this approach is adopted.

As well as choice of pouching system there are numerous products which can enhance stoma management and improve quality of life. Skin protection products may be used routinely or if and when problems develop. Use of rings, wafers and adhesive paste can be beneficial in preventing skin excoriation, achieving longer wear periods and increasing security. Skin damage may also be minimized by the use of barrier creams, skin sealants and gel. Introduction of these products into care regimens should be based on individual assessment.

In the UK ostomy equipment can usually be supplied on prescription. Individuals who have a stoma formed can apply for a certificate of exemption from prescription charges.

Some individuals who have a colostomy raised and exude solid faecal material may prefer to use irrigation techniques to manage elimination. This approach requires a degree of dexterity and motivation, takes approximately 35–40 minutes to perform, and is usually necessary once every 24–48 hours depending on gut motility. Lavage of the terminal colon using 1 litre of warm tap water is involved and slight discomfort may be experienced. This strategy is very popular in the USA but less commonly utilized in the UK.

SPECIAL PROBLEMS ASSOCIATED WITH CANCER TREATMENTS

Treatment following stoma formation either of a curative or palliative nature may involve delivery of radio- or chemotherapy. Both approaches can have an effect on gut functioning and may require adaptation of usual stoma care. The general implications of both modalities are the same as for any individual undergoing these treatments and these are discussed in Chapters 5 and 6. However, the ostomist may experience specific problems which may be resolved or minimized by thoughtful intervention. These are dealt with in detail in specialist texts such as Topping (1991, pp. 301–4) and Breckman (1981).

Problems such as diarrhoea can be encountered with chemotherapeutic agents such as adriamycin, 5-fluorouracil and methotrexate, and radiotherapy where fields including the gut are irradiated. The ostomist who uses irrigation should be advised to change to a drainable pouching system. A belt may be useful in providing extra support and reassurance. Also dietary modifications, such as including egg, cheese, and banana, may lengthen transit times. If severe the prescription of antidiarrhoeal agents may be warranted. Signs of electrolyte disturbance and dehydration should be monitored.

Patients undergoing radiotherapy should clean skin with water alone and avoid rubbing. Trauma should be minimized, therefore the use of a skin-sparing appliance which will allow long wear times may be appropriate, such as a two-piece system. Any skin reddening, itching, burning or pain should be reported. Self-administration of skin creams, solvents or sprays should be avoided unless allowed by the radiotherapist.

NUTRITION AND THE SURGICAL CANCER PATIENT

The relationship between cancer and malnutrition is only partially understood but from experience health care professionals recognize that the two often go together (Cushman, 1986). Nutritional abnormalities can result from the tumour itself or the treatment programme, or a combination of both. It should be remembered that any individual undergoing surgery faces increased metabolic demands from perioperative catabolism. In the cancer patient these may be increased by poor nutritional status prior to surgery, augmented by fatigue, pain, psychological distress, gastrointestinal disturbance, loss of appetite, etc., although a vast number of patients undergoing primarily curative surgery are 'uncomplicated' and face similar demands to those of the non-malignant surgical candidate.

The individual undergoing cancer surgery may also face periods of prolonged fasting due to diagnostic tests and/or preparation. This is followed by the actual surgery itself and subsequent post-operative period. Complications may prolong this further. Individuals who undergo resection of the gastrointestinal tract or head and neck region may experience difficulties in relation to ingestion, digestion or absorption, delaying recovery (Grant, 1986).

Strategies to assess, implement and evaluate care in relation to nutritional support are discussed in other work (Hunter and Janes, 1988; Pritchard and Mallett, 1992). Whatever approach is incorporated it is recommended that the following measures should be used to monitor outcomes (Jones, 1991):

- regular weighing of the patient;
- fluid intake and output;
- electrolyte balance;
- monitoring of food input and preference.

The importance of recognizing and anticipating problems in relation to nutrition cannot be over-emphasized. Early involvement of dietitians as members of the multidisciplinary team can be valuable in preventing complications of surgery and promoting well-being and recovery. This may include referral to community-based services prior to admission for surgery and continued community-based support following discharge.

INTENSIVE NUTRITIONAL SUPPORT

The use of intensive nutritional management in the form of total parenteral nutrition (TPN) or enteral nutrition remains controversial. Issues concerning 'feeding the tumour', complications associated with administration outweighing the therapeutic benefits, and whether ultimate outcome is influenced, are often debated both in cancer care and intensive care settings (Irwin, 1986; Endacott, 1993). Ollenschlager *et al.* (1988) advocate two indications for intensive nutritional support. These are:

1. Apparent malnutrition
   - body weight $< 90\%$ of ideal body weight;
   - weight loss $> 10\%$ in six months; $> 5\%$ in one month;
   - Serum albumin $< 3.5\,g/100\,ml$.
2. Imminent malnutrition
   - inadequate intake $< 60\%$ of requirements for longer than one week;
   - sepsis;
   - intensive antineoplastic treatment.

The issue of benefit resulting from intensive and potentially expensive nutritional support deserves consideration. Grant (1986), reviewing a meta-analysis of 11 prospective controlled randomized trials of perioperative administration of TPN, proposes that the following individuals may benefit:

- severely malnourished individuals prior to surgery;
- well-nourished individuals who develop complications which result in inadequate nutritional intake, e.g. prolonged ileus;

- well-nourished individuals who will experience long periods of nutritional inadequacy.

PSYCHOLOGICAL AND SOCIAL INFLUENCES

The diagnosis of cancer, particularly solid tumours, is usually determined by biopsy. This procedure in surgical terms can be minor and could be performed in out-patients under local anaesthetic. This minor physical intervention should not be viewed as minor in terms of psychological importance. Research findings have consistently found that the diagnostic period is one of profound anxiety, with individuals and their relatives experiencing severe anxiety (Jamison *et al.*, 1978; Derogatis *et al.*, 1983). Although anxiety is a normal response to threat, symptoms such as nausea, anorexia, diarrhoea and vomiting can be produced by worries and fears, and prolonged anxiety can lead to depression and other psychological morbidity (Maguire *et al.*, 1980).

Although more recent research has challenged the prevalence of anxiety and depression (McCorkle and Benoliel, 1983; Cassileth *et al.*, 1983) and the importance in relation to recovery (Salmon, 1993), work does suggest that psychological problems have been overlooked by health care professionals and that there has been a lack of systematic assessment (Maguire, 1985). Other researchers have explored the relationship between information and anxiety and subsequent recovery. It is suggested that information giving, reassurance and relaxation technique training may all enhance outcome from surgery when measured in terms of length of hospital stay, use of analgesia and infection rates (Boore, 1978; Flaherty and Fitzpatrick, 1978; Hayward, 1978).

Feelings of hopelessness and helplessness have also been associated with cancer. The influence of these feelings on recovery has yet to be fully researched, but studies have shown high levels of anxiety associated with psychological disturbance (Maguire *et al.*, 1980; Donovan, 1986).

RECOVERY AND ADAPTATION

Whether the surgical intervention has been major or minor, most patients will require supportive care and a period of rehabilitation. The diagnosis and management of malignancy can produce feelings of vulnerability and awareness of mortality which can be psychologically demanding. Although an individual's cancer may be minor in medical terms it may become all-important to the individual. Likewise an individual with widespread disease and a potentially poor prognosis may be more accepting and stoical. No two individuals respond similarly. For the nurse this means individual assessment and recognition of possible ongoing difficulties resulting from surgery or cancer.

Immediately following surgery the patient is not usually concerned with body image changes but physical healing, functioning and survival. Once transient limitations are removed and physical recovery established, other concerns may emerge. Learning to cope with long-term limitations, disabilities and/or disfigurement resulting from the surgical intervention may be a lifelong process of adaptation.

In studies exploring recovery and client needs, three to six months following treatment has been shown to be a particularly difficult point for many individuals and their partners (Oberst and Scott, 1988; Northouse, 1989; Scott *et al.*, 1983). This is often a time of physical recovery and re-emergence into the social world: return to work, social activities, etc. This juncture is also a time when some individuals may fully consider the impact of living with cancer or the unknown of 'cure'. Supportive interventions at this time may be valuable, although this is often a time when services are being withdrawn.

BODY IMAGE: WHAT IS IT?

Body image – the mental picture of ourselves which we hold in our mind – can be seriously altered by cancer and cancer treatments. This mental picture develops from birth and is constructed from sensory and motor stimuli and our exploration of the world. Through exploration we perceive or gain awareness of size, function and sensation. We also learn and value parts of the body in different ways. We recognize that some parts may be dirty (or, more correctly, may be perceived as such), or private; we also learn how to enhance aspects that we value. Much of this learning is through social interaction with others.

Research since the 1950s has recognized that illness or treatment which results in altered body image can result in temporary, and for some permanent, distress. This may be manifested as social isolation, anxiety, depression, sexual or marital difficulties; all these have been associated with cancer.

Price (1990) proposes that body image is made up of three parts: body reality, body ideal, and body presentation. Table 7.3 describes these in more detail. In normal circumstances individuals integrate or balance these three parts whilst redefining the whole in response to influences. Body image should therefore be seen as a dynamic construct. However, within the context of threat such as surgery for cancer an individual's body image requires considerable redefinition. In effect, surgical disfigurement can produce disequilibrium in body reality and reinforce dissonance with body reality. This may be manifested in behaviour by an individual being unwilling to resume prior social activities, e.g. refusing to go out of the home.

Table 7.3 Component parts of body image*

	Description	Process
Body reality	As the body exists and functions	Changed abruptly by surgery. May take time to reorientate
Body ideal	Is the 'ideal' picture in our heads of how we look and present ourselves	Seriously affected by altered body reality
Body presentation	Vehicle by which we present ourselves and balance ideal with reality	Can be hampered by altered abilities and visual appearance

* Adapted from Price (1990).

For example, a man who has undergone head and neck surgery is forced by that event to include the change as part of his body image. His ideal is intactness of his face without scars. This ideal is reinforced constantly by seeing others who are intact, by the media, advertising, etc. Behaviour such as refusing or being unwilling to participate in care which would result in social interaction or even to wear outdoor clothing could be indications of difficulties in the area of body image.

Body image is related to self-concept, self-esteem and personal identity. Schain and Howards (1985) see self-concept as having four elements: **the body self** – body image; **the interpersonal self** – interactions with others; **the achieving self** – aspirations and goals; and **the identification self** – values, beliefs and prejudices. All these elements can be affected by cancer. Self-esteem is said to be the sum of all these aspects which together make up our personal worth. So loss, change or damage to any of these aspects can result in feelings of worthlessness and a devaluation of personal esteem.

For the clinician the issue is what that means in terms of patient problems or pathology. Research has established a correlation between poor self-esteem and negative feelings towards altered body image. Leading on, there is an established relationship between altered body image, poor self-esteem and psychological morbidity demonstrated as depression and anxiety states in individuals with cancer (Jamison *et al.*, 1978; Maguire *et al.*, 1980; Watson *et al.*, 1988).

Alongside the effects of body image change, individuals may be experiencing alteration in sexual functioning. Cancer and cancer treatments have long been recognized as having an impact on aspects of sexuality, including role, functioning and frequency of sexual activity, relationships, etc. (Dyk and Sutherland, 1956; Bransfield, 1982/3; Fisher, 1983; Follick *et al.*, 1985; Metcalfe and Fischman, 1985; Blackmore,

Table 7.4   Sexuality and body image implications of cancer surgery

Site/purpose of surgery	Sexuality consequences	Body image implications	Strategies or help agencies
Head and neck	Usual kissing and love-making positions may be compromised	Changes may be permanently on view	Advice on prosthetics Opportunity to discuss feelings Discussion of alternative positions for love-making Information about self-help groups*
Breast	Loss or 'alteration' of erogenous zone Potential inhibition with partner Vaginal dryness Menopausal changes Effects on fertility and/or contraceptive management	Change in body contour Physical sensation of loss: 'phantom breast pain'	Opportunity to discuss options and participate in informed decision-making Discussion of feelings about self and relationships Involvement of partner Strategies to reduce menopausal symptoms Prosthetic advice Contraceptive advice Suggestions for love-making Discussion of reconstructive surgery as appropriate Information about self-help groups*
Bowel or bladder (where stoma or internal reservoir formed)	Loss of self-esteem Disgust with altered elimination Difficulties in love-making due to applicances, impotence, sensory loss or alteration, or altered anatomy Effects on fertility	Change in body contour although can be concealed from public view In men: possible dysfunctional external genitalia	Discussion about feelings in relation to self and others Discussion of potential sexual problems and actual problems if they emerge Advice regarding alternative positions for love-making, prosthetics and possible surgical intervention for impotence Advice on clothing Information about self-help groups*
Pelvis (uterus, ovaries, vulva, vagina)	Depending on type of surgery: menstruation, fertility, treatment-induced menopause, altered internal and/or external anatomy Loss of femininity, fears of effects on partners Psychosocial impact of: complications of treatment (e.g. fistulae, impaired healing); recurrence; fungating lesions; discharge, etc.	May be minimal external scarring other than abdominal wound Radical surgery may result in altered genital anatomy Chronic lesions with (or without) odour discharge, pain, etc.	Discussion of feelings about self and relationships Advice on contraception, hormone replacement therapy, as appropriate Advice regarding reconstructive surgery Creative wound care strategies Information regarding support agencies and self-help groups*

Table 7.4   contd

Site/purpose of surgery	Sexuality consequences	Body image implications	Strategies or help agencies
Testes	Treatment may reduce desire, activity and satisfaction with performance Para-aortic node dissection may result in ejaculatory problems Previously undetected spermatic difficulties, e.g. low motility may be discovered	Unilateral orchidectomy results in empty scrotal sac on affected side Prosthetic repair may result in an 'unnatural' appearance Discovery of infertility may negatively affect self-image	Discussion of feelings about self and relationships Advice regarding surgical insertion of prosthesis Pre-treatment sperm banking should be offered with information Supportive sympathetic interventions Advice regarding return of spermatogenesis
Limb	May effect love-making positions, relationships Impact on self-esteem Potential difficulties emerging with development, e.g. ageing	Possible implications of loss of mobility and intactness	Strategies to deal with phantom pain Involvement of other members of the health care team: physio, occupational therapist, prosthetic service, etc.
Devices (for supplementary nutrition, pain, chemotherapy)	Fear of closeness which may result in displacement Inhibition with partner	Feelings of loss for altered functions, e.g. eating. Feelings of fragility Weight loss	Strategies to value other social interactions Discussion and advice regarding positions for love-making Opportunities to express feelings

Sources: Blackmore (1989a); Harvard and Topping (1991); Schover (1991a, 1991b).
* See Chapter 17, Where to get help.

1989b; Topping, 1990) Table 7.4 outlines some of the possible implications in terms of sexuality and body image, and strategies which may be employed to address this dimension.

PROMOTING ADAPTATIVE RESPONSES

Adaptation is a long if not a lifelong process. The full impact of a change may not be felt until full healing has occurred, or following discharge or on return to work. For some it may be when they are beginning new relationships, and for others when they wish to resume sexual activity. The basis of any intervention in this area must be a trusting and non-judgemental relationship. These dimensions are personally constructed and in usual circumstances private, therefore sensitivity and tact are invaluable. Negative beliefs can easily be reinforced by the unsure or uncomfortable care giver. An informed carer who can educate clients may reduce anxiety, assist in reorientating to body image change, and enhance feelings of personal autonomy (Burns and Holmes, 1991; Richardson, 1992; Topping, 1992).

Concerns in relation to body image and sexuality can result in profound distress. The nurse's role may be to promote expression of concerns, refocusing of investment in certain characteristics, or to give information and advice. Any efforts should be performed against a recognition of one's limitations and values. If in encouraging discussion a scenario or cluster of difficulties emerges which would be best managed by another professional then referral with appropriate informed consent should be the course of action. Professional experts such as clinical psychologists, psychiatrists, specialist nurses or relationship counsellors may be more effective if involved early. The health professional who encourages clients to expose concerns must recognize that this may lead to the expression of long-repressed or hidden events which require more expert intervention and may force questioning of one's own values.

An individual's social network – family, friends and colleagues – are important and some would suggest instrumental in promoting adaptation. Occasionally a partner may also be experiencing real difficulties and therefore be unable to offer support. Guilt is not an uncommon reaction, particularly in relation to cancers where the sexual organs are affected. Inhibition and rejection are responses which have been reported. The partner may be under considerable stress maintaining family, home and work. Also relationships may have been problematic prior to diagnosis and treatment. Alongside that, individuals with cancer do not come with an empty history: they have had experiences or hold beliefs which may impinge on their adjustment.

The aims of care in this area would be to assess how the individual perceives body image changes, encourage expression of feelings and facilitate the building of a healthy body image. The actual process can be time consuming, demanding and sometimes unsuccessful. The following may be useful pointers to care management in relation to body image and sexuality:

- Assess individual's (and partner's if appropriate) feelings about changes, understanding and level of knowledge about condition and treatment and how it may impinge upon self.
- Give permission to be open and frank.
- Acknowledge expressed feelings as valid.
- Encourage verbalization of feelings by partner in a safe, supportive, environment.
- Assist the individual to attain realistic levels of presentation. This may include advice or referral to specialists for prosthetics or aids.
- Praise efforts.

Table 7.5   Successful outcomes to body image change

Verbalization of concerns regarding body image and sexuality changes
Demonstration of healthy coping abilities
Resumption of former lifestyle, including relationships, style of dress,
employment, social activities, etc.
Willingness to resume sexual activity
Ability to incorporate changes in order to take part in satisfying activities, work,
sex, hobbies, etc.
Ability to touch, look at and reveal altered body site(s)
Expression of high self-esteem
Ability to discuss and consider reconstruction

Sources: Burns and Holmes (1991); Topping (1992).

- Suggest strategies which provide opportunities for success, thereby demonstrating self-worth.
- Provide information about support agencies and self-help groups.
- Promote self-autonomy and value participation in planning care and decision-making.

Failure to cope may diminish quality of life. Table 7.5 outlines some of the behaviours which may indicate successful adjustment. We are as yet a long way from establishing which strategies are most valuble or effective in this sensitive area of care. The future hopefully will bring greater insight; there is a major need for research in this area. Collaborative work between clinicians and researchers may help us gain the much-needed understanding of the world of patients and their partners.

REFERENCES

Ames, F.C. (1986) in *Fundamentals of Surgical Oncology* (eds R.J. McKenna and G.P. Murphy), MacMillan, New York, pp. 40–55.

Beattie, E.J. (1984) Surgical treatment of pulmonary metastases *Cancer*, **54**, 2729–31.

Blackmore, C. (1989a) Nursing patients with testicular tumours, in *Oncology for Nurses and Health Care Professionals*, Vol. 3, 2nd edn (eds D. Borley and R. Tiffany), Harper Collins, London, pp. 372–6.

Blackmore, C. (1989b) Altered images. *Nursing Times*, **85**(12), 36–7.

Boore, J. (1978) *Prescription for Recovery*. Royal College of Nursing, London.

Bown, S.G., Barr, H., Matthewson, K. *et al.* (1986) Endoscopic treatment of inoperable colorectal cancers with Nd YAG laser. *British Journal of Surgery*, **73**, 949–52.

Bransfield, D.D. (1982/3) Breast cancer and sexual functioning: a review of the literature and implications for future research. *International Journal of Psychiatry in Medicine*, **12**(3), 197–211.

Breckman, B. (1981) *Stoma Care*. Beaconsfield Publishers, Beaconsfield.

Brennan, S.S. and Leaper, D.J. (1985) The effect of antiseptics on the healing wound: a study using the rabbit ear chamber. *British Journal of Surgery*, **72**, 780–2.

Burns, N. and Holmes, B.C. (1991) Alterations in body image, in *Cancer Nursing: A Comprehensive Textbook* (eds S. Baird, R. McCorkle and M. Grant), Saunders, Philadelphia.

Cassileth, B.R., Lusk, E.J., Miller, D.S. *et al.* (1985) Psychological correlates of survival in advanced malignant disease? *New England Journal of Medicine*, **312**, 1551–5.

Chvapil, M. and Koopman, C.F. (1982) Age and other factors regulating wound healing. *Otolaryngologic Clinics of North America*, **15**(2), 259–70.

Coloplast Ltd (1987) *Ostomy and Ostomy Patients: An introductory Guide for Nurses*. Medicine Group (UK) Ltd, Oxford.

Cumming, J., Worth, P.H.L. and Woodhouse, C.R.J. (1987) The choice of suprapubic continent catheterisable urinary stoma. *British Journal of Urology*, **60**, 227–30.

Cushman, K.E. (1986) Symptom management: a comprehensive approach to increasing nutritional status in the cancer patient. *Seminars in Oncology Nursing*, **2**(1), 30–5.

d'Angelo, T.M. and Gorrell, C.R. (1989) Breast reconstruction using tissue expanders. *Oncology Nursing Forum*, **16**(1), 23–7.

Derogatis, L.R., Morrow, G.R., Fetting, J. *et al.* (1983) The prevalence of psychiatric disorder among cancer patients. *Journal of the American Medical Association*, **249**, 751–7.

Devlin, H.B., Plant, J.A. and Griffin, M. (1971) Aftermath of surgery for anorectal cancer. *British Medical Journal*, **3**, 413–18.

Donovan, M. (1986) Symptom management: the nurse is the key, in *Issues and Topics in Cancer Nursing* (eds R. McCorkle and G. Hongaladarom), Appleton-Century-Crofts, Newark, CT.

Dudas, S. (1983) Rehabilitation concepts of nursing. *Journal of Enterostomal Therapy*, **11**(1), 6–15.

Dudas, S. (1986) Psychological aspects of patient care, in *Ostomy Care and the Cancer Patient* (eds D.B. Smith and D.E. Johnson), Grune & Stratton, Orlando, FL.

Dyk, R.B. and Sutherland, A.M. (1956) Adaptations of spouse and other family members to the colostomy patient. *Cancer*, **9**, 123–38.

Endacott, R. (1993) Nutritional support for critically ill patients. *Nursing Standard*, **7**(52), 25–8.

Ferguson, M.K. (1982) The effect of antineoplastic agents on wound healing. *Surgery, Gynaecology and Obstetrics*, **154**, 421–9.

Fisher, S. (1983) The psychosexual effects of cancer treatments. *Oncology Nursing Forum*, **10**(2), 63–8.

Flaherty, G.G. and Fitzpatrick, J.J. (1978) Relaxation technique to increase comfort in postoperative patients. *Nursing Research*, **27**(6), 353–5.

Follick, M.J., Smith, T.W. and Turk, D.C. (1985) Psychosocial adjustment following ostomy. *Health Psychology*, **3**(6), 505–17.

Fortner, J.M. (1984) Multivariate analysis of a personal series of 247 consecutive patients with liver metastases from colorectal cancer. *Annals of Surgery*, **199**, 306–16.

Gallucci, B.B. (1985) Selected concepts of cancer as a disease: from the Greeks to 1900. *Oncology Nursing Forum,* **12**(4), 67–71.

Grant, M. (1986) Nutritional Interventions: increasing oral intake. *Seminars in Oncology Nursing,* **2**(1), 36–43.

Grant, M. and Ropka, M.E. (1991) Alterations in nutrition, in *Cancer Nursing: A Comprehensive Textbook* (eds S. Baird, R. McCorkle and M. Grant), Saunders, Philadelphia.

Havard, K. and Topping, A. (1991) Surgical oncology, in *Cancer Nursing: A Comprehensive Textbook* (eds S. Baird, R. McCorkle and M. Grant), Saunders, Philadelphia.

Hayward, J. (1978) Preoperative factors affecting postoperative recovery, in *Proceedings of the Nursing Mirror International Cancer Conference.* Nursing Mirror, London.

Hunter, M. and Janes, E.M.H. (1988) Nutrition in cancer care, in *Oncology for Nurses and Health Care Professionals.* Vol. 2: *Care and Support* (eds R. Tiffany and P. Webb), Harper & Row, Beaconsfield.

Hurney, C. and Holland, J. (1985) Psychological sequelae of ostomies in cancer patients. *Cancer,* **35,** 170–83.

Irwin, M.M. (1986) Enteral and parenteral nutrition support. *Seminars in Oncology Nursing,* **2**(1), 44–54.

Jamison, K.R., Wellisch, D.K. and Pasnau, R.O. (1978) Psychosocial aspects of mastectomy. I. The women's perspective. *American Journal of Psychiatry,* **133**(4), 432–6.

Jones, E. (1991) Nursing patients having cancer surgery, in *Oncology for Nurses and Health Care Professionals.* Vol. 2: *Care and Support* (eds R. Tiffany and D. Borley), Harper & Row, Beaconsfield.

Luthert, J. and Robinson, L. (1993) *Manual of Standards of Care.* Blackwell Scientific, Oxford, pp. 127–30.

Maguire, P., Tait, A., Brooke, M. *et al.* (1980) The effect of counselling on the psychiatric morbidity associated with mastectomy. *British Medical Journal,* **281,** 1454–6.

Maguire, P. (1985) Improving the detection of psychiatric problems in cancer patients. *Social Science and Medicine,* **20,** 819–23.

McCorkle, R. and Benoliel, J. (1983) Symptom distress: current concerns and mood disturbances after diagnosis of life threatening disease. *Social Science and Medicine,* **17,** 431–8.

Messer, M.S. (1989) Wound care. *Critical Care Nursing Quarterly,* **11**(4), 17–27.

Metcalfe, M. and Fischman, J. (1985) Factors affecting the sexuality of patients with head and neck cancer. *Oncology Nursing Forum,* **12**(2), 21–6.

Morgan, D.A. (1990) *Formulary of Wound Management Products.* Academic Pharmacy Practice Unit, Mold, Clwyd and BritCair Ltd.

Northouse, L. (1989) A longitudinal study of the adjustment of patients and husbands to breast cancer. *Oncology Nursing Forum,* **16**(4), 511–16.

Oberst, M.T. and Scott, D.W. (1988) Postdischarge distress in surgically treated cancer patients. *Research in Nursing and Health,* **11,** 223–233.

Ollenschlager, G., Konkal, K. and Modder, B. (1988) Indications for and results of nutritional therapy in cancer patients. *Recent Results in Cancer Research,* **108,** 172–84.

Price, R. (1990) A model for body-image care. *Journal of Advanced Nursing* **15**(5), 585–93.

Pritchard, A.P. and Mallett, J. (eds) (1992) *Manual of Clinical Nursing Procedures*. Blackwell Scientific Publications, London.

Richardson, A. (1992) *Manual of Core Care Plans for Cancer Nursing*. Scutari Press, Harrow, pp. 104–5.

Salmon, P. (1993) The reduction of anxiety in surgical patients: an important nursing task or the medicalization of preparatory worry? *International Journal of Nursing Studies,* **30**(4), 523–30.

Schain, W.S. and Howards, S.S. (1985) Sexual problems of patients with cancer, in *Cancer: Principles and Practice of Oncology*, 2nd edn (eds V.T. DeVita Jr, S. Hellman and S.A. Rosenberg), Lippincott, Philadelphia, pp. 2066–82.

Schover, L. (1991a) *Sexuality and Cancer for the Woman with Cancer and her Partner*. American Cancer Society, New York.

Schover, L. (1991b) *Sexuality and Cancer for the Man with Cancer and his Partner*. American Cancer Society, New York.

Scott, D.W., Oberst, M.T. and Bookbinder, M.I. (1983) Stress-coping response to genito-urinary carcinoma in men. *Nursing Research,* **33**(6), 325–30.

Stevens, L.A., McGrath, M.H., Druss, R.G. *et al.* (1984) The psychological impact of immediate breast reconstruction for women with early breast cancer. *Plastics and Reconstructive Surgery,* **73**(4), 619–26.

Szopa, T.J. (1987) Surgery in *Core Curriculum for Oncology Nurses* (ed. C.R. Ziegfeld), Saunders, Philadelphia, pp. 199–206.

Thomas, S. (1992) *Handbook of Surgical Dressings*. Surgical Materials Testing Laboratory, Bridgend, Mid Glamorgan.

Topping, A.E. (1987) The urostomy experience. Unpublished thesis, University of Surrey/North-East Surrey College of Technology.

Topping, A.E. (1990) Sexuality and the stoma patient. *Nursing Standard,* **4**(41), 24–6.

Topping, A. (1991) Nursing patients with tumours of the gastrointestinal tract, in *Oncology for Nurses and Health Care Professionals*. Vol. 3: *Cancer Nursing* (eds R. Tiffany and D. Borley), Chapman & Hall, London.

Topping, A.E. (1992) The trauma of burns. *Wound Management,* **2**(3), 8–9.

Torrance, C. (1985) Wound care in accident and emergency. *Nursing,* **2**(4), (Suppl.), 1–3.

Turner, T.D. (1983) Absorbents and wound dressing. *Nursing* (2nd series Suppl. 12), 1–7.

Turner, T.D., Schmidt, R.J. and Harding, K.G. (1986) *Advances in Wound Management*. Wiley, Chichester.

Wade, B. (1989) *A Stoma is for Life*. Scutari Press, London.

Watson, M., Denton, S., Baum, M. and Greer, S. (1988) Counselling breast cancer patients: a specialist nursing service. *Counselling Psychology Quarterly,* **1**, 23–32.

Westaby, S. (1981) Wound care healing: the normal mechanism 2. *Nursing Times,* 25th November (Suppl.).

Westaby, S. (1985) *Wound Care*. Heinemann, London.

Westbury, G. (1988) Surgical oncology, in *Oncology for Nurses and Health Care Professionals*. Vol. 1: *Pathology, Diagnosis and Treatment* (eds R. Tiffany and P. Pritchard), Harper & Row Beaconsfield.

Williams, D.L., Dykes, P.J. and Marks, R. (1985) Effects of a new hydrocolloid dressing on healing of full thickness wounds in normal volunteers, in *An Environment for Healing: The Role of Occlusion* (ed. T.J. Ryan), Royal Society of Medicine, London.

Wilson, E. and Desruisseaux, B. (1983) in *Patient Teaching* (ed. J. Wilson-Barnett), Churchill Livingstone, Edinburgh.

Wilson-Barnett, J. and Bateup, I. (1988) *Patient Problems: A Research Base for Nursing Care.* Scutari, Harrow.

FURTHER READING

Brunner, L. (1990) *Lippincott Manual of Medical-Surgical Nursing.* Chapman & Hall, London.

David, J. (1986) *Wound Management: Comprehensive Guide to Dressing and Healing.* Martin Dunitz, London.

Denton, S. (ed.) (1995) *Breast Cancer Nursing.* Chapman & Hall, London.

Price, R. (1990) *Body Image: Nursing Concepts and Care.* Prentice Hall, London.

Royal College of Nursing (1992) *Stoma Care Nursing: Standards of Care.* Scutari Press, London.

Thompson, J.K. (1993) *Body Image Disturbance.* Prentice Hall, London.

USEFUL ADDRESSES

British Association of Skin Camouflage, Jane Goulding, 25 Blackthorne Drive, Silkstone Common, Barnsley S75 4SD

Changing Faces (Workshop and Counselling Service), 27 Cowper Street, London EC2A 4AP

Let's Face It (network for the facially disfigured), Christine Piff, 10 Wood End, Crowthorne, Berkshire RG11 6DQ

See also Chapter 17: Where to get help

8 Biological and hormonal therapy

Jaqualyn Moore

INTRODUCTION

This chapter will address the areas of biological and hormonal therapy both of which are recent additions to the armoury of weapons against cancer. Biological therapy involves using and manipulating various components of the immune system and so the role and function of the immune system will be discussed before looking at how biological therapy works and how it is currently being used in cancer treatment. The side-effects of treatment will also be examined along with suggestions of how to manage treatment toxicities. In the same way that biological therapy is based on the immune system so hormonal therapy relies upon the endocrine system. This system will therefore be reviewed before discussing how hormones work in cancer therapy. The side-effects of treatment will be discussed and suggestions given for managing treatment toxicities.

BIOLOGICAL THERAPY

Biological therapy for the treatment of cancer is not new but relies on the concept of immunotherapy, which is based on several observations. In the late nineteenth century William Coley, a New York surgeon, noticed that some patients experienced remissions of their cancer following bacterial infection. Other patients experienced spontaneous regressions. More recently it has been noted that immunosuppressed patients often exhibit an increased incidence of certain types of cancer and that pathological examination of tumour specimens have shown infiltration with immune cells. The observations that interactions take place between the immune system and malignant cells has led to the development of therapies which mimic and manipulate this process.

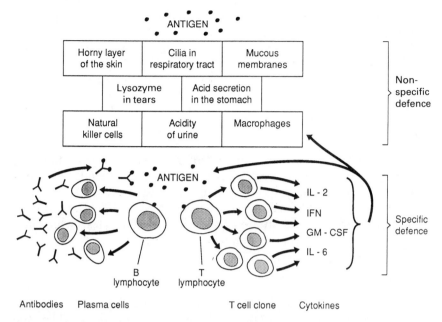

Figure 8.1 Non-specific and specific mechanisms in the immune system.

The many developments in biotechnology over the last decade have led to a greater understanding of the immune system and the identification of a host of chemical mediators which exert their effects on various immune cells, thereby regulating the immune response.

Over the past 5–10 years biological therapy has become increasingly used in the treatment of cancer to a point where it is now sometimes referred to as the fourth treatment modality. It stands apart from chemotherapy in that it works in a completely different way, recruiting the body's own immune system cells to attack the cancer.

THE IMMUNE SYSTEM

In order to appreciate how biological therapy works it is important to understand how the immune system functions. The immune system comprises two main mechanisms of defence which enable the body to resist and fight infection and disease, these are (1) non-specific defence and (2) specific defence (Figure 8.1).

Non-specific defence

Non-specific defence is involved in preventing the entry of pathogens into the body and includes the skin, mucous membranes, the cilia and mucous lining of the respiratory tract, which filter out or trap inhaled pathogens and acid secretions in the stomach, all of which prevent the entry of pathogens into the body. Monocytes, macrophages and other phagocytic cells are also non-specific in that they show no inherent specificity for foreign material, and any phagocyte is potentially able to recognize and respond to any foreign cell or particle.

Specific defence

Specific defence is the responsibility of lymphocytes, the primary function of which is to recognize the presence of non-self material which has entered the body, such as bacteria, viruses, transplanted cells, etc. Two broad classes of lymphocytes are recognized: B lymphocytes, which are responsible for humoral immunity; and T lymphocytes, which are responsible for cell-mediated immunity.

B lymphocytes

B lymphocytes, which constitute about 15% of circulating lymphocytes, differentiate into antibody-secreting plasma cells when stimulated by the binding of an antigen. Antibodies are secreted into the circulation and are capable of interaction with the antigen at a distance from the cell in which they were produced. An expanded population of B lymphocytes which can react against the original and stimulating antigen remain in the body as memory cells and undergo fewer mitotic divisions to produce secretory plasma cells upon second exposure to the same antigen. Therefore a rapid antibody response will ensue.

T lymphocytes

T lymphocytes when stimulated by an antigen increase in size and multiply by mitosis. They differentiate into a series of subtypes, some of which are involved in the regulation of other cells, e.g. helper and suppressor subsets, and some which have an action on other cells, e.g. cytotoxic and delayed-type hypersensitivity subsets. This is known as cellular immunity. Activated T lymphocytes give rise to a large number of genetically identical cells (clones). These cells release cytokines, which control the development of the immune response. Cytokines are chemical messengers which are secreted by and act on the immune system cells. They can be regarded as local hormones which by little-understood mechanisms cause changes in cell behaviour, including proliferation, and activation of lymphocytes and phagocytes. They can also act as cytotoxins. Many cytokines have more than one action and different cells produce different combinations of cytokines. Together cytokines form part of a complex network where production of one cytokine influences

Table 8.1   Cytokines and their principal actions

Cytokine	Principal actions
Interferons	
alpha (α-IFN)	Antiviral, antiproliferative, increases natural killer cell activity
beta (β-IFN)	Antiviral, antiproliferative
gamma (γ-IFN)	Activates macrophages
Interleukins	
IL-1	Activates neutrophils, induces cytokines, T cell stimulation, cytotoxic to some tumour cells
IL-2	Proliferation of T and B lymphocytes
IL-3	Proliferation of neutrophils, macrophages, eosinophils, basophils, megakaryocytes, erythrocytes
IL-4	Differentiation of B lymphocytes
IL-5	Regulation of eosinophils
IL-6	Stimulation of antibody production by B cells
Tumour necrosis factor	
TNF-α (cachectin)	Cytotoxic to some tumour cells, induces cytokines, enhances B cell proliferation, alters vascular epithelium, activates neutrophils
TNF-β (lymphotoxin)	As above
Colony stimulating factors	
Granulocyte– macrophage (GM-CSF)	Stimulates production of neutrophils, macrophages, eosinophils, megakaryocytes and erythrocytes
Granulocyte (G-CSF)	Stimulates neutrophil production
Macrophage (M-CSF)	Stimulates macrophage production
Multi (multi-CSF)	See IL-3

production of or response to other cytokines. This complex, integrated network is responsible for immunological homeostasis and it is these regulators of immune response which are used in biological therapy.

Principles of biological therapy

The wide use of biological agents over the last 10 years has seen the emergence of certain principles of biological therapy. First, unlike chemotherapy, where it has generally been found that the higher the dose of drug administered the greater the tumour kill, i.e. the greater the response to treatment, too high a dose of a biological agent may suppress a desired response and too low a dose fail to induce a response. Second, rapid and obvious responses are often seen following chemotherapy, but response to biological therapy may take several weeks or months to become evident (Balkwill, 1989).

A growing number of cytokines have now been identified and characterized and include the interferons, interleukins, tumour necrosis factor and haemopoietic growth factors (Table 8.1).

INTERFERON

Interferon (IFN) was first discovered in 1957 by Alec Isaacs and Jean Lindenmann. It is a substance produced by the cells of the body upon infection by a virus. The infected host cell is instructed to synthesize interferon by the genetic mechanisms of the cell. IFN is then released to protect surrounding cells from invasion by the virus (Patel, 1988).

It is now well established that IFN is not a single protein but a group of molecules with similar, but distinct, properties that may be classified into three types: (1) α-interferon, produced by leucocytes; (2) β-interferon, produced by fibroblasts; (3) γ-interferon, produced by T lymphocytes.

Using recombinant DNA technology, vast quantities of IFNs can be produced and this has allowed biological studies and clinical trials of IFN to take place in order to evaluate its therapeutic value. There appear to be three main areas where IFN exerts an important action. First, IFN has the ability to inhibit viral growth. Although it cannot protect or cure the infected cell in which it is first produced, IFN serves to protect other cells from invasion by the virus. Second, IFN can also inhibit proliferation of cancer cells and in this way halts the growth of the tumour or even gives a reduction in its size. Third, it is thought that IFN enhances the host's immunity by increasing the cytotoxic activity of natural killer (NK) cells. These NK cells specifically kill virus-infected and tumour cells. IFNs are also thought to activate macrophages, increasing their phagocytic activity (Smith, 1987), and may enhance the host's ability to recognize and respond to the presence of non-self cells such as cancer cells.

IFN has been extensively investigated in a wide range of cancers. Early work in human malignancies was carried out in acute leukaemia and osteogenic sarcoma, since both of these cancers were considered to have a viral aetiology. As a result of these studies, the effect of IFNs on other malignancies was also assessed and significant activity was noted in tumours such as the malignant lymphomas, multiple myeloma and breast cancer. The cumulative results from many studies of the effects of IFN on various tumour types has shown that IFN has a major role in the treatment of hairy cell leukaemia, chronic myeloid leukaemia, low-grade non-Hodgkin's lymphoma and cutaneous T cell lymphoma where a significant number of patients have a major response to treatment (Hancock and Dorreen, 1987). Less important clinical activity has been observed in malignant melanoma, renal cell carcinoma and multiple myeloma.

The most commonly employed route of administration for IFN is the subcutaneous route, although it can also be given intravenously and intramuscularly. It is produced as a solution or as a white powder which is reconstituted with water for injection prior to administration. The dose given will depend on the disease being treated and can range from 3–36 million units per day. However, most patients will be receiving 3–10 million units of IFN three times a week.

The side-effects of IFN are dose, route and schedule dependent, with the most severe toxicities accompanying the intravenous administration of high doses of interferon on a daily schedule. Low doses of IFN given by the subcutaneous route, on a three times weekly schedule, are generally well tolerated, with patients experiencing few side-effects.

Toxicities appear to be similar for all the IFNs and include an acute flu-like syndrome (FLS) consisting of fever, chills, arthralgias, myalgias and headache, and these will be experienced to some degree by most patients. Less common side-effects include anorexia, nausea, vomiting, diarrhoea, fatigue, suppression of blood counts (i.e. haemoglobin, white cells and platelets) and elevation of hepatic enzymes. Rarely, patients may experience central nervous system (CNS) and cardiovascular toxicities. CNS toxicities have included anxiety, agitation, somnolence, altered cognitive function and seizures. Cardiovascular toxicities have included cardiac arrhythmias, cardiomyopathy, myocardial ischaemia, acute myocardial infarction, hypotension and hypertension. The CNS and cardiovascular toxicities are generally induced by high doses of IFN, i.e. doses exceeding 20 million units daily. Tachyphylaxis, or tolerance adaptation, to the acute side-effects occurs with regular, repetitive dosing and is normally induced within two weeks of commencing treatment. Fatigue, however, often occurs after a few weeks of treatment and may not improve.

INTERLEUKIN 2

Interleukin 2 (IL-2) was licensed in the UK in 1992 for the treatment of renal cell carcinoma and is currently widely used in the treatment of this disease and also in other cancers in the clinical trial setting.

IL-2 was first described in 1976 as a growth factor for T lymphocytes (Morgan *et al.*, 1976). When a T lymphocyte is activated by interacting with an antigen specific to itself it secretes IL-2 and also expresses receptors for IL-2 on its cell surface. Interaction of IL-2 with its receptor stimulates the T cell to divide and a clone of T cells specific to the stimulating antigen is produced. Some other cells also possess receptors for IL-2, and IL-2 molecules secreted by the activated T cells bind to IL-2 receptors on these cells. Examples of such cells are NK cells, killer cells which become activated by the IL-2 and become lymphokine-activated killer (LAK) cells, and macrophages which are stimulated to increase their cytotoxic activity. These cells play an important role in the destruction of tumour cells. B cell growth and differentiation are stimulated by the binding of IL-2 molecules to receptors which appear on the outer surface of activated B cells. IL-2 also stimulates proliferation of oligodendrocytes in the CNS. The binding of IL-2 to the T cell receptor also induces the secretion of other cytokines including tumour necrosis factor (TNF), IFN and lymphotoxins (LT) from the T cells.

Like the IFNs, IL-2 is now available as a recombinant DNA product and therefore large quantities are available for biological studies and clinical trials. The continuing evaluation of the therapeutic value of IL-2 is of great importance.

Clinical trials of IL-2 began in 1984 and its effect on various diagnostic groups including renal cell carcinoma, melanoma, colorectal cancer, breast cancer, non-Hodgkin's lymphoma, mesothelioma, squamous cell carcinoma of the head and neck region and post-bone marrow transplantation have been studied. Most trials, however, have concentrated on evaluating the effect of IL-2 on renal cell carcinoma and malignant melanoma, as both of these solid tumours have been shown to be immunoresponsive. As well as being given as a single agent, IL-2 has also been given in combination with other cytokines such as IFN; with adoptive immunotherapy, i.e. the transfer of cells with specific anti-tumour activity, e.g. LAK cells; and with chemotherapeutic agents such as cisplatin and dacarbazine. This has been in an attempt to increase tumour response to treatment, which has varied considerably depending on the combinations used and the doses given. Cumulative results have shown that IL-2 has an important role to play in the treatment of renal cell carcinoma and malignant melanoma, where complete regression of tumour has been seen in 10% of patients and partial responses, i.e. at least 50% reduction in the tumour, in 15–20% of the patients. This is an improvement on results achieved with standard treatment, e.g. chemotherapy.

IL-2 is produced as a white powder which is reconstituted with water for injection before use. Although it has been given by most routes in the clinical trials setting, the most commonly employed routes of administration for IL-2 are the intravenous route, and by subcutaneous injection. As previously mentioned, IL-2 is licensed for the treatment of renal cell carcinoma and when used for this disease is most commonly given by continuous intravenous infusion at a dose of 18 million IU/m² body surface area per day (18×10^6 IU/m² per day). When given in this way at this dose IL-2 gives rise to a host of toxicities which can effect every body system (Table 8.2). However, as IL-2 has a relatively short half-life, any toxicities which have developed during treatment quickly resolve once the IL-2 has stopped. Therefore patients are often discharged home while still recovering from the side-effects of IL-2. Toxicities commonly seen with intravenous administration of IL-2 include:

Table 8.2   Toxicities of high-dose and low-dose interleukin-2

System	High-dose (i.v.) IL-2	Low-dose (s.c.) IL-2
Cardiovascular	Hypotension, weight gain, oedema, ascites, arrhythmias, myocardial infarction, increased cardiac output	Palpitations, dizziness
Respiratory	Dyspnoea at rest, pulmonary oedema, pleural effusion, respiratory distress syndrome	Dyspnoea
Gastrointestinal	Anorexia, nausea, vomiting, diarrhoea, weight loss	Anorexia, nausea, vomiting
Oral	Dry mouth, taste changes, mucositis, oral candida	Dry mouth
Skin	Erythematous rash, pruritus, dry exfoliation, moist desquamation, oedema	Dry skin, erythema, oedema
Renal	Oliguria, proteinuria, elevated serum creatinine	Oliguria, proteinuria
Haematological	Anaemia, thrombocytopenia, lymphopenia, eosinophilia	Lymphopenia, eosinophilia
Neuropsychiatric	Mood alterations, confusion, disorientation, hallucinations, psychoses	Difficulties with concentration, forgetfulness
Hepatic	Elevated liver enzymes and bilirubin	Elevated liver enzymes
Miscellaneous	Chills, fever, rigors, arthralgia, myalgia, malaise, fatigue, headache, nasal congestion	Chills, fever, rigors, arthralgia, myalgia, fatigue, headache, nasal congestion

Adapted from Batchelor and Snoek-Liefrink (1991).

FLS, pruritus, skin desquamation and capillary leak syndrome (see below); also nausea, vomiting, diarrhoea, anorexia, weight loss, anaemia, leucopenia, thrombocytopenia and elevation of liver enzymes. Occasionally patients may become confused and disorientated or develop psychosis. Rarely, cardiac arrhythmias and myocardial infarction may occur (Table 8.2).

Capillary leak syndrome is a well-documented toxicity of high-dose IL-2 treatment. It is characterized by hypotension, tachycardia, oliguria, fluid overload and weight gain. The mechanisms of this side-effect are not fully understood, but it appears that IL-2 causes a leak of protein from the intravascular system into the interstitial tissues. The protein is accompanied by water, which means that there is depletion of fluid in the intravascular space. Intravascular dehydration results in oliguria, hypotension and tachycardia. The increase of water in the tissues is seen as a generalized oedema and the patient gains weight. The management of these physiological changes is a challenge to both the nurse and the physician, and an understanding of the syndrome is essential if this is to be done effectively. Correction of the hypoproteinaemia is necessary in order to raise the concentration of protein in the intravascular space. This will have the effect of drawing fluid back across from the tissues, reducing the oedema and weight gain. Once IL-2 has ceased the syndrome resolves fairly quickly, but patients are often discharged home with a certain amount of oedema which will continue to resolve spontaneously.

As with IFN, the development and severity of side-effects of IL-2 are dependent on the dose given, the route of administration and the dosing schedule, with most severe toxicities experienced when high doses of IL-2 are given by intravenous bolus injection. Consequently when IL-2 is given in smaller doses by the subcutaneous route it is much better tolerated and commonly given as out-patient treatment. However, the patient will still experience some toxicities and these will most likely include FLS, fluid retention, fatigue, pruritus, skin erythema, and redness and induration at the injection site. Tachyphylaxis for some side-effects does not occur in the same way as it does for IFN.

HAEMOPOIETIC GROWTH FACTORS

Haemopoietic growth factors (HGFs) are becoming more frequently used as supportive therapy for patients receiving cancer treatment. They are used for their ability to stimulate the production of blood cells by bone marrow which has been suppressed by the administration of cytotoxic chemotherapy, especially high dose, and radiotherapy.

All blood cells are derived from a population of stem cells which are resident in the bone marrow and which give rise to all mature red cells, neutrophils, basophils, eosinophils, monocytes, lymphocytes and platelets (Figure 8.2). Their production is subject to complex and strict regulation so that constant blood levels are maintained in health and a rapid alteration in levels can be made in response to trauma or infection. This regulation is the function of the HGFs which are more specifically known as colony-stimulating factors (CSFs). To date six different CSFs have been identified: stem cell factor (SCF), granulocyte colony-stimulating factor (G-CSF), granulocyte–macrophage colony-stimulating factor (GM-CSF), macrophage colony-stimulating factor (M-CSF), multipotential colony-stimulating factor (Multi-CSF, IL-3) and erythropoietin (EPO). Some CSFs exert their effects on more than one cell line, for example GM-CSF and IL-3, while EPO, G-CSF and M-CSF are lineage specific, predominantly stimulating the growth of erythrocytes, granulocytes and macrophages respectively (Vahdan-Raj, 1989).

As with the cytokines discussed previously, the recent developments in biotechnology and genetic engineering have allowed the identification of the gene encoding for each HGF and led to the production of recombinant forms of these proteins, so that they are now available for clinical use.

The HGFs have obvious therapeutic value and three (G-CSF/

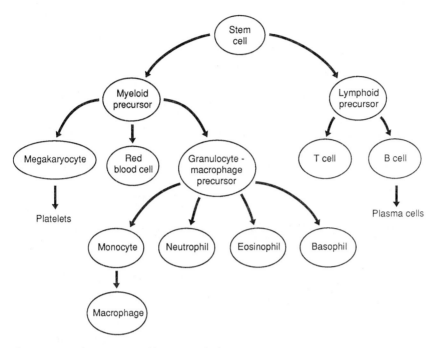

Figure 8.2   The process of haemopoiesis.

Neupogen; GM-CSF/Leucomax; EPO/Epoetin) have already been licensed, while they and others continue to be evaluated in clinical trials for
their therapeutic potential.

Granolocyte and granulocyte–macrophage colony-stimulating factors

Of most note in relation to cancer therapy is the ability of G-CSF and
GM-CSF to accelerate leucocyte production in a manner that mimics the
normal process of haemopoiesis. When given after chemotherapy administration these HGFs can, by stimulating the production of neutrophils,
significantly reduce the period of neutropenia. The risk of infection is
therefore reduced and this allows for better adherence to the chemotherapy regimen (Haeuber and DiJulio, 1989).

Both G-CSF and GM-CSF have been used to accelerate myeloid
recovery in patients following autologous or syngeneic bone marrow
transplant. Some clinical trials have also shown that it is possible to
stimulate the release of primitive stem cells from the bone marrow into the
peripheral blood, making it possible to collect cells for transplant by
leucophoresis rather than by bone marrow harvest (Scarffe, 1991).

HGFs are most commonly given as a subcutaneous injection although they can also be given by the intravenous route. Doses and schedules will vary depending on both the HGF used and the patient's response to treatment. It is important to note that neither G-CSF nor GM-CSF should be administered within less than 24 hours of completing cytotoxic chemotherapy. Also, patients will need more frequent blood tests to ensure that leucocytosis (increased number of leucocytes in the blood) is not developing. If the absolute neutrophil count rises above 50×10^9 per litre (normal range = $2.2–7.5 \times 10^9$ per litre) the treatment should be stopped. The leucocyte count will generally return to normal levels within one to seven days.

G-CSF and GM-CSF are generally well tolerated, with mostly mild toxicities experienced. With G-CSF mild to moderate bone pain, thought to be caused by the expansion of the bone marrow cell population or by release of cells from the bone marrow, is experienced by some patients. Liver enzymes may also be elevated and occasionally skin rashes and dysuria occur. With GM-CSF the most common side-effects include fever, nausea, dyspnoea, diarrhoea, rash, rigors, injection site reaction (with subcutaneous injections), vomiting, fatigue, anorexia, musculoskeletal pain and asthenia. Less frequently non-specific chest pain, stomatitis, headache, increased sweating, abdominal pain, pruritus, dizziness, peripheral oedema, paraesthesia and myalgia may occur. Rare side-effects include anaphylaxis, bronchospasm, cardiac failure, capillary leak syndrome and cerebrovascular disorders.

Erythropoietin

A recombinant form of erythropoeitin (Epoetin), the growth factor for red cells, is licensed for the treatment of patients with anaemia due to chronic renal failure. However, many cancer patients suffer what has been termed anaemia of chronic disease (ACD) which can be made worse by the administration of cytotoxic chemotherapy. Clinical trials to determine the therapeutic value of administering Epoetin to patients with ACD have found that anaemia can be corrected and blood transfusion requirements reduced.

Epoetin comes in injection form and is most commonly administered as a subcutaneous injection three times a week, although it can also be given as an intravenous infusion. It is generally well tolerated with few side-effects, which may include an increase in blood pressure, FLS, convulsions, skin reactions and oedema. Rarely myocardial infarction or anaphylaxis may occur. As with G-CSF and GM-CSF administration the patient will require more frequent blood tests to ensure that erythrocytosis is not developing.

The routine use of HGFs is not yet commonplace as they are relatively

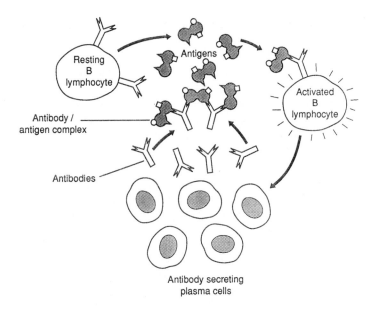

Figure 8.3   The production of antibodies and the formation of antigen–antibody complex.

expensive. However, once the results of a number of cost analysis studies have been assessed the use of HGFs is likely to become more frequent.

MONOCLONAL ANTIBODIES

Cancer therapy targeted at specific cells has been a long-term research goal. Monoclonal antibodies (MoAbs) have the potential of making targeted therapy a reality by carrying a cytotoxic substance to the cancer cell directly. In order to appreciate the potential for this type of therapy and, indeed, how it can be accomplished, it is useful to review the production and function of antibodies in the immune system.

Antibodies are produced when a B lymphocyte binds to an antigen (e.g. a bacteria, virus, transplanted cell or cancer cell) which has invaded the body. The binding of antigen to the antigen combining site on the cell surface of a particular B lymphocyte leads to activation of the B lymphocyte and causes it to divide rapidly, with some differentiating into antibody-secreting plasma cells. The secreted antibodies which have antigen combining sites identical to those on the B lymphocyte are then able to bind with the antigen to form an antigen–antibody complex (Figure 8.3), which can be inactivated and destroyed by various components of the immune system. The antigen combining site on the B lymphocyte binds to a particular site on the surface of the antigen called an epitope. The specific chemistry and shape of the combining site are complementary to the chemistry and shape of the epitope. Several epitopes together form the antigen determinant and it is this which makes an antigen recognizable as a specific antigen which can be named.

MoAbs are identical antibodies (a clone) which have been produced in the laboratory against a specific epitope on the antigen using a procedure first described by Kohler and Milstein (1975). Non-human MoAbs are made by injecting an animal, such as a mouse or rat, with an antigen, such as a cancer cell. The animal's immune system produces antibodies against the antigens. The spleen is then removed and spleen cells are fused with immortal myeloma cells, which are immunoglobulin-secreting cells that replicate indefinitely in culture. Antibody by itself is rarely cytotoxic but can engage chemical and cellular components of the immune system which will damage the cell. Scientists have devised ways to attach (conjugate) cytotoxic substances such as radioactive isotopes, chemo-therapeutic agents or toxins directly to the MoAb. By administering a MoAb with a radioactive conjugate it is possible to trace localization of the isotope throughout the body in much the same way as a bone scan yields 'hot spots', or to deliver a dose of radiation to the tumour site. When conjugated to chemotherapeutic agents or toxins the MoAb will deliver the substance to the target cells (cancer cells), sparing the normal surrounding cells.

A major limitation to the use of MoAbs is that they are a non-human protein and the subject injected will mount an immune response against them. Multiple exposures to a murine (mouse) or rodent (rat) MoAb can sensitize the patient and allergy or anaphylaxis may occur. Scientists are now beginning to develop human or part-human MoAbs to overcome this problem.

Treatment toxicities can be related to the antibody and/or the substance conjugated to the antibody.

GENE THERAPY

Gene therapy can be defined as the transfer of new genetic material to the cells of an individual with resulting therapeutic benefit to that individual (Morgan and French-Anderson, 1993). It is estimated that 4000 human diseases, including some cancers, have a genetic component. Some diseases stem from a single misplaced base in a single gene; others are caused by a number of defective genes in combination. The genetic components of deoxyribonucleic acid (DNA) are gradually being identi-fied, as are the sequencing codes for various proteins, and gene therapy seeks to exploit such discoveries by replacing, substituting, deleting or adding genes to the DNA. In this way potentially cytotoxic material can be carried to the site of a tumour (e.g. the addition of an IL-2 gene) or harmful genetic alterations, which may lead to the malignant transformation of a cell, can be blocked. The discovery of a genetic defect, however, does not necessarily mean finding the cure although it may guide scientists to focus their work on a particular area.

There have been several studies in the USA involving the use of gene therapy which have included small numbers of cancer patients, but gene therapy for cancer is still in its infancy and it is too early to assess how successful this form of treatment will be. It does, however, hold great promise.

OTHER BIOLOGICAL THERAPIES

This chapter has so far looked at the most frequently used and well-known biological agents and approaches. There are, however, an increasing number of others which have entered or are about to enter clinical trials. It is therefore useful to mention, briefly, what these substances are and their biological actions. Currently there are studies evaluating the effects of IL-1, IL-3, IL-4, IL-6, IL-8, β-IFN, γ-IFN and TNF.

IL-1 is produced by a variety of cells in response to infection, inflammation, tissue injury and physiological stress. Its secretion can also be stimulated by the presence of other cytokines. IL-1 activates neutrophils and is cytotoxic for some tumour cells. It also works in conjunction with other cytokines to stimulate B cell growth and differentiation and with the CSFs to promote haemopoiesis. Side-effects resemble those of other cytokines and include flu-like syndrome, tachycardia, nausea, vomiting, anorexia, headache, hypotension and erythema at the injection site (Tewari *et al.*, 1990).

IL-3, also known as multipotential colony-stimulating factor (multi-CSF), belongs to the family of haemopoietic growth factors responsible for regulating haemopoiesis. IL-3 acts on cells early in the differentiation pathway. Several studies have been undertaken to evaluate the effects of IL-3 and results indicate that it is a stimulus for thrombopoiesis, granulopoiesis and, to a lesser extent, erythropoiesis. Side-effects related to IL-3 administration include fever, headache, myalgia, fatigue, watery eyes, local erythema, pruritus, bone pain and generalized flushing (Teplar *et al.*, 1992).

IL-4 is produced by activated T lymphocytes and has a variety of actions, including stimulation and activation of B lymphocytes and regulation of T cells, granulocytes, mast cells and megakaryocytes. IL-4 also enhances the activity of cytotoxic T cells and therefore has potential as a cancer therapy. There have been a small number of studies involving

IL-4. Side-effects have included nausea, vomiting, diarrhoea, nasal congestion, dyspnoea, headache, fatigue and capillary leak syndrome.

IL-6 is produced by activated T and B lymphocytes, fibroblasts, monocytes and endothelial cells. It stimulates antibody production by B lymphocytes and the production of acute-phase proteins by hepatocytes. IL-6 is also involved in the activation of T lymphocytes and the production of IL-2. The role of IL-6 in cancer has not yet been elucidated.

β-IFN is produced by fibroblasts and some of its actions are similar to those of α-*IFN*, including the protection of cells from viruses, inhibition of normal and transformed cell growth and the enhancement of NK cell activity. It has been used in several clinical studies where it has been found to have similar activities to α-IFN, but it appears to be less toxic.

γ-IFN is produced by T lymphocytes and has a variety of actions. It influences cell differentiation, enhances cell recognition factors, activates macrophages and enhances NK cell activity. It is also antiviral and antiproliferative.

TNF is mainly produced by activated macrophages. A wide variety of infectious and inflammatory stimuli are capable of triggering TNF synthesis. TNF interacts with many cell populations, including endothelial cells, fibroblasts, adipocytes, keratinocytes, osteoclasts, T and B cells, neutrophils, eosinophils and macrophages. The mechanisms of action of TNF are unclear but it may have an effect on endothelial cells, thereby causing intravascular damage which may result in loss of blood supply to the tumour and thus necrosis due to hypoxia. Antitumour activity may also be due to the activation of neutrophils, monocytes and NK cells. Side-effects include fever, moderate to severe rigors, hypotension, anorexia, fatigue, weight loss, elevation of hepatic enzymes, leucopenia and thrombocytopenia.

SCF controls the primitive stem cells in the bone marrow. It is thought to act in synergy with G-CSF and may be responsible for stimulating the stem cells to leave the bone marrow and circulate for brief periods in the peripheral circulation. It may therefore play an important role in making stem cells available for collection and transplantation.

M-CSF is produced by fibroblasts, monocytes and macrophages themselves and stimulates the production of macrophages. M-CSF also affects the activity of mature macrophages and induces various cells of the immune system to secrete cytokines, including IL-3, G-CSF and TNF. The role of M-CSF in the clinical setting is as yet undefined.

CARING FOR PATIENTS RECEIVING BIOLOGICAL THERAPY IN THE COMMUNITY

Biological therapy is now moving away from being predominantly in-patient therapy and becoming more frequently administered by the patient in his or her own home. It is therefore important that those nurses caring for and supporting patients in the community are well informed about the treatments the patients are receiving. The well-informed and educated nurse can more confidently support patients and their families and can continue to teach them and inform them about the disease being treated and the therapy being given. Although the patient will already have received such information during a hospital stay or at an out-patient visit, it is unlikely that he or she will have fully understood or appreciated all the information given to him or her. It is necessary to reinforce what has been said as well as provide new information as the need arises or the patient requests it. Information leaflets and booklets designed specifically for patients are becoming more readily available and act as a valuable resource (see below).

As biological agents such as IFN, IL-2 and the growth factors are all proteins, it is not possible to administer them by mouth and so the patient receiving biological therapy at home will self-administer or be given the treatment by injection. As previously stated, the injections are most commonly administered by the subcutaneous route, but it is as well to check the route of administration before commencing treatment as this will sometimes vary. Where patients are self-administering treatment they may need constant reassurance that they are doing this correctly and, indeed, even where patients appear confident in managing the treatment regime and report that they are competent in self-injection it is as well to make an assessment. This should be done in a way that will affirm the patient rather than undermine his confidence. Family members or friends also need constant reassurance and support, especially when directly involved in giving a treatment which is causing unpleasant side-effects. They may feel personally responsible for causing any treatment toxicities.

Handling of biological agents

Biological therapy is not harmful in the same way that chemotherapy agents are, as it consists not of chemicals but of natural proteins. It can therefore be handled quite safely, although it is advisable to wear gloves to ensure that no local sensitivity reaction occurs.

Storage

Storage will vary depending on the agent and also the manufacturer. For example, α-IFN made by Schering Plough Ltd (Intron A) is stored in the refrigerator, while α-IFN made by Roche Products Ltd (Roferon A) is stored at room temperature.

Recording side-effects

Most biological agents are still undergoing clinical trials to determine both their efficacy and toxicity. It is therefore useful to keep a record of any side-effects experienced by the patient. This information will be useful, not just in terms of collecting helpful data about the drugs, but will also help the investigating doctor to determine how the patient is tolerating treatment and if dose adjustments need to be made. If the patient experiences any unexpected side-effects, this should be reported to the investigating doctor or research nurse/assistant immediately to ensure that the patient is not put at risk.

Managing treatment toxicities

The side-effects of biological therapy are many and varied. They are dependent on the biological agent, the route of administration, the dose and the schedule. It is exceptional for a patient not to have any side-effects from the treatment and most patients will experience several of the more common toxicities for the agent they are receiving. Severity of toxicities will vary among patients and courses of treatment. Certain criteria are used for the grading of toxicities and applied to each study to gain a commonality between study centres. An example of this is the World Health Organization (WHO) toxicity grading criteria. With this measurement tool toxicities are graded from 0 to 4, where 0 denotes absence of toxicity and 4 denotes a toxicity of life-threatening proportions.

Although the toxicities vary greatly according to the agent used, dose, route and schedule, a number of side-effects are particularly common. Table 8.3 gives suggestions as to how these can be managed by the patient at home.

HORMONE THERAPY

In the seventeenth century, William Harvey observed that prostatic atrophy occurred following castration and this led to the earliest treatments for cancer. In 1876 Beatson observed that oophorectomy resulted in regression of an established breast cancer and many years later Huggins demonstrated that metastatic prostate cancer would regress following orchidectomy or the administration of oestrogens. However, a rational basis for the hormonal treatment of cancer has only been possible in recent years as an understanding of how hormones act on cancer cells has been gained. It is therefore appropriate to review the endocrine system and the function of hormones in the body before discussing various hormonal therapies.

Table 8.3   Management of biological therapy-related toxicities

Toxicity	Comment	Intervention
Chills	Common to most biological agents; more apparent with the first few injections	Dress warmly and/or cover with blankets
Fever	Common to most biologicals; high temperatures tend to accompany the first few injections but tend to improve with time. NB: fever may denote infection	Paracetamol 500 mg should be taken 30 min pre- and 2 h post-injection Where paracetamol is ineffective naproxen 250–500 mg b.d. may be used
Pruritus/erythema	Frequently seen with IL-2, especially high dose	Apply aqueous cream with menthol Antihistamines
Dry skin/exfoliation	Common with higher doses of IL-2 and may take several days to improve post-treatment	Apply moisturizing cream, e.g. Diprobase Add Diprobath to all washing water
Erythema/induration at injection site	Very common with subcutaneous administration of IL-2	Avoid using alcohol swabs to clean the skin Apply topical lignocaine if painful Apply calamine or other soothing ointment
Anorexia	Often persistent for those patients who experience it	Advise to take small, frequent meals Obtain dietary supplements NB: steroids should not be used to stimulate appetite as they may interfere with treatment efficacy
Nausea/vomiting	Can be managed in the same way as chemotherapy-related nausea and vomiting	Give dietary advice on fluid intake and eating small meals Carbonated drinks, e.g. ginger ale Antiemetics
Diarrhoea	Commonly experienced with high-dose IL-2 but also with other agents	Ensure fluid intake is adequate Give antidiarrhoeal agents
Dry mouth	This, accompanied by taste changes, is common	Encourage frequent mouthwashes Fizzy drinks, e.g. mineral water or soda water Suck ice cubes/fruit drops Inspect for signs of infection
Fatigue	Common to most biological agents and may worsen throughout treatment	Teach patient energy-conserving strategies Advise periods of rest Dose adjustment may be necessary

THE ENDOCRINE SYSTEM

The endocrine system is composed of ductless glands and enables the body to adapt to the changing demands of the internal and external

Table 8.4   Principal endocrine glands, their hormones and target tissues

Gland	Hormone	Target tissue
Posterior pituitary	Antidiuretic hormone (ADH)	Kidney tubules, arterioles
	Oxytocin	Smooth muscles, especially uterus and breasts
Anterior pituitary	Growth hormone (GH)	Bone, muscle
	Prolactin	Mammary glands
	Thyroid stimulating hormone	Thyroid gland
	Adrenocorticotrophic hormone	Adrenal cortex, skin, liver, mammary glands
	Luteinizing hormone	Ovaries, testes
	Follicle stimulating hormone	Ovaries, testes
Thyroid	Thyroxine	Most cell types
	Triiodothyronine	
	Calcitonin	Bone, kidneys, other cells
Parathyroids	Parathormone (PTH)	Bone, intestine, kidneys, other cells
Adrenal cortex	Glucocorticoids	General
Adrenal medulla	Adrenaline	Heart, smooth muscle, arterioles, liver, skeletal muscle
Pancreatic islets (beta cells)	Insulin	Muscle, liver, adipose tissue
Pancreatic islets (alpha cells)	Glucagon	Liver
Ovaries	Oestrogens	Reproductive system, other parts of body
	Progesterone	Uterus
Testes	Androgens (testosterone)	Reproductive system, other parts of body
Placenta	Oestrogens	Ovaries, mammary glands, uterus
	Progesterone	
	Human chorionic gonadotrophin	

environment, thereby maintaining homeostasis. These adaptive changes are brought about by hormones – chemical messengers synthesized and secreted by the endocrine glands. They are transported in the circulation to distant target tissues where, at very low concentrations, they elicit a response. Hence they affect growth, development, metabolic activity and function of tissues and can, in fact, be considered as growth factors. The principal endocrine glands in man are the hypothalamus, pituitary, thyroid, parathyroids, adrenals, pancreatic islets, gonads and placenta (Table 8.4). Hormones and hormone-like substances are also produced in the heart, kidney, liver, lung, pineal gland, thymus and certain cells of the gastrointestinal tract.

To elicit a response in a target cell the hormone must first be 'recognized'. Recognition takes place by the binding of a hormone to a specific receptor which may be located in the plasma membrane, cytoplasm or nucleus of the target cell. The interaction between the hormone and its receptor modifies DNA activity, bringing about a change in the cell attributable to the specific hormone. For example, oestrogen will bind to a specific receptor in the cytoplasm of the cell. This initiates a conformational change in the receptor which exposes a DNA binding site, allowing interaction with oestrogen-sensitive genes and this leads to an increase in the production of proteins that alter cell function. There is also evidence that the synthesis of the receptor proteins is promoted by the hormone to which they bind and that other hormones can reduce the synthesis of receptor proteins (Souhami and Tobias, 1986).

An understanding of the concepts of hormone action has allowed the development of several strategies for modifying tumour growth: first, reduction in the plasma levels of stimulating hormones; second, prevention of hormone and receptor binding; and third, prevention of the binding of the hormone/receptor complex to the nucleus.

There are several cancers which are responsive to hormonal therapy. They are, of course, those which occur in organs that are under the control of the endocrine system such as the breast, prostate and endometrium. Certain other cancers such as renal cell carcinoma, leukaemia, lymphoma and melanoma may also respond to hormone therapy.

HORMONE THERAPY FOR BREAST CANCER

Each year in the UK approximately 25 000 women are diagnosed as having breast cancer and about 15 000 women die as a direct result, accounting for the largest number of cancer deaths in women. It has a variable natural history, being rapidly progressive in some women, leading to early death, while in others it may lie dormant for many years following initial therapy.

Hormones play a significant part in the development and maintenance of normal breast tissue. The hormone-dependent cells contain receptors in their cytoplasm for each hormone, influencing their growth and function. The specific hormones are oestrogen and progesterone. In pre-menopausal women oestrogens are secreted by the ovaries, with a small amount being converted from androgens by the enzyme aromatase. In post-menopausal women, where the ovaries no longer produce oestrogens, the adrenal glands remain the major source of circulating androgens, which are then converted to oestrogens in the peripheral tissues.

In the same way that hormones influence the development of normal cells in the breast they can also influence the cellular function and growth of breast cancer cells. It has been found that some breast cancers are oestrogen dependent and that progesterone is synthesized in the cell in response to the presence of oestrogen. Approximately one-third of all breast cancers are hormone dependent and reported as being oestrogen receptor (ER) or progesterone receptor (PR) positive. The levels of oestrogen or progesterone receptors strongly predict response to hormone manipulation, and absence of an oestrogen receptor suggests a lack of response, whereas high levels of receptor are indicative of probable response.

Thirty per cent of women with breast cancer will respond to hormonal manipulation. Whereas in the past surgery was used to change the hormonal environment, drugs have now been developed which can produce the same effect. Examples of these are tamoxifen, which blocks the oestrogen receptors and therefore has the same effect as oophorectomy; and aminoglutethimide (AG), which inhibits the conversion of androgens to oestrogens by blocking the enzyme aromatase. This has the same effect as adrenalectomy.

Hormone therapy is now the treatment of choice for women with advanced breast cancer because although there have been many advances in this disease, metastatic breast cancer remains incurable. The aim of treatment is the palliation of disease-related symptoms without undue treatment-related toxicity. Chemotherapy is effective for approximately 60% of patients but response duration is only about nine months and treatment is accompanied by various unpleasant toxicities. Although only 30% of patients will respond to hormone therapy the response tends to be longer (approximately 18 months) and the treatment has fewer side-effects. Those patients who respond after first-line endocrine therapy have about a 50% chance of responding to a second-line treatment. Antioestrogens, progestins and aromatase inhibitors are all used in the endocrine therapy of breast cancer.

ANTIOESTROGENS

Tamoxifen is the most well-known and frequently used antioestrogen. It binds with oestrogen receptors in the cell and the formation of the tamoxifen–oestrogen complex blocks oestrogenic activity.

Tamoxifen as a 20 mg dose taken orally, daily, is usually the first-line treatment for women with advanced breast cancer and the overall response rate is reported to be 34%, with duration of response ranging from two to 24+ months (Litherland and Jackson, 1988). A further 20% of patients have stabilization of their disease.

Side-effects of tamoxifen are seen in approximately 3% of patients and include mild indigestion or nausea, alterations in the menstrual cycle (pre-menopausal women), hot flushes, vaginal discharge and slight weight gain. Pruritus vulvae, vaginal soreness and dyspareunia may occur as a result of vaginitis due to oestrogen deprivation. Rarely, thrombocytopenia, retinal and corneal damage with visual loss may occur. In approximately 4% of patients a 'tumour flare' will be seen – a reaction which consists of a temporary worsening of the disease occuring one to three weeks after initiation of hormone therapy. Manifestations of this may include increased pain, swelling and erythema in metastatic soft tissue deposits or skin disease, increased tumour size and hypercalcaemia, which are usually short lived, lasting one to two weeks.

PROGESTINS

Progestins such as medroxyprogesterone acetate (MPA) and megesterol (MA) are commonly used as second-line treatments. They have a direct effect on the progesterone receptor and subsequently reduce the cells' sensitivity to oestrogens. The overall response rate for both MPA and MA when used as a second-line treatment is approximately 30%, with responses lasting about six to nine months.

MPA is usually given orally as a dose of 400–800 mg daily and MA is given as a dose of 160 mg daily in four divided doses. Side-effects of both drugs include weight gain (up to 20–30 kg in 8% of patients), hot flushes, vaginal bleeding, fluid retention, depression and 'tumour flare'.

AROMATASE INHIBITORS

The conversion of androgens to oestrogens in the subcutaneous tissues is brought about by the aromatase enzyme complex. The administration of aromatase inhibitors such as AG blocks this effect. This is important in post-menopausal women, where the principal source of oestrogen is through the conversion of androgens by the enzyme aromatase. As well as blocking this enzyme AG will also block adrenal synthesis of steroid hormones, so glucocorticoid replacement therapy must be given for the duration of AG therapy.

The side-effects of AG include a macropapular rash which usually appears after 7–14 days of commencing therapy and often resolves spontaneously. Drowsiness, depression and ataxia have also been reported. AG can alter the rate of metabolism of drugs such as anticoagulants, oral diabetic drugs and synthetic steroids, and caution should be taken as patients taking these drugs may need a dose adjustment while on AG (Jones, 1990).

HORMONE THERAPY FOR PROSTATE CANCER

The prostate gland, a male endocrine gland which forms part of the reproductive system, is situated at the base of the bladder, surrounding the bladder neck and the first part of the uretha into which its secretions pass. These secretions consist of a thin, slightly acidic, milky fluid containing enzymes, citric acid and calcium and is responsible for the odour of semen. The growth and maintenance of normal prostate tissue and the production of normal prostatic secretions depend upon the presence of testosterone, which is secreted by the testes.

Each year in the UK approximately 8500 men develop prostatic cancer and 3500 die as its direct result. Its incidence increases with age and it is thought to be associated with dietary and smoking habits and influenced by sexual factors, environment and race. Clinically, prostate cancer may vary from a small latent lesion found accidentally at prostatectomy to a rapidly progressive tumour which produces multiple and widespread metastases. Patients usually present with bone pain, urinary obstruction or general symptoms relating to malignancy.

As with normal prostatic tissue the growth and multiplication of prostate cancer cells also depend on testosterone. Small amounts of oestrogen produced by the adrenal gland and testes also modify prostatic activity. Since Higgins and Hodges (1941) demonstrated that orchidectomy and oestrogen therapy caused regression in prostate cancer, a rational basis has developed for the different methods of endocrine therapy employed in the management of carcinoma of the prostate. More recent research has shown that normal and malignant prostatic cells are composed of three populations: hormone dependent, hormone sensitive and hormone independent. Hormone-dependent cells die when androgens are withdrawn and hormone-sensitive cells stop dividing until resupplied with androgens. Hormone-independent cells do not require hormones to stimulate their activity.

The main source of testosterone is the testis, and a small amount of androgen produced by the adrenal cortex is converted into testosterone in the peripheral tissues, so the most effective way of reducing testosterone levels is by bilateral orchidectomy. In patients with metastatic disease this is associated with rapid relief of symptoms, reduction in size of the primary lesion and a fall in prostatic specific antigen (PSA), which acts as a marker for the disease status. Although this treatment is effective it is unacceptable to many patients and not always the treatment of choice. Oestrogen administration in the form of stilboesterol or diethylstilboesterol results in a rapid decline in testicular testosterone production and is one non-surgical alternative to castration. However, they are now used less often because of the side-effects, which include nausea, fluid retention, venous and arterial thrombosis, gynaecomastia, loss of libido and impotence. The cardiovascular complications can occasionally be fatal and have limited the success of this therapy. Also, impotence and gynaecomastia are generally unacceptable to the patient.

Analogues of gonadotrophin releasing hormone (luteinizing hormone releasing hormone: LHRH antagonists) enhance the gonadotrophic drive to increase testosterone output from testicular tissue. However, long-term administration results in a paradoxical failure of the pituitary to secrete luteinizing hormone (LH), which leads to reduced synthesis of testosterone in the testes. The initial increase in testosterone levels can result in a 'tumour flare' which may increase bone pain or result in spinal cord compression. Therefore an antiandrogen such as cyproterone acetate will usually be given for the three days prior to LHRH administration in order to block this 'tumour flare' effect. Gonadotrophin releasing hormone analogues such as goserelin (Zoladex) are administered as a subcutaneous injection every 28 days into the anterior abdominal wall. Side-effects include 'tumour flare', hot flushes, decreased libido, urticaria and rarely gynaecomastia. The antiandrogen cyproterone acetate may cause fatigue, weight changes, alterations in hair pattern and, with continued use, gynaecomastia. The use of LHRH antagonists along with antiandrogens is effective at blocking testicular testosterone and that produced by conversion of androgens from the adrenal gland and is therefore considered by some as being more effective than orchidectomy.

Orchidectomy and/or hormone therapy remain the most effective way of reducing androgen levels and are associated with a response rate of around 80%. Response is associated with rapid relief of symptoms, especially pain from bone metastases, but duration of response tends to be short, with over half of patients relapsing within three years.

HORMONE THERAPY FOR ENDOMETRIAL CANCER

The endometrium is a mucous membrane which lines the uterus. Under the influence of oestrogens endometrial cells proliferate and increase in vascularity. Progesterone causes the endometrium to thicken, engorge and become enriched with glycogen-based mucous. Oestrogenic stimulation without the influence of progesterone causes hyperplasia and malignancy.

Endometrial cancer is the most common and the most curable gynaecological cancer. It most frequently occurs in women 50–70 years of age and it is usually diagnosed early because the presenting symptom is commonly that of post-menopausal bleeding. Early diagnosis combined with the fact that endometrial cancer is relatively slow growing and well localized accounts for the low mortality rate.

Treatment is based on the stage of disease, with surgery and radio-therapy being the primary forms of treatment. Hormonal therapy is used for palliation of advanced disease. Approximately 30% of patients will respond to treatment with progesterone, for example medroxyprogesterone acetate or megestrol.

HORMONE THERAPY FOR RENAL CELL CARCINOMA

Renal cell cancer (RCC) is the third most common urological cancer and there are approximately 3500 new cases per year in the UK. Environmental, hormonal, cellular and genetic factors have all been implicated in the aetiology of RCC.

The response to all treatment modalities for disseminated RCC is poor. Hormone therapy using medroxyprogesterone acetate gives a response rate of approximately 10%. It is well tolerated, with mild side-effects of salt and water retention. Weight gain may occur in patients whose appetite is stimulated by the drug. Other patients have a general sense of well-being.

GLUCOCORTICOID THERAPY IN CANCER

Glucocorticoids such as hydrocortisone, prednisolone and dexamethasone are frequently given to the cancer patient, where they have a wide range of uses which fall into two broad categories: (1) treatment and (2) symptomatic relief.

Treatment

Glucocorticoids are an importrant part of cytotoxic chemotherapy regimens, especially in the treatment of many forms of leukaemia and lymphoma, where they add to the efficacy of the therapy. Response to glucocorticoids is via steroid receptors in the cytoplasm of the cell and all major categories of normal lymphoid and myeloid cells contain glucocorticoid receptors. The mechanisms of action of glucocorticoids is not fully understood but they exert effects on virtually all types of haemopoietic cells, including the killing of certain cell populations, the inhibition of the growth of others and the inhibition of certain specialized cellular functions.

Symptomatic relief

Glucocorticoids are frequently used for their ability to treat and control disease-related symptoms. They are given for the treatment of conditions such as hypercalcaemia, spinal cord compression and oedema associated with cerebral metastases. Dexamethasone will usually be prescribed to prevent the development of oedema during spinal cord or cerebral radiotherapy. Glucocorticoids, especially dexamethasone, are also commonly prescribed for the control of chemotherapy-related nausea and vomiting and tend to be given only during the administration of treatment.

Glucocorticoids are also useful in the treatment of symptoms related to advanced malignant disease such as painful bony metastases and dyspnoea, and have also been found to stimulate appetite and give the patient a general feeling of well-being.

The side-effects of glucocorticoid therapy are considerable and especially significant when the drugs are given in high doses or for a protracted length of time. Then the classic signs of Cushing's syndrome may become evident. This syndrome is characterized by muscle wasting, thinning of the skin which subsequently bruises more easily, thinning of the hair, facial hirsutism, acne, thin extremities with truncal obesity, 'buffalo hump', abdominal striae, moon face and red cheeks. Wound healing is poor. Patients taking low doses of glucocorticoids may also develop some of these symptoms.

The use of glucocorticoids to alleviate some of the side-effects related to biological therapy is generally contraindicated because of their depression of some aspects of the immune response.

CARING FOR PATIENTS RECEIVING HORMONE THERAPY IN THE COMMUNITY

Virtually all hormonal agents are administered orally and patients will therefore be taking these medications at home. Response is often slow, with treatment continuing for months or even years, and it is important that the patient appreciates the need for continued therapy and is aware of how and where to obtain further supplies of the drug. Patients need to be informed about the nature of the treatment they are receiving, the side-effects they may experience and what can be done to alleviate these symptoms. It is especially important to warn women receiving tamoxifen, medroxyprogesterone acetate or megestrol, or men receiving Zoladex (gonadotrophin releasing hormone analogue) that they may experience a 'tumour flare'. An increase in tumour size or worsening of disease symptoms can be very frightening for the patient, who may feel that the treatment is making the disease worse. Much reassurance needs to be given that this reaction is quite normal within the first weeks of therapy and that it does not mean that treatment will not be effective. Hypercalcaemia, while rare, is often a part of the 'tumour flare' reaction and may be caused by increased bone resorption of calcium following temporary acceleration of bone metastases. Patients and their families need to be aware that a sudden change in mental status such as reduced memory or shortening of attention span, accompanied by nausea, constipation, thirst and polyuria, indicate the development of hypercalcaemia and the doctor should be informed immediately so that appropriate remedial action can be taken.

Many of the side-effects of hormone therapy are short lived and patients will need encouragement to persevere with the treatment, especially where they are deriving symptomatic benefit from their cancer. Where weight gain is a problem the nurse, through dietary advice, needs to help the patient to maintain weight at an acceptable level throughout treatment.

It is important to ensure that patients taking steroid replacement because of aminoglutethimide therapy or taking glucocorticoids as a part of their chemotherapy or for symptomatic relief understand why these drugs are necessary and that they should only be stopped on medical advice. If the patient is unable to take the medications because of gastrointestinal upset or for any other reason this should also be reported to the doctor as this may lead to low circulating levels of steroid hormones and result in weakness, weight loss, diarrhoea, vomiting and hypotension. During certain situations such as infection the body's requirement for steroids increases and it may therefore be necessary to adjust the dose of steroids the patient is taking. The nurse must ensure that patients carry a card which states that they are taking steroid therapy, the name of the drug and the dose. Patients should also be advised to seek medical advice early if they become unwell in any way.

Many patients receiving hormone therapy are afraid of the effects this treatment may have on their normal masculine or feminine characteristics and of developing those associated with the opposite sex. It is important to ensure that the patient is fully aware of the side-effects that might be expected from the particular drugs prescribed and understands that most do not have virilizing or feminizing effects. Where these changes are associated with therapy the patient must be reassured that these can be minimized. The management of these and other toxicities associated with hormone therapy are outlined in Table 8.5.

CONCLUSION

The fields of biological and hormonal therapies are continuing to develop as new discoveries are made concerning the immune system, the endocrine system and the presence of receptors on tumour cells. Biological therapy, in particular, is constantly changing as new cytokines are discovered and their function in the immune system elucidated. The complex nature of the immune system and the frequent discovery of new cytokines and other immune modulators means that it is impossible to

Table 8.5   Management of hormone therapy-related toxicities

Symptom	Hormone	Intervention
Hot flushes	Antioestrogens Progestins	Wear loose clothing Rest during flush Use a hand-held fan Give clonidine if severe
Weight gain	Antioestrogens Progestins	Reduce intake of starches and sugars Increase fruit and vegetable intake
Oedema	Progestins Oestrogens	Avoid added salt in food Check weight and blood pressure regularly Observe for signs of heart failure
Vaginal discharge	Antioestrogens Progestins Oestrogens	Encourage frequent washing with mild soap and water Observe for yellow/green discharge (indicates infection) Observe for unpleasant odour (indicates infection)
Vaginitis	Antioestrogens	Oral antihistamines may be helpful Topical hydrocortisone cream if severe
Gynaecomastia	Oestrogens	Radiotherapy if given to the male breast prior to commencing oestrogen can prevent this
Impotence	Oestrogens	Acknowledge symptom and be ready to listen Refer for sexual counselling if appropriate

provide more than an overview of the subject in a chapter such as this and the reader is therefore encouraged to do their own further reading.

Where treatment is not yet established but is still undergoing evaluation in the research setting it is important not to lose site of the patient but always to ensure that he or she is receiving the best possible care and treatment and that this goal is not compromised by the need for scientific knowledge. This is particularly relevant where patients are receiving biological therapy as this is still largely experimental. Even though hormone therapy is better established as a treatment option patients may still be invited to participate in research studies to evaluate new hormonal preparations. If nurses see themselves as patients' advocates they must ensure that patients are fully aware of the implications of therapy.

This is an exciting era as far as the development of new therapies for cancer is concerned and nurses need to avail themselves of the opportunities for learning about these current developments and their possible implications for patients.

REFERENCES

Balkwill, F.R. (1989) *Cytokines in Cancer Therapy*. Oxford University Press, Oxford.

Batchelor, D. and Snoek-Liefrink, J. (1991) The immunotherapy unit. *Interferons and Cytokines,* **6** (Nursing Suppl. 6–9).

Haeuber, D. and DiJulio, J.A. (1989) Haemopoietic colony stimulating factors. *Oncology Nursing Forum,* **16**(2), 247–55.

Hancock, B.W. and Dorreen, M.S. (1987) Interferons in the therapy of human cancer: a review. *Interferon,* **2**, 19–25.

Higgins, C. and Hodges, C.F. (1941) Studies on prostatic cancer. 1: The effects of castration, of oestrogen and of androgen injection on serum acid phosphatase in metastatic carcinoma of the prostate. *Cancer Research,* **1**, 29.

Jones, A.L. (1990) Hormonal treatment of breast cancer. *Therapy Express,* **59**, 1–4.

Kohler, G. and Milstein, C. (1975) Continuous culture of fused cells secreting antibody of predefined specificity. *Nature,* **256**, 495–6.

Litherland, S. and Jackson, I.M. (1988) Antioestrogens in the management of hormone dependent cancer. *Cancer Treatment Reports,* **15**, 183–94.

Morgan, R.A. and French-Anderson, W. (1993) Human gene therapy. *Helix,* **2**(1), 27–36.

Morgan, D.A., Ruscetti, F.W. and Gallo, R.C. (1976) Selective in vitro growth of T lymphocytes from normal human bone marrows. *Science,* **193**(4257), 1007–8.

Patel, F. (1988) An introduction to interferons. *Interferon,* **3** (Nursing Suppl. 10–12).

Scarffe, J.H. (1991) Emerging clinical uses of GM-CSF. *European Journal of Cancer,* **27**(11), 1493–504.

Smith, I. (1987) The biological actions of interferon. *Interferon,* **2**, 4–6.

Souhami, R. and Tobias, J. (1986) Systemic treatments for cancer, in *Cancer and its Management* (eds R. Souhami and J. Tobias), Blackwell Scientific Publications, Oxford.

Teplar, I., Elias, A., Young, D. *et al.* (1992) Use of recombinant Interleukin-3 after chemotherapy for non-small cell lung cancer: effects on haematologic recovery. *Proceedings ASCO,* **11** (abstract 990), 296.

Tewari, A., Buhles, W.C. and Stares, H.F. (1990) Preliminary report: effects of interleukin-1 on platelet counts. *Lancet,* **335**, 712–14.

Vahdan-Raj, S. (1989) Clinical applications of colony stimulating factors. *Oncology Nursing Forum,* **16**(6) (Suppl.), 21–6.

FURTHER READING

Balkwill, F.R. (1989) *Cytokines in Cancer Therapy*. Oxford University Press, Oxford.

Furr, B.J.A. (ed.) (1982) *Clinics in Oncology: Hormone Therapy*. Saunders, London.

Ganong, W.F. (1989) *Review of Medical Physiology*, 14th edn. Appleton & Lange, East Norwalk, CT, USA.

Reeves, G. and Todd, I. (1991) *Lecture Notes on Immunology*, 2nd edn. Blackwell Scientific, London.

Souhami, R. and Tobias, J. (1986) *Cancer and its Management*. Blackwell Scientific, London.

Waxman, J. and Coombes, R.C. (eds) (1987) *The New Endocrinology of Cancer*. Edward Arnold, London.

RESOURCES

BIOLOGICAL THERAPY

Biological Therapy Nurses Association UK (a national group of nurse experts in biological therapy), correspondence c/o The Secretary: Ms K. Shaw, Clinical Nurse Specialist in Oncology, Institute of Cancer Studies, St James' University Trust, Beckett St., Leeds LS9 7TF.

'Interferon-Alpha: Your Guide to Treatment' (video), produced by Roche Products Ltd.

'Interferon and Self-Administration', produced by the Royal Marsden Hospital.

'Intron A: A Practical Guide for Patients' (ed. Sister G.A. Pout), produced by Schering-Plough Ltd.

'Neupogen: A Practical Guide for Health Care Professionals', produced by Amgen Ltd.

'Roferon A: A Patient Guide to Self-Administration', produced by F. Hoffmann-La Roche Ltd.

HORMONE THERAPY

'Tamoxifen: What It Is and What It Does', produced by the Jeannie Campbell Breast Cancer Radiotherapy Appeal, 29 St Lukes Avenue, Ramsgate, Kent CT11 7JZ.

9 Communication

Susie Wilkinson

INTRODUCTION

Communication is the imparting or exchange of information, ideas or feelings. Whenever two or more individuals are together, communication is taking place. Cassee (1975) believes effective communication is achieved when open two-way communication takes place and patients are informed about the nature of their illness and treatment and are encouraged to express their anxieties and emotions.

Communicating openly with cancer patients is considered a vital aspect of nursing care, which some nurses find very satisfying, but there are others who find communication with patients very difficult.

As long ago as 1972, Quint, an American nurse, described how nurses when asked a direct question by cancer patients used one of four different ways to handle such questions. Nurses either did not answer the question or referred the patient to another health professional, changed the subject, ignored the question and remained silent or made stereotyped statements such as 'We all have to go sometime'.

In the UK the same nurse behaviours with cancer patients were first noted by Bond in 1978; since then most research findings concerning nurse–patient communication have reached the same conclusions that the amount of communication cancer patients receive is limited and mostly related to physical tasks that have to be carried out. Little communication between cancer patients and nurses is related to a patient's diagnosis, prognosis, or how he or she is feeling about the illness, and nurses continue to use avoidance behaviours when the going gets tough and they are faced with difficult questions.

PATIENT NEEDS FOR OPEN COMMUNICATION

This lack of open communication clearly distresses cancer patients. A number of studies show that up to one in four patients will have significant problems and would benefit from help (Greer, 1985; Maguire, 1985).

Furthermore, up to 80% of psychological problems in cancer patients go unrecognized and therefore untreated (Bond, 1982).

Staff sometimes assume that patients will always disclose any psychological problems they have and that there is no need for them to enquire. Some doctors and nurses are reluctant to enquire because they fear that patients will reveal strong emotions such as anger or depression which they feel unable to handle.

Patient satisfaction research also continues to indicate cancer patients are not satisfied with the information they receive regarding their treatment and nursing care (Maguire, 1976; Anderson, 1988; Karani and Wilshaw, 1986). It would seem that most patients with cancer would prefer to know if they have a diagnosis of cancer (Cancer Relief Macmillan, 1988). It also seems clear that **most** patients appear to benefit from open truthful communication with health professionals, as active seeking of information about the disease and its treatment has been identified as a coping mechanism (Weisman, 1979) to help people gain control over their situation (Friedman, 1980). Open communication also appears to reduce anxiety and depression in patients with cancer (Hames and Stirling, 1987; Morris and Royle, 1987).

There is as yet no evidence to suggest that open communication or information giving has the detrimental effect of increasing anxiety or depression in those cancer patients who **want** to be fully informed about their disease. The key issue in giving information to patients, therefore, is not so much whether to tell or not to tell but to identify just how much information patients require, so tailoring it to individual needs.

Nurses in hospitals and in the community are in the forefront of care during the period when patients may want to discuss their diagnosis or prognosis, and yet regardless of an emphasis on communication skills training over recent years the majority still appear to use the avoidance behaviours described by Quint more than 20 years ago (Wilkinson, 1991). Why is this still happening?

DIFFICULTIES NURSES EXPERIENCE

One reason could be because research has not focused on nurses' opinions and feelings regarding this area of care or identified exact details of the difficulties that nurses experience. With this in mind, 54 nurses were interviewed and asked whether they had any difficulties with communication with patients in general – to which 63% of nurses said 'no' and 37% of nurses said 'yes'. When the question was asked specifically about cancer patients the picture was very different. There was a major shift in response, with 81% of nurses believing they had difficulties communicating with cancer patients with only 19% believing they had no difficulties.

The nurses were asked to describe their specific difficulties. Their answers created nine categories, the first three of which were related to handling those difficult questions. The difficulties were as follows.

TO TELL OR NOT TO TELL

Thirty-three (61%) nurses described how, having been told they could tell a patient the diagnosis or prognosis if asked, they were unable to interpret for sure whether patients really wanted to know. Nurse W described such a situation.

> Mr T was a police inspector you know, a very intelligent sort of man who had been diagnosed Ca oesophagus six months ago and had had the works. He came in again as there was nothing more they could do. He knew what was wrong and that he had cancer but we never discussed openly about dying. I just couldn't make out whether he wanted to discuss it or not, we did in a roundabout way when I said we're going to try as a last resort to put this tube in and if it doesn't work really there isn't any more we can do. He knew where he was up to and it was like sort of playing a game and I just couldn't fathom out whether he wanted to talk openly or not. Should I play along with his game or not? I felt very uncomfortable.

If nurses did fathom out whether a patient wanted to talk openly, many felt they did not know how to tell the patient the truth.

NOT A CLUE HOW TO TELL

Nurses described how they were 'frightened to death' because they didn't know the best way of levelling with patients about their situation – what to say, or how to say it. The biggest fear they disclosed was the patient's reaction to the bad news and how they would best cope in that situation, as in the next category.

SUPPORT AFTER TELLING: WHAT NEXT?

The greatest difficulty in this category was the nurses' feeling that they had no idea of what to say if the patients broke down and cried, or the kind of things they could say or how to support a patient who has been given bad

news. A particular theme that ran through this category was the nurses'
feeling that they had to be able to **do** something. Nurse X explains:

> What can I say that will help the patients? There is no point in saying
> anything unless it is constructive and can help the patients. I just feel
> that I have got to come up the whole time with an answer for patients
> – due I'm sure to the nursing process. They say find the problem, plan
> the care and that should solve the problem, but how can you in such a
> situation? So what on earth do you do? No one has ever given us even
> guidelines of how to support patients after receiving bad news, and
> doctors are always leaving us in a situation of having to console
> patients.

Nurses confided that they felt failures if patients cried; many felt just
listening was not enough and if they couldn't do more than that they had
failed.

So how can nurses handle such difficult situations without feeling a
failure, or getting into trouble with doctors or patients' relatives, who
often do not wish patients to be informed of their diagnosis?

The UKCC's advisory document on 'Exercising Accountability' states:
'If it is accepted that the patient has a right to information about his
condition it follows that the professional practitioners involved in his care
have a duty to provide information'. This statement indicates that if
nurses have assessed a patient's desire for information they have the duty
to give it.

To facilitate this process, it is perhaps necessary in the first place for
nurses in any health care setting to try and negotiate with the doctors with
whom they work that they can discuss openly a patient's diagnosis and
prognosis if they are asked to do so, and then make sure the rest of the
nursing staff are aware of the results of such negotiations. The working
environments where such negotiations have taken place clearly have the
benefit of improving nurses' open communication with cancer patients
(Wilkinson, 1991).

Secondly, the key to handling all those situations the nurses found
difficult is good assessment skills. Since the introduction of the nursing
process approach to care, assessment has become a crucial aspect of
nursing care. It is vital in identifying patients' problems and needs and in
providing good emotional support. Good assessment is achieved by having
knowledge of appropriate verbal and non-verbal communication skills.

NON-VERBAL COMMUNICATION

This can be divided into two elements

1. vocal, e.g. sighs and grunts;
2. body language.

There are many forms of bodily communication; the most important ones include the following.

FACIAL EXPRESSIONS

These include frown lines, position of the eyebrows and eyelids, size of pupils, shape of mouth and use of nose. Facial expressions display emotions and can be used as an interaction signal; more importantly they can conflict with or support the spoken word.

EYE CONTACT

Making eye contact is important in building satisfying relationships; it tells us how people feel about us. Avoiding eye contact can signal feeling uncomfortable or disinterest.

POSTURE

Posture can be related to mood; it demonstrates attitudes and emotions and can support or conflict with the spoken word.

GESTURES

These include anything from small movements, like raising a finger, to large movements, for example raising a clenched fist. Gestures are used as signals, they illustrate speech and express emotions; for example, increased hand movements may indicate anxiety, or minimal hand movements may indicate depression.

TOUCH

Research has demonstrated the importance of touch in formulating loving, caring relationships and as a therapeutic agent for some groups of patients. It can also express emotion.

PERSONAL SPACE

This is an area or zone around our body. If this area is intruded by some people it makes us feel uncomfortable; it can therefore tell us how people feel about us.

VERBAL COMMUNICATION

The language we use may vary according to nationality. There will be cultural variations in how language is used.

Verbal communication can be divided into elements:

1. **Language** The words we use – what is said.
2. **Paralanguage** How it is said – e.g. tone of voice, volume, pitch, clarity, rate.

REQUIRED VERBAL SKILLS

Listening

This is an active skill which requires great concentration if patients' cues are to be picked up.

Acknowledgement

This involves utterances which indicate the patient is being heard and taken notice of, e.g. 'uuh', 'yes', 'mmh'.

Encouragement

This is a more active skill compared with acknowledgement. It is important for the maintenance of the interaction. By actively showing interest and understanding it encourages patients to continue, e.g. 'Really? That is interesting; please do go on.'

Picking up of cues

Patients often drop hints of problems. The skill is in listening and being able to pick up the cues about problems, and establishing they do want to talk about them. For example:

Nurse: 'Is there anything you want to ask me about?'
Patient: 'No, I'm fine really, it's the family that have been upsetting me.'

The cue is 'the family have been upsetting me'. The way of dealing with this cue is to use the skill of reflection.

Reflection

This encourages people to talk about a topic or problem they have raised and may want to discuss further. The words are reflected back to the

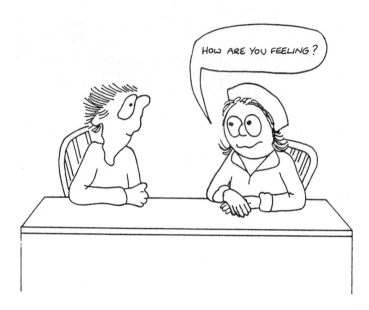

patient, e.g. 'The family have been upsetting you? In what way have they been upsetting you?'

Open questions

These are questions which elicit how patients are feeling and provide patients with an opportunity of expressing how they are feeling, e.g. 'How do you feel today? How have you been sleeping?'

Clarification

This involves statements or questions which either make sure the patient's meaning is understood, for example:

Patient: 'I'm feeling non-plussed today.'
Nurse: 'What do you mean by that?'

or questions which enable more detailed information of problems to be elicited, giving more accurate data on which to plan nursing care, for example:

Nurse: 'You said that you have not been sleeping. Can you tell me exactly what is happening with your sleep pattern?'

Empathy

This involves statements which demonstrate understanding from the patient's point of view which will encourage the patient to go into more depth. This is not saying that you understand from your point of view ('I know how you feel.') but that you feel how it must be for him/her, for example: 'It sounds as if it has all been very hard for you lately'; or 'Gosh, from what you have said, I get the feeling that you have been feeling pretty low.'

Confrontation/challenge

Questions or statements may challenge discrepancies in what patients say, e.g. 'You said you are feeling fine and had no worries but you have just said that you are feeling anxious. Can you tell me a bit more about this?' or 'You say you want to go home as quickly as possible, but you have also said that you cannot be on your own and your daughter cannot help. Can we talk about this?'

Information giving

Patients should only be given information they require; assessment of patients' informational needs should be done before giving information. Patients are only able to retain small amounts of information at a time, which should be given slowly without using jargon or technical terms. Unfortunately research indicates that many nurses block patients from revealing their problems. This in many instances is because few nurses have received education or training in identifying blocking behaviours. As a result many nurses use them without realizing that what they say can actually be detrimental to open communication.

EXPLANATION OF BLOCKING BEHAVIOURS

NORMALIZING, BELITTLING AND STEREOTYPED COMMENTS

Comments given automatically tend to convey either lack of understanding from the patient's point of view, or that the patient's experiences are not unique or important. Such comments usually shift the focus away from the patient.

Normalizing

Patient: 'I'm very anxious about this operation.'
Nurse: 'Everyone feels anxious when they have an operation – it's normal.'

Whereas in fact the nurse needs to focus on what is causing the patient to feel anxious.

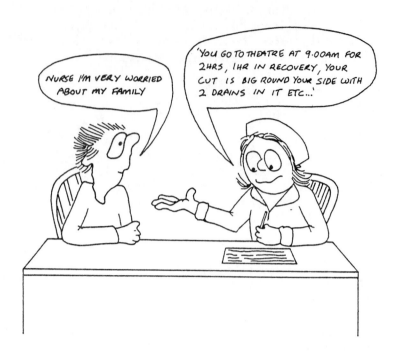

Belittling

Patient: 'I'm a bit apprehensive about my operation.'
Nurse: 'It's quite natural to feel as you do but it is just a routine operation.'

Or

Patient: 'This treatment I'm having doesn't sound very nice.'
Nurse: 'The treatment you are having is nothing compared to some of the treatments we give.'

Stereotyped

Patient: 'I really feel that this treatment isn't going to work.'
Nurse: 'Oh, where there is treatment, there is always hope.'

PREMATURE/FALSE REASSURANCES

These are remarks or comments made to the patient (without having identified the reasons for the concern) which are more positive than are warranted in the circumstances, or which could become untrue. For example:

Patient: 'I must say I'm concerned about the biopsy this time.'
Nurse: 'Don't worry about it, it was all right last time. I'm sure it will be this time.'
Patient: 'Will I have any pain?'
Nurse: 'No, you won't have any pain because we will give you some painkillers.'

Such comments, because they are not realistic, can often cause patients to lose their trust in their carers.

INAPPROPRIATE ADVICE

The patient's decision-making is taken over by imposing one's own opinions and solutions rather than assisting patients to explore ways of arriving at conclusions. For example:

Patient: 'I don't know whether to have this treatment.'
Nurse: 'Well, I would if it was me.'

Or the patient may be given too much or too detailed information to assimilate.

LEADING/CLOSED/MULTIPLE QUESTIONS

A leading question is one asked in a way that could influence or predetermine the patients response, e.g. 'You are looking very well, you must be feeling well,' or 'Your bowels are all right aren't they?'

A closed question is one asked in a way that restricts the range of possible responses by the patient usually to 'yes' or 'no'; it does not allow the patient to express how he or she feels, e.g. 'Any problems with your sleep?'

Multiple questions are those asked without waiting for a reply, either by asking another question or responding oneself to the question, e.g. 'So how did you feel? Did you go to the doctor?' or 'Your lump, how did you find it? Monthly examinations?'

PASSING THE BUCK

Because a question is uncomfortable it is suggested the patient asks someone else, which can often alter a relationship as the patient has entrusted the question to the nurse in the first place. For example:

Patient: 'I'm worried this lump could mean cancer.'

> Nurse: 'Have you asked the doctor about this? Do when you next see him.'

REQUESTING AN EXPLANATION

The patient is asked to immediately analyse and explain feelings or actions usually using a stark '*why?*' question which can intimidate or annoy a patient. For example:

> Patient: 'I think I will never get used to the loss of my breast.'
> Nurse: 'Why won't you get used to it?'

Or:

> Patient: 'I didn't sleep well last night'.
> Nurse: 'Why didn't you sleep well?'

APPROVING/AGREEING

The nurse makes remarks or gives an opinion which shifts the focus to the nurse's values, standards or feelings, imposing on the free expression of the patient. For example:

> Patient: 'My husband says there is more to living with a woman than two breasts, but I don't feel like that.'
> Nurse: 'Well, like your husband, that's just what I think.'

Or:

> Patient: 'They couldn't remove my lung. I wasn't too happy about that. My appetite went and I lost weight but my appetite has improved a lot.'
> Nurse: 'Well to me I think you certainly look well.'

Or:

> Patient: 'My family have been worrying me.'
> Nurse: 'You must stop worrying about your family and concentrate on getting better.'

CHANGING THE TOPIC/IGNORING THE SELECTIVE ATTENTION TO CUES

Changing the topic

A new or unrelated topic is introduced, taking the lead in the conversation from the patient (often by ignoring a cue or question from the patient);

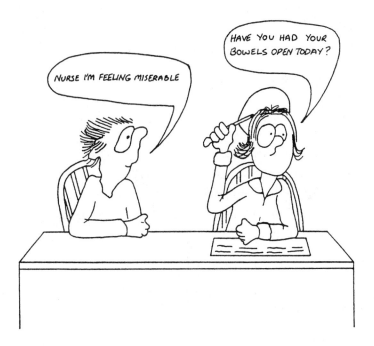

the patient may not make a further attempt to make his or her feelings known. For example:

Patient: 'I don't know how I am going to feel after the operation.'
Nurse: 'Well, you will be going down to theatre at 9.00 a.m.

Or:

Patient: 'I have not been sleeping well – worrying you know.'
Nurse: 'How has your appetite been?'

Selective attention to cues

In this avoidance technique if cues or questions are given, the selected reply will be to discuss the cue or question related to physical aspects rather than emotional aspects. For example:

Patient: 'My appetite has improved but I still get quite low at times.'
Nurse: 'I am pleased your appetite is better.'

Change of focus from patient to relative

In discussion with the patient about his or her problems, the focus is switched from how the patient feels to how his or her relatives feel or think. For example:

Patient: 'I think I am going to find it very hard managing the colostomy.'

Nurse: 'What does your husband think about it?'

Jollying along

In an effort to help patients who have good reason to feel upset or down, jollying along tactics are employed in the hope that they will make the patient feel better. Instead such remarks make the patient feel uneasy in stating how they really feel. For example:

Nurse: 'Mrs C, don't look so glum. Give me a smile. It is a gorgeous day outside.'

Personal chit-chat

Personal irrelevant chat about oneself moves the focus from the patient and his or her real problems.

ASSESSING PATIENTS' PROBLEMS

If good verbal and non-verbal communication skills are used, assessment of patients' problems is made much easier. However, to facilitate this process fuller it is often helpful to have a structure to follow.

STRUCTURE FOR TAKING A NURSING ASSESSMENT

1. **Introduction of self, name and position.** Patients see many health care professionals and can get confused with uniforms, etc. It is therefore important to state exactly who you are and what you do.
2. **Give a clear purpose for the interaction.** For example, if you will be looking after the patient, and to help you plan care, it is necessary to identify the problems and difficulties the patient may be experiencing.
3. **Check this is all right with the patient** – by asking if he or she would be willing to talk to you about his or her concerns.
4. **Patients' agenda: identify patients' problems.** First, allow patients to identify problems they feel they have or are experiencing. The areas to cover are indicated below.
5. **Nurses' agenda.** Obtain information for the care plan. Once patients' problems have been identified from their perspective, it is often

necessary to obtain more information in order to complete the nursing assessment sheet.

6. **Summarize problems.** It is important to do this only after patients have expressed their concerns. Once all a patient's problems have been identified, it is useful to summarize what appear to be the most important problems and check this out with the patient to see if what you have understood is correct.

7. **Patients' questions.** Ask patients if they want to ask any questions or if they need any information.

8. **Address patients' problems: give information.** Where possible give patients realistic information of how you are going to try to manage their problems.

9. **Consultation over plan of action.** Ask patients how they feel about how you are going to try and help them with their problems.

10. **Close interaction.** Assure patients that you will be continually assessing their progress and that if at any time they feel they need further help or clarification you will be pleased to try and answer their queries.

AREAS TO COVER WHEN UNDERTAKING A NURSING ASSESSMENT

1. **Patients' understanding of admission.** Establish patients' understanding of why they have been admitted.

2. **Patients' perception of diagnosis/prognosis.** Establish **patients'** understanding (not just what the doctor has said) of their diagnosis by asking what they understand is wrong with them.

3. **Patients' history of illness.** Establish when and how the patients first realized they had a problem, what they did about it, how they felt about it and what treatment they have had to date.

4. **Patients' previous medical history.** Establish reasons for previous admissions and the outcomes and any previous medical conditions.

5. **Physical assessment.** Identify whether the patient has any problems and the extent of any problem – exactly how much the problem is affecting the patient's normal activities of daily living.

6. **Social assessment.** Establish:
   (a) with whom the patient has a meaningful relationship; the extent of support from the relationship;
   (b) satisfaction with their sexual relationship (if appropriate);
   (c) the patient's home conditions and ability to cope with household chores;
   (d) the patient's hobbies or leisure activities.

7. **Mental assessment.** Establish patients' present mood states, in

terms of how the illness is affecting them. Pick up on any clues as to how the patient has been feeling in terms of anxiety and depression.

Assessment is such an important part of nursing care and can be improved with practice. One way of improving assessment techniques is to tape-record interviews with patients and listen to the recording using the above criteria as a guide for self-analysis. This technique has been used successfully in both medical student (Ramirez, 1992) and nurse training (Wilkinson, 1992). It is obviously important to gain consent from patients to record your interaction and assure them that all the information will be treated in confidence. Most patients are willing to help nurses improve their communication skills by allowing them to tape-record their assessment skills, but if patients do not want to have their assessment recorded they must be assured it will in no way affect their future care.

If in-depth assessments are carried out, invariably patients do ask difficult questions, such as 'Have I got cancer?' or 'Am I dying?' The next section of this chapter will focus on possible ways of handling such questions.

HANDLING DIFFICULT QUESTIONS

To illustrate how this could be done, take as an example a situation that nurses state often occurs when working with cancer patients. The nurse visits a patient – Mr R. – who is receiving only palliative care for an inoperable cancer with metastatic spread and during the visit the patient turns to the nurse and says, 'Am I dying, nurse?'

For the visiting nurse the tummy turns over, the heart misses a beat and the feeling is, what on earth do I say?

Initially it is important to assess and ascertain what the patient thinks is happening, what has happened for the patient to ask such a question and whether he really wants the truth.

This can be done by saying something like, 'I'll be happy to answer your question, but first perhaps you could give me some idea as to what has made you feel you might be dying?'

Invariably the patient will give such reasons as 'I'm feeling weaker. I just don't think I'm getting better. I'm losing weight.' Such a reply suggests that the patient may have come to the conclusion in his own mind that he is dying and now wants verification that he is.

However, human nature being what it is, people often ask questions that, when they have asked them, they wish they had not. To guard against this occurring and to make doubly sure the patient really does want to know if he is dying, it is often helpful to err on the side of caution and get more information from the patient to clarify that he really does want to know the truth. This can be done by acknowledging the reasons that the patient has already given and see if there are any more reasons, by saying something like 'Right. I understand the reasons you have given me might make you think you may be dying, but are there any other reasons?' This gives the patient the opportunity of opting out and not having his worst fears confirmed if he is not truly ready to receive that information.

A very few patients reply saying something like 'No not really, it is just me being silly, I've had a bad day today, and I've felt a bit down, but I'm sure I'll be back to my old self tomorrow.'

This reply indicates that perhaps the patient is not quite ready to have his worst fears confirmed. If the patient makes that kind of response he invariably leads the conversation to a safer subject, thus indicating he does not want to continue talking about his prognosis.

It would seem reasonable to accept his decision as usually the patient returns to the subject of his prognosis in the very near future when he has decided he can cope with having his worst fear confirmed.

However, most patients respond to this question along the lines of 'I just feel as if I am, I am so tired and weak and a friend down the road had the same operation as me and he went downhill like me and died and I feel I'm going the same way.' Such responses indicate that the patient has reached the decision in his own mind and now wants his suspicions confirmed. When such statements are made it seems only right that the patient is given the confirmation he obviously wants. This can be done by saying something similar to 'Yes, I can see that you yourself have come to the conclusion that you are dying and I'm afraid that your suspicions are right. I am sorry.'

Sometimes, but not always, the patient understandably becomes distressed and cries. The key point here is to let the patient cry and comfort him physically if it seems appropriate and not rush in immediately with what can be done in terms of pain and symptom control, but rather pause, and wait with the patient to see if he raises any issues.

If he does not, empathy can be very useful in these situations. For example: 'I can see this is very distressing for you. Would you like to talk to me about how you are feeling or any worries or concerns that you have that we may be able to help you with?'

The reason for not rushing in regarding pain and symptoms is because any information that the patient wants should be tailored to his needs, and it is necessary to find out what they are so they can be dealt with appropriately. If information is given which the patient has not raised as a concern, there is the possibility that further worries or fears may be created which the patient had not been concerned with.

The most common concerns patients seem to raise are:

- How long have I got?
- Will I have pain?
- How will I tell my wife/husband?

The key to answering these questions is to be as honest as possible. 'How long have I got?' is a very difficult question and all too often it is very tempting to try and give the patient some indication, but one of the most honest and satisfactory ways of handling this seems to be: 'I wish I could tell you, but I honestly don't know. So often if we do try to tell patients we get it wrong, but I can appreciate this is not a very satisfactory answer for you and I'm sorry I can't be more helpful.' Patients often seem to realize this questions can't be answered and may have said things like 'I know you can't really but I thought I'd ask anyway.'

If pain is a worry it is reassuring to the patient to know that many medications exist to relieve pain and that they will be given. A response to the pain question could be something like 'It is important that if you are in pain you tell us immediately. We have a whole range of medications that we can use to hopefully relieve any pain you may have. We will do our very best to relieve any pain you have if pain does become a problem for you.'

The patient is often worried about how he will tell his loved ones that he is not getting any better and is dying. So it is important to check out whether he feels able to tell them himself or whether he wants some help. A response to that question could be: 'Is telling your wife something you find very worrying?' If the response is 'Yes', it is appropriate to offer to help or tell the patients' wife if the patient wants that, so a reply could be: 'Would you like to tell your wife or shall we do it for you?'

There are of course many other concerns that the patient may have and these are just a few examples. The key point is to allow the patient to talk about them and offer honest help without being drawn into giving premature or false reassurances, such as 'We can control any pain or vomiting that you may have'.

It is important to give realistic information because honesty at this time will help to build up a trusting relationship, giving the patient hope that he will not be abandoned and that there are people around him whom he can confide in and trust.

When all the patient's concerns have been addressed and the patient has had the opportunity to ask any further questions, he may want the nurse to remain with him or to be left alone. If he does want to be left alone it is important that he has the reassurance of continued support if he needs it, and this can be offered by saying something like 'If at any time you feel you have any queries or you feel like having a chat, please just let me know.'

If a difficult question is handled in this way it has the benefit of allowing nurses in all honesty to inform the doctor or relatives that when they were talking to the patient he said that he thought he was dying and gave the reasons why he felt he was dying. Experience suggests that dealing with situations in this way does not seem to cause relatives to be angry or distressed. In most instances relatives have been relieved: the difficulties of pretending are no longer necessary and it allows the patient to share with them his thoughts, worries and concerns.

DEALING WITH PATIENTS' FEELINGS

In many circumstances, like handling difficult questions, nurses are faced with patients expressing feelings which they feel inadequate to deal with. These are often situations which cannot be solved by anyone, but allowing patients to express how they are feeling has been shown to be very beneficial (Maguire *et al.*, 1980).

The following steps illustrate how it is possible to help patients express feelings such as anxiety.

RECOGNITION

The nurse recognizes either from what patients say or their body language that they are anxious.

ACKNOWLEDGEMENT

The nurse acknowledges that the patient may be anxious by saying 'I can hear from what you are saying that you are anxious' or 'I can see you are anxious'.

PERMISSION

The nurse gives the patient permission to be anxious by saying 'It is all right or OK for you to be anxious'.

UNDERSTANDING

The nurse gives patients the opportunity to find out what is making them anxious by saying 'I would like to try and find out what is making you anxious'.

EMPATHIC ACCEPTANCE

The nurse reiterates from the patient's point of view that he or she is anxious by saying 'From what you have said, you are anxious because . . .'.

ASSESSMENT

The nurse then tries to establish just how much the feelings of anxiety are affecting the patient and whether these feelings of anxiety are present all the time and preventing the patient from carrying out normal activities.

ALTERATION (IF APPROPRIATE)

It is not always possible to alter someone's anxiety, but if it is possible to remove the cause of the stress this should be carried out. Alteration of anxiety is sometimes possible by boosting past coping strategies or offering relaxation or massage, for example. If these are not appropriate, it is often appropriate to refer patients for medication.

Although the problem may not be solved by using these steps, the patient has been allowed to voice his or her feelings to someone who accepts those feelings and does not try to suppress them, which relatives and friends frequently try to do.

To put into print examples of how such a difficult question and patients' feelings might be handled seems very banal and stereotyped, but the examples are only intended to demonstrate principles and give guidelines that do appear to make a very difficult situation easier. Obviously everyone has their own words that they feel comfortable with and might use within these guidelines. Many doctors and nurses attending workshops, and nurses undertaking the ENB Oncology Course and the Continuing Care of the Dying Patient and the Family Course, have had the opportunity to practise these principles using role-play and audio/video tape-recordings with feedback (see Chapter 16). The written evaluations seem to suggest that this way of handling a difficult question is helpful and leads individuals to feel more confident in handling situations that can be very stressful. Obviously this is not the only technique that can be used in such situations. However, it may be worth trying out, if there is a possibility of creating open communication with those patients, and only those patients, who indicate they wish to be fully aware of their diagnosis or prognosis and discuss their feelings.

See also Chapter 10: 'Ethical Pathways in Cancer and Palliative Care'.

REFERENCES

Anderson, J. (1988) Coming to terms with mastectomy. *Nursing Times*, **84**(43), 41–4.

Bond, S. (1978) Processes of communication about cancer in a radiotherapy department. Unpublished PhD thesis, University of Edinburgh.

Bond, S. (1982) Communications in cancer nursing, in *Cancer Nursing* (ed. M. Cahoon), Churchill Livingstone, Edinburgh.

Cancer Relief Macmillan Fund (1988) *Public Attitudes and Knowledge of Cancer in the UK*. Cancer Relief Macmillan Fund, London.

Cassee, E. (1975) Therapeutic behaviour, hospital culture and communication, in *Sociology of Medical Practice* (eds C. Cox and A. Mead), Collier-Macmillan, London.

Friedman, B.D. (1980) Coping with cancer: a guide for health care professionals. *Cancer Nursing*, **3**(2), 105–10.

Greer, S. (1985) Cancer: psychiatric aspects, in *Advances in Psychiatric Aspects* (ed. G. Grossman), Churchill Livingstone, Edinburgh.

Hames, A. and Stirling, E. (1987) Choice aids recovery. *Nursing Times*, **83**(8), 49–51.

Karani, D. and Wilshaw, E. (1986) How well informed? *Cancer Nursing*, **9**(5), 238–42.

Maguire, P. (1976) The psychological effects of cancers and their treatment, in *Oncology for Nurses*, Vol. 2 (ed. R. Tiffany), Allen & Unwin, London.

Maguire, P. (1985) For debate: barriers to the psychological care of the dying. *British Medical Journal*, **219**, 1711–13.

Maguire, P., Tait, A., Brooke, A. *et al.* (1980) The effect of counselling on the psychiatric morbidity associated with mastectomy. *British Medical Journal*, **ii**, 1454–6.

Morris, J. and Royle, G.T. (1987) Choice of surgery for early breast cancer; pre and post operative levels of clinical anxiety and depression in patients and their husbands. *British Journal of Surgery*, **74**, 1017–19.

Quint, J.C. (1972) Institutionalised practices of information control, in *Medical men and their Work* (eds E. Friedson and J. Lorber), McGraw-Hill, New York.

Ramirez, A. (1992) Teaching medical students to communicate. Paper delivered at the Marie Curie Conference, *Communicating with the Seriously Ill: Training, Assessment and Evaluation*. Kings Fund, London.

Weisman, A.D. (1979) *Coping with Cancer*. McGraw-Hill, New York.

Wilkinson, S. (1991) Factors which influence how nurses communicate with cancer patients. *Journal of Advanced Nursing*, **16**(6), 677–88.

Wilkinson, S. (1992) Teaching psycho-social skills: a symposium for nurse educators. *Eighth International Conference on Cancer Nursing, Vienna*. Scutari, London.

10 Ethical pathways in cancer and palliative care

Kevin Kendrick

INTRODUCTION

Ethics is a strange and ambiguous word which conjures up different meanings for different people. It may be that you think of ethics as an abstract subject which has no relevance to the real world but belongs in the rather 'stuffy' realm of academe. Conversely, you may view ethics as being concerned with major dilemmas which seem extremely complex and, often, unresolvable. You may have been involved with debates or discussions with colleagues and friends about issues which have an ethical dimension. These may have centred around abortion, euthanasia, nuclear arms, the environment or a vast range of other subjects which have a strong ethical content. Everybody seems to hold a valid opinion and this is often expressed with the firm conviction that the only 'right' answer is the one which we personally assert. This means that debates often seem to go around and around in ever-decreasing circles until arguments cancel each other out and we are left with neither consensus nor agreement. All of this describes experiences which we can identify with – the passionate exchange of sharply different perspectives with neither side managing to gain the higher moral ground.

So what can we deduce from this? Is it reasonable to presume that, ultimately, ethics is just a matter of personal opinions, values and beliefs? It is certainly valid to see these attributes as important influences upon ethical reasoning – but do they tell us the whole story? In this chapter we will explore some of the major elements involved with the word 'ethics'. It is a word which is becoming increasingly prevalent in the everyday language of nurses and other health professionals. If we can demystify the confusion which surrounds much of ethics then it can provide us with a valuable tool to help clarify many of the difficult issues which we meet in practice.

NURSING AND THE MORAL MAZE

Nursing involves a vast range of tasks and activities; most practitioners now accept that giving care goes over and beyond dealing with the client's needs. The ethos of modern nursing places a great deal of emphasis upon caring for all aspects of the human condition. This approach is sometimes called 'holistic' care because it is concerned with the needs of the 'whole' person – this unites the physical, emotional and spiritual elements of being human and gives them equal prominence. All of this places demands upon our skills which bring us into contact with a potentially vast array of circumstances and questions. Sometimes this will involve issues of a clinical nature, for example: 'Is it time for me to have my bed bath?' or 'Can you give me something to take away the horrible taste in my mouth?' These are the types of enquiry which we often face in practice; they are usually straightforward and our experience allows us to deal with them with reasonable ease. However, what do we do when issues are raised which have a moral and ethical dimension? We all know how uncomfortable and disconcerting it is to be faced with a dilemma which doesn't seem to have a solution.

Caring for people who have cancer raises a host of ethical issues and moral questions. Perhaps one of the biggest dilemmas we have to face is when medical intervention fails to cure a cancer and the client asks the question 'Nurse, am I going to die?' Such an enquiry asks for much more than a purely clinical response; if we are to show true understanding and empathy then we must search for the ethical insights to underpin our answer.

You will have learnt many skills since joining the profession of nursing. When nurses recall their early days of training it becomes apparent that many rich and diverse experiences occur on the road to becoming a competent practitioner. Like other professions, nursing has its own language which is totally alien to the novice: 'MI', 'CVA', 'COAD', 'CA'. These abbreviations are commonly used and create distinct mental images for us as qualified staff. We know that 'MI' means that somebody has had a myocardial infarction; moreover, it probably evokes clearly defined themes which must be addressed when formulating a care plan. However, think how foreign these terms were as you started your first placement on a medical ward. Everybody around you seemed to exude a nonchalant air and discussed these mystical issues with a confidence which probably made you want to retreat further into a corner. Yet we usually survive such traumas and go on to display the same casual tendency with those words and terms which had once terrified us.

Like all of the other skills which you have developed, ethical analysis can be encouraged and advanced to improve the moral insights which you bring to the process of care giving. During this chapter we will examine a number of ethical themes and issues which relate directly to nursing. If you have never studied ethics before then some of the language may seem a little strange – this will become less so as we apply theory to situations which have probably occurred in your practice. The main focus is to introduce the essential elements of ethical theory in a way which helps you reflect upon the moral difficulties and scenarios which occur in professional settings. A number of different approaches can be used to help us achieve this. This will involve the inclusion of various 'activities' designed to help you gain insight and confidence in the use of ethics. Whilst you are under no obligation to do the activities, completing them will certainly make the theory seem more 'real' and of relevance to similar situations which you may have encountered in the past, or, indeed, may meet in the future.

The practice of nursing demands that we are familiar with and competent to use certain 'tools'. This may be as simple as reading a thermometer or using a fob watch to take a pulse. However, sometimes we meet new technology which challenges us to gain a different and often demanding set of skills and insights. An example of this might be the increasing prevalence of information technology in health care today. Many of us find the prospect of computer-based care planning both daunting and highly complex; yet people who have mastered the skill tell us it is merely a 'tool' which, when used properly, can make professional life much easier.

We hope that by the end of this chapter you will have begun to see ethics as a 'tool'. Ethics is not a panacea for all moral ills; however, it can offer you a pathway for reasoned thought in the search for possible solutions.

So far the case has been made for why ethics should play an important part in the nurse's inventory of skills. Now we shall move on to apply ethics to a range of issues and problems commonly encountered in the care of people who have cancer. This will involve an analysis and investigation of how the following areas can be informed by ethical reasoning and clarification:

- truth-telling
- consent
- relationships and power.

It would be impossible to cover every aspect of ethical relevance in a single chapter dealing with moral issues in cancer care. However, what we have tried to do is present you with key areas which relate directly to situations which occur frequently in practice. This perspective is informed by repeated requests by students on specialist courses to deal with these subjects in an ethical context. The first area we will cover deals with the subject of truth-telling; it is a central theme in all human relationships and finds particular relevance in the complex scenario of caring for people with cancer.

SHOULD NURSES ALWAYS TELL THE TRUTH?

Nursing is highly influenced by the notion of duty. There is almost a military theme underpinning so much of our practice: we call time away from work 'off-duty'; this work is performed wearing a uniform; and the notion of a 'duty' to care for patients is drummed into us from the very earliest days of our training. Moreover, practice is led by principles imbued in the *Code of Professional Conduct*. Given all this, we can hardly be surprised that most of us involved in nursing find it difficult to think that lying could ever be justified in the process of caring. Everything about our professional training and conditioning asks us to deal with the 'truth'. However, what do we do in circumstances where telling the truth creates more harm than good? For example, if you saw a woman running down the street looking totally distraught, followed immediately by a man waving a long-bladed knife who asks which way she has gone, would telling him the truth be the most moral and appropriate action? It may be that the man's reasons for wanting to find the woman are innocent and that carrying the knife is purely incidental – but is it worth taking such a risk if it may endanger the woman's safety? Straight away we can see that the concept of truth is highly complex, rarely showing itself in 'black and white' terms but often in a murky grey which leaves us confused about the best way to proceed. We hope that this section will help you to think about and clarify many of the difficulties which surround truth-telling in every day practice. By the end of the section you will:

- be familiar with the debate about 'truth' and its significance to practice;
- be aware of the risks, hazards, harm of truth-telling or of lying to patients or their families;
- be aware of the challenges involved in truth-telling.

TWO PERSPECTIVES IN THE TRUTH-TELLING DEBATE

Like all other academic subjects, ethics has different perspectives and approaches which can be used to help analyse certain issues or situations – these are sometimes called 'schools of thought'. People have, for centuries, used a variety of ethical methods in searching for clarification when dealing with issues which have a moral dimension. We shall consider two of these methods in relation to truth-telling:

1. **Deontology**. This school of ethical analysis maintains that being moral entails acting from a sense of moral duty, respecting others' rights and honouring one's obligations.

2. **Utilitarianism.** This approach argues that actions are morally right when they result in happiness or pleasure for the majority of people.

Let us now look more closely at the major elements involved in deontology.

MOTIVES AND DUTIES

Deontology is most closely associated with the philosopher Immanuel Kant; he was a prolific writer and advocate of the notion that people had intrinsic worth and value. Moreover, he argued that a vital tenet of being human was the innate ability to use reason in deciding upon the moral worth of an action. For Kant, this ability invariably found itself rooted in a sense of duty.

We have already seen that nursing has a long tradition of emphasizing the importance of one's duties. A major principle emerging from this is that nurses should be concerned with the pursuit of truth. However, truth does not always stand alone as an isolated principle; most of us would agree that, as a general rule, it is right to tell the truth – but other principles of duty inform our professional accountability and responsibility. Consider the two following principles:

1. A duty to do good (beneficence)
2. A duty to do no harm (non-maleficence).

Do these two principles mean the same thing? We always try to ensure that our actions are of benefit to clients, but does that mean that harm never results from them? Here are some examples of actions intended to promote good but which can also cause harm:

- An intravenous drip can result in tissue damage.
- Antibiotics can cause an irritating rash.
- Chemotherapy can cause excessive nausea, alopecia and diarrhoea.
- Aspirin can cause gastric erosion.
- Excessive radiotherapy can cause cancer.
- Psychoactive drugs can cause Parkinson-type features.

This list shows that many of the actions nurses are involved with daily can produce harm. You have given many injections – every time a syringe is introduced into a muscle it causes pain. In caring for people with cancer we often give diamorphine or other opiate derivatives through this route. However, we legitimate the moral worth of the action by referring to its therapeutic value. In other words, the pain of the injection is validated by the relief which the client obtains. The key issue is that a subtle balance exists between the amount of benefit or harm which an action generates.

These themes can be applied to truth-telling: if telling the truth leads to harm should we tell a lie to try and promote beneficence?

Reflect on this for a few minutes and then write down an example from your own practice where telling the truth has resulted in some harm being done.

It is impossible for us to comment upon the very individual example which you have given. However, we did ask some other nurses the same question. Here are their replies.

'When I was a newly qualified staff nurse, a man with advanced cancer of the lung asked me if he was going to die. It came as a real shock to me – I hadn't known him long yet he looked me straight in the eye and asked 'Is this cancer going to kill me? I've a right to know and everyone's evading the issue.' Anyway, I told him he would die. Later that morning a student nurse went into the room and found him dead; he had taken a massive overdose of tablets which had been brought in from home. The man's wife and two children were absolutely devastated – I later learnt that they had asked that he be spared the truth about his prognosis, fearing that he could not take it. My role in bringing truth to that man has haunted me for 12 years.' (Kevin: a charge nurse in a hospice).

'What immediately springs to mind is the occasion when a young 17-year-old girl was admitted to the surgical ward where I had just got a junior sister's post. She had recently had a biopsy which revealed that the bony prominence on her knee was a malignancy – a sarcoma. I know that the surgical team had decided to treat the cancer aggressively and perform an above-knee amputation. My concern was the medical team seemed to be less than honest with the girl; nobody had told her that the tumour was cancer. Words like 'growth', 'lump' and 'tumour' were used but nobody had mentioned cancer or the above-knee amputation. The girl was at ballet school and had been given a provisional offer to join a local company. It was her life – 'all that really mattered' is how she put it. One afternoon she asked me some very straight questions and I gave her similar answers. I told her about the cancer and about the operation; she thanked me for being so open and honest, adding that the doctors had been unclear in their explanation. I left with a warm feeling in my stomach – the type you get after a 'job well done'. The trouble is that the girl discharged herself that evening and refused outright to even contemplate surgery. We never found out what happened to her but the prognosis was roughly six months maximum without treatment. I felt devastated – but I still believe she had the right to know the truth.' (Pauline: senior lecturer in cancer nursing).

Both Pauline and Kevin have experienced major traumas through being open and honest with patients. However, from a deontological perspective the actions they both took were valid. Explaining this further, a deontologist is concerned that duty, whatever that may be, is always carried out – irrespective of consequences. Thus, if somebody believes that there is a strict duty **always** to tell the truth then this must be abided by. The philosopher Kant would almost certainly reassure Kevin and Pauline that they had been perfectly ethical and moral in being honest with patients. Moreover, he would probably argue that, having been truthful, they could not then be responsible or accountable for the actions of other people. As we saw earlier, Kant believed that a central facet of being human was the ability to know intuitively what was the most moral way to proceed. This gives people a certain degree of licence in choosing the way to act – both of the patients in Kevin's and Pauline's vivid experiences had followed this path in reaching their decisions.

So far we have looked at the possible risks, hazards and harm which can emerge from telling the truth. Bok (1978) cites studies and empirical evidence to support the notion that 80% of patients preferred to be told the truth about their condition. This still leaves us in the moral quandry of realizing that 20% of patients do **not** want to know about their condition. Nurses may reveal the truth to clients with the firm conviction that they are promoting good; unfortunately, as we have seen with Pauline's and Kevin's experiences, this can sometimes lead to harmful results. We seem to find ourselves in a 'catch-22' situation: a duty to do good seems intrinsically linked to truth-telling yet the harm which can result contradicts the other duty of non-maleficence. Hebblethwaite (1991) offers us a lifeline in this complex dilemma by citing the work of Moutsopoulos (1984) and Haring (1974).

Moutsopoulos argues that we search in vain for the elusive concept of perfect truth – it simply does not exist. In logical sequence, if truth cannot be found in a perfect form then it cannot be given to clients in a perfect way. Building upon this theme, Haring argues that the patient should always be introduced to truth in a humane manner – this places a moral obligation upon the practitioner to ease the patient into a gentle awareness of a poor prognosis. This does not mean that a naive stance has been taken about the traumas which truth-telling can bring; as Hebblethwaite (1991) states: 'There is a recognition that "the truth" will almost inevitably be painful and nothing can make it painless, but we must be careful not to underestimate anyone's inner resources.'

So far we have considered the essence of truth-telling from a deontological perspective. This places emphasis upon duty as a means for considering the moral worth of action. We have seen this graphically illustrated by looking at the conflicting issues which arise between a duty to do good/do no harm. The glaring omission of deontology is that it isolates duties from their possible consequences. To argue that a nurse should always tell the truth, irrespective of the consequences, is to give an unbalanced viewpoint in the moral equation. Now we will examine the main themes of utilitarianism: a method of moral analysis which assesses the worth of an action by the amount of happiness it generates for the majority of people.

TRUTH-TELLING AND THE MORAL MAJORITY

Unlike deontology, with its emphasis upon individual duty, utilitarianism argues that a moral action is one which promotes happiness for as many people as possible. Conversely, an action can be said to be immoral if it fails to promote happiness for the majority. Initially, this seems like a tenable method of ethical analysis; it would be impossible to please everybody in every situation. For example, read the following scenario and decide what you think would be a utilitarian solution.

Raj is a charge nurse on a busy surgical ward. An anonymous benefactor has donated £500 to be spent on the purchase of item(s) which will bring pleasure to patients. A suggestion box was left outside the nurses' station asking for proposals as to what the money should be spent on. There are 15 permanent staff on the ward and the final count of suggestions was: 10 in favour of a new television; five in support of a video recorder. Raj thought that the problem had been dealt with in a democratic manner – clearly the money should be spent on a television, which was the wish of the majority of staff. Mary, a staff nurse who voted in favour of a video recorder, asks for a quiet word with Raj and states: 'We've only had the present TV for six months. The video is five years old and has needed repairing twice in the last month; why should the choice of the majority of our staff automatically make it the right one?' Raj realizes that his problems are far from solved on this particular issue.

If we consider the above scenario solely from a utilitarian perspective then a television should be purchased. This is clearly indicated because the majority of staff voted for it. However, Mary raised a very valid point in asking whether the majority decision should automatically be accepted as the right one. Most of the nurses feel it would give the patients pleasure if a television is bought – but is this a prudent action given Mary's misgivings about the video recorder? If the benefactor's wishes are to be followed then whatever is bought must bring pleasure to patients.

What seems to be fundamental to this problem is deciding which item will actually promote happiness and pleasure. This pinpoints a major flaw with utilitarian thinking, as Kendrick (1992a) states: 'Utilitarianism is fine as a method for deliberating over what action should be taken to maximize happiness – once it has been decided and agreed what that "happiness" or "good" should be. A great deal of time and energy can be spent in debating what the most moral course of action should be in terms of the amount of happiness it would generate.' Even though the staff cannot agree on what to spend the £500 on, at least they have only two items to choose between. We have seen that a utilitarian decision would undoubtedly lead to the purchase of a television – irrespective of the concerns or wishes of the minority of staff. The existing video is unreliable, old and frequently in a state of disrepair. You may feel that it is a little unjust and unfair to buy a new television when the existing one is perfectly adequate, especially given the condition of the video recorder. However, such considerations would not enter utilitarian reasoning; the only pressing concern is that the happiness of the majority is promoted through actions or decisions – an action is moral when it achieves this end.

Utilitarianism underpins many of the decisions which we make in both our professional and private lives. We can all identify with the difficulties involved in trying to finalize the destination for a family holiday. It seems that somebody is always unhappy with the final choice, but the decision will almost certainly go in favour of majority preference. Sometimes, this means we have the company of a malcontent who shows displeasure with every suggestion and activity throughout the vacation. This points to another important aspect of utilitarian thinking – once the majority decision has been made then all people must abide by it. Returning to the family member who is unhappy, we may reassure the individual that next year's holiday will be more in keeping with his or her personal choice. In the meantime, 'stop complaining and get into the holiday spirit'.

Similar themes can be applied to the Christmas off-duty – everybody feels that they have good reason to be granted the off-duty which they have requested; Kendrick (1993) discusses this issue in the following way: 'There is much heated debate and many changes are made before the absolute version is finalized. The person who plans, adapts and finally implements the off-duty would like to agree with each individual appeal but recognizes this as impractical. This inevitably leads to most people being reasonably happy with their festive off-duty whilst a small number remain totally dissatisfied.' All of this illustrates that utilitarianism plays a central role in the decision-making processes involved in our everyday lives.

So far in this chapter we have considered the major differences between the moral theories of deontology and utilitarianism. This has led us to see deontology as a method of analysis which is based firmly upon the duties and motives which underpin an action. In relation to truth-telling, a person who identifies with the edicts of deontology would find it difficult to lie; this is particularly so with nursing, where a very strong moral agenda exists to the point where caring is almost synonymous with truth-telling. However, we have also seen that telling the truth at all costs can have detrimental results. This highlights a problem with deontology: basing moral worth solely upon duties/rules does not necessarily guarantee positive outcomes. Conversely, utilitarianism is concerned solely with the notion that outcomes must lead to an increase in happiness. If the moral worth of an action is based solely upon the amount of happiness it creates then it gives us a completely different perspective in the truth-telling debate. Telling the truth is acceptable to the utilitarian only when it will maximize happiness or goodness for the majority of people involved with it. It would equally be an affirmation of the utilitarian theme if it became essential to lie in order to foster happiness. Spend a few moments reading the following scenario from practice.

Rodger is 32 years of age and has been admitted for the investigation of a testicular neoplasm. It has been there for three months but he thought it was a result of the rough and tumble involved in rugby. The surgical team have told Rodger that he may lose the testicle because all the clinical signs point towards cancer. However, pre-surgical investigations have shown widespread metastases indicating that Rodger will have to lose both testicles and undergo an intensive regimen of both chemotherapy and radiotherapy. Even given these treatments, the aggressive nature of the tumour means that the prognosis is poor.

Rodger's wife has been told of his condition and, subsequently, has shared this information with his parents. All three people have asked the team not to tell Rodger about the poor nature of his prognosis, believing that he would be unable to cope with such news. Members of the team feel very awkward about this request; after all, what would happen if Rodger clearly asks for the whole truth about his condition – surely it would be morally indefensible to keep anything from him? This is put to Rodger's family but they remain resolute, arguing that the truth about the prognosis must be kept from him – even if this means lying. Rodger's wife emphasizes the feelings of the family by stating: 'Look, we know Rodger better than you could ever hope to. His Mum and Dad nurtured him and I've been married to him for 12 years. So I think we should know more about what he can take than strangers who have only just met him. Rodger's going to need every ounce of will and strength if he's to have any hope of beating this thing. If that means lying then at least it will protect him from the horrid truth about how far the cancer has spread – rather that than to be crushed by the truth. Honesty isn't always the best policy.'

We have seen that deontology and utilitarianism can give different perspectives in the subject of truth-telling. Imagine that you are a nurse involved with this case; given the family's strong feelings, what do you think would be the most appropriate and moral response to a direct enquiry from Rodger about his prognosis?

Most nurses involved with cancer and palliative care will have encountered situations similar to this one. It is traumatic for all concerned when a client's relatives wish, for all the best intentions, to protect their loved one from the truth of a poor prognosis. In reality, we often spend a great deal of time counselling relatives in such cases. It is right to acknowledge that we can never know a client in the intimate fashion of a dear friend or relative – but professional experience and empathy indicate that openness, whilst initially painful, often clears a path for discussion based upon insight and understanding rather than fear and possible resentment.

When we consider Rodger's situation in terms of an ethical analysis then it reveals interesting themes about utilitarian thought. It is essential that an action promotes happiness for the majority of people – if we limit the moral equation to Rodger and his family then the ratio is three to one in favour of the family's wishes, namely, that the truth about the prognosis is kept from him. However, we have to remember that utilitarianism relies upon the **net** result of an action resulting in overall happiness for most people; Rodger will almost certainly find out about his prognosis at some stage – knowing that the truth had been kept from him might lead to anger, bitterness and possible rage. This would contradict utilitarian principles because it would also mean that his family are very upset with the emotional turmoil involved with having denied Rodger access to the truth. Moreover, we must also include the health care team who would, almost certainly, have felt worried that Rodger would ask a pointed question about the future outlook of his condition. Given all these pointers and indications, it becomes evident that the truth should be told if the happiness of nearly all those involved is to be ultimately preserved. Therefore, we can conclude that a utilitarian solution to Rodger's situation would advocate a gentle introduction to as many aspects of the truth as he wanted to have.

A deontological solution is slightly less involved. As nurses, our duty of care lies primarily with the client – the wishes of friends and family must come secondary to this. In keeping with this theme, if Rodger asks a direct question about his prognosis then we have a duty to deal with it in an open and sensitive manner. Truth-telling and honesty are sometimes called 'veracity' and are an essential aspect of the nurse–client partnership: it implies that truth exists and can be accepted by both persons within the relationship. Once trust has been established it must never be abused or violated – if Rodger had been denied the truth then any hope of reciprocal openness with members of the health care team would have been irredeemably lost. This is a price which no health professional can ever afford to pay – honesty forms the cornerstone of the relationship which we have with clients and should never be underestimated or damaged.

CONSENTING TO THE TRUTH

We have seen that truth-telling is a central feature in the relationships which exist between ourselves and clients. However, it is also intrinsically linked to the notion of consent. As nurses, we are used to clients being asked to give consent for treatment or a specific intervention. However, a key issue surrounds the nature of **informed** consent – clients may give permission to have a procedure performed upon them, but do they really have sufficient information to make a decision based upon an understanding of all the relevant information? Indeed, is it right that we should expect clients to consider information which may be frightening just so that all the possible ramifications of a procedure have been explained?

The nature of consent is very broad and is not limited to examples related to surgery or situations in which a consent form would be used. This can be directly applied to our everyday practice; you would probably ask for a client's consent prior to giving a bedbath or intramuscular injection – but should this be done each time we take a blood pressure or pulse? When we think about the issues involved with consent a plethora of ethical questions start to emerge. The next section will help you deal with these and develop a method of thinking which can be applied to your own area of work. By the end of this section you will:

- be able to define consent;
- be able to understand the way consent acts as a mechanism to protect a patient's autonomy against paternalism;
- be able to discuss the concept of informed consent as a basis for the nurse–client partnership.

CLIENTS AND THE ENABLEMENT OF CONSENT

The mutual exchange of information is an essential part of all human communication. This is especially important in relation to consent; only when a dialogue takes place between a nurse and client can issues be discussed and informed decisions made about care. However, the amount of information which should be given to clients remains a contentious and much debated issue amongst health professionals. Kendrick (1992a) argues that there are two opposing views on this subject:

- **The paternalist view.** This view holds that the nurse has the necessary insight and professional knowledge to judge when the giving of certain information would be harmful to the patient/client.
- **Freedom of information.** This perspective argues that patients/clients should have free access to every conceivable issue involved in their treatment or care. This is based on the belief that a patient/client who is aware of both the positive and the negative aspects of treatment or care will be able to make an informed and valid consent.

    Both of these perspectives portray viewpoints which are diametrically opposed to each other. We saw in the previous section that complete honesty can sometimes be harmful – should we divulge everything about a nursing intervention when such information may cause psychological trauma? Conversely, what right do we have to withhold information from people which is pertinent and of relevance to them?

    For example, some of the known complications associated with male catheterization are:

- infection

- irritation of the bladder
- ruptured urethra
- blood in the urine (haematuria)
- urinary incontinence.

Which of these complications would you tell a patient/client about prior to a catheterization and what reasons do you have for that choice?

Once again, it must be emphasized that clients need information before an informed choice can be made. People who hold the view that all the negative possibilities should be put before the client would probably argue that every complication should be discussed. The justification for this would be that only following an opportunity to enquire and ask questions can a client reach a considered and balanced decision. However, how many of us would tell a client about the possibility of a ruptured urethra? In the section on truth-telling we discussed the principles of beneficence and non-maleficence; not only do we have a duty to do good but a positive duty not to do harm. It would be highly unlikely that a client's already vulnerable position would be enhanced by the news of a possible urethral perforation. In reality, we tend to deal with the complications of treatment as they arise and use every preventive measure to stop their occurrence.

This example will have given you an opportunity to think about the nature of consent in relation to your own work setting. Catheterization is something nearly all of us come into contact with in our professional work. However, this example could equally well have been about other procedures which we regularly perform, for example passing a nasogastric tube or giving an intramuscular injection. They both have complications which can harm.

We are still left in the precarious position of wondering how much information should be given before an informed consent can be achieved. Given these difficulties, it is important that nurses have their own working definition of consent which can then be used in the practice setting. Reflect on this for a while and when you are ready try writing down a personal definition of consent which you feel could be applied to your working situation.

It is not easy to define consent. There are so many variables and factors which we need to consider; even when we finally think we have solved the problem something will happen in practice which makes our personal definition look decidedly 'wobbly'. To highlight this point, you may have written that consent should be concerned with giving as much information as possible without causing harm – then you will meet a client who argues vehemently that all information should be divulged because it is not **your** body to be deciding what is and is not harmful. However, despite these pitfalls, Raanan Gillon (1986), a qualified doctor and philosopher, defines consent in the following way:

a voluntary unco-erced decision, made by a sufficiently competent or autonomous person, on the basis of adequate information and deliberation, to accept rather than reject some proposed course of action that will affect him or her.

How can the themes of this definition be applied to our practice as nurses? Ultimately, the amount of information which we give to clients depends upon their individual needs and the relationship which we have with them. The experience which we have earned during our years in practice can provide a firm foundation for indicating how much information a client needs. This does not mean that we deny people freedom of choice or treat them in a paternalistic fashion – but it does give us a certain insight into situations where only the bare minimum of information should be divulged. Conversely, it can also help us to realize when certain people need and wish to know everything; they gain a sense of security from having access to all the facts – including the negative ones.

The key issue here is that clients should be given options – whether they need all or a little of the information about care is a matter for discussion and discernment. We have already seen that the notion of perfect truth is highly elusive, which makes it virtually impossible to present truth in a perfect way. Given that the human condition is far from perfect, there will be times when we misjudge the amount of information which a client requires. In terms of the old adage we can say 'to err is human' and mistakes are something which we all make; this is not to be confused with lying. To make a mistake about the amount of information which somebody requires is an inevitable part of being a nurse – nobody gets it right all of the time. Moreover, denying a client access to the full truth about the complications which may follow a procedure is not to tell a lie. To tell a lie involves making an intentionally false statement; this is completely different from misjudging the amount of information a client needs. Taking this to its logical conclusion, telling a lie is something which is done knowingly and with intent; mistakes are errors of judgement which are not based on intent and lack malice.

Perhaps one of the most important areas we need to facilitate as nurses is an atmosphere in which the client feels safe to make active and open enquiries about their care. When this happens it enables the client to become an active participant in the decision-making process; this is at odds with the traditional image of the client as a passive recipient of nursing care. All of this fits in with the notion of client/patient autonomy: the contemporary health care climate encourages individuals to be assertive about their particular needs and expectations concerning treatment. Enabling clients to give an informed consent can do much to enhance this process, promoting client autonomy and guarding against the negative theme of invasive paternalism.

AUTONOMOUS CONSENT

Autonomy is something of a 'buzz word' at the moment; we hear of client autonomy and are expected to fulfil the role of an autonomous practitioner; moreover, nursing is now spoken of as an autonomous profession. All of this can lead to different perceptions and ideas about what autonomy means – it is a difficult concept to understand clearly and can lead to confusion at the 'cutting edge' of health care practice.

In its purest form, the term 'autonomy' is used to mean 'self-government'. Beuchamp and Childress (1982) present the following interpretation of what the essence of autonomy involves:

> The autonomous person determines his or her course of action in accordance with a plan chosen by himself or herself. Such a person deliberates about and chooses plans and is capable of acting on the basis of such deliberations, just as a truly independent government is capable of controlling its territories and policies.

We can see, from this definition, that autonomy is concerned with the expression of self-determination. It is an idea which cannot operate in isolation – to accept people's right to autonomy means accepting their equality as people and their rights to dignity, privacy and control. When we seek to help a client give a full and informed consent it acknowledges the importance of these two themes. At the start of this section we said that perspectives about consent can be broadly split into two camps: those health professionals who firmly believe that they hold the expert knowledge to decide what is best for the client to know; and those professionals who believe that clients should have complete freedom to as much information as possible. Most of us tend to practise somewhere between these two extremes. However, the first of these viewpoints is sometimes called the 'paternalist' approach because it disempowers the client to a point which is analogous with the passivity of a child.

Informed consent is intrinsically linked to empowerment and provides a vision of nursing which actively encourages clients to become involved in their own care; it is the baseline from which other themes – such as autonomy, individuality and freedom of choice – are developed.

Faulder (1985) has written with great insight into the whole issue of informed consent. She places this concept at the very epicentre of health care practice and displays an erudite enquiry into the harm which can result when health professionals do not seek to give clients insight and understanding about issues concerning their bodies. This does not limit itself to consent to treatment but includes every aspect of health care which demands a client's informed permission – including research trials. An informed consent is very different from a client merely giving permission: the one demands a full explanation of what the client is consenting to; the other just means the client has said 'yes'; as Faulder (1985) states: 'informed consent enables us to say no as well as yes'.

When clients give an informed consent it enables them to take an active involvement in the caring process (Figure 10.1).

Clients need to feel safe and secure about an active involvement before they can engage in one. In this section, you will have seen that this can be achieved through a relationship with clients which is based on empowerment, listening and dialogue. All of these can help to create a powerful instrument for influencing change, challenging structure and enabling clients. This brings us neatly to our final section in which we will consider relationships and power in health care.

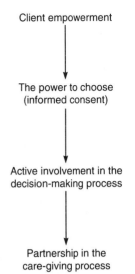

Figure 10.1 Patient involvement in the caring process.

THE POWER BASE IN CARING

The three key individuals most often portrayed as central to the health care equation are the doctor, nurse and patient. However, the power which is held by each of these differs considerably. Chadwick and Tadd (1992) discuss this in relation to the doctor–nurse–patient relationship and state: 'Characteristically the doctor has been portrayed as "all knowing" and powerful; the nurse as caring, unselfish, obedient and submissive; and the patient as helpless and utterly trusting.' Although this traditional picture is being challenged by the continued emergence of nursing as an autonomous profession and by clients increasingly exercising their rights as 'consumers' of health care, medicine still enjoys the most influential power base in the health care scenario.

In this final section we will examine a number of different concepts which can be incorporated to help achieve a balance in the power relationships which exist in health care settings. By the end of this section you will be able to:

● define power;
● explore the influence of power upon decision-making;
● define and explore the concept of advocacy.

WHY DO PATIENTS DO WHAT HEALTH PROFESSIONALS SAY?

If somebody stopped you in the high street and asked 'Good morning, how are your bowels?' you would probably make a hasty retreat, and with good reason. However, we ask this question as an accepted part of everyday practice – of course, the amount of opiates used in cancer treatment and palliative care, together with nutritional factors, do provide a rationale for such an enquiry. The amazing thing is that clients very rarely ask us to qualify the question – they are usually more than willing to give us detailed answers. This has got more than a little to do with the power which we hold as a profession – it may be less than that held by doctors or lawyers, but to a vulnerable client a nurse holds power.

Spend a few moments here writing down what you already understand by the word 'power'.

Much has been written in social science and social psychology about power in interprofessional relationships. Early writers such as French and Raven (1959) refer to this as expert social power and use it to describe the level of knowledge which a professional may have, and how this can influence and produce a position of private acceptance in either individuals or groups. Penner (1978) argues that professionals are perceived as having a strong knowledge base and, therefore, 'an expert has social power because they are perceived as correct'. There is a great deal of mystique surrounding medicine and nursing; we have a professional language which is jargonese to the layperson. Turner (1987) argues that the inaccessibility of these themes maintains the status quo and reinforces the power regimes in the health care equation. All of this reinforces the client's sense of vulnerability and disempowerment.

Think what factors you have observed in the case of clients with cancer which contribute to their feeling disempowered.

When a person is diagnosed as having cancer or, indeed, that there is no real chance of a cure, then the unthinkable suddenly becomes a violent reality. Emotions are sent into a swirling vortex as the frailties of mortality become much too evident. Kubler-Ross (1979) writes that it is impossible to internalize the idea of our **own** death: 'in simple terms, in our conscious mind we can only be killed, it is inconceivable to die of a natural cause or of old age'. There may be no greater cause of disempowerment than to be confronted with the news that life is near to an end or under very real threat. Every client whom we meet in cancer or palliative care will have been violated by at least one of these devastating themes.

We have already seen that the use of our everyday professional language can serve only to frighten and alienate our clients. As with any other institution, care settings need some form of routine and, in cancer or palliative care, this sometimes means that we ask clients to wear their night attire during the day (for certain procedures or therapies); but this does not mean that this has to become the accepted norm. The factors which contribute to the disempowerment of clients are highlighted in Figure 10.2.

All of these factors impinge upon clients and stop them from even approximating towards a position of parity in any of the discussions involved in the caring process. As well as these environmental and situational considerations, we also need to reflect upon the effect of the combined forces of the nurse and doctor on the client.

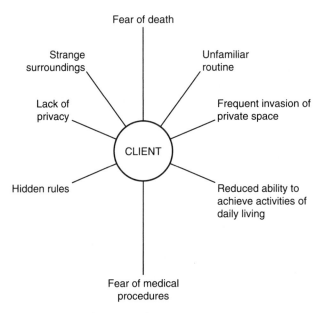

Figure 10.2   Factors contributing to disempowerment.

THE POWER OF PARENTALISM

You have probably heard said of some people that they behave in a paternal or maternal fashion. The paternalist label is usually fixed to men who behave in a fatherly fashion to colleagues. Conversely, the image of the matriarch is usually preserved for women who act in a motherly way towards colleagues and subordinates. Whilst the intentions of people who behave in this way can be beneficent, the effect it can have upon those around them can be patronizing and terribly 'dwarfing'. Coupling both these male and female images together can give us a set of 'parents' – in organizations where these traits exist in mutual duplicity this form of behaviour is called 'parentalism'.

The characteristics of parentalism are heavily imprinted upon the traditional picture of the relationship between doctors, nurses and **their** patients. Resulting from this image of the 'pseudo-family' is a completely disempowered patient who passively conforms to the dominant wishes of 'mother' and 'father'. This is illustrated in Figure 10.3.

This triangular relationship is based upon inequality and power; it should have no place in contemporary health care and is ethical anathema to those who feel client empowerment should be the focus of skills and care giving. We will now consider the notion of advocacy as a powerful mechanism for breaking the shackles which have traditionally held clients in a passive and unassertive role.

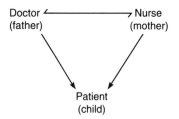

Figure 10.3   Parentalism in health care.

ADVOCATING EMPOWERMENT

We have spent a lot of time looking at client empowerment and the various factors which can either enhance or reduce this process. As nurses, advocacy demands that we represent the 'best interests' of the clients in our care. This does not necessarily mean that we decide alone what constitutes 'best interests' but actively seek to find what the client's wishes are and help to achieve them. Sometimes this can be a straightforward request, such as getting in touch with a minister of religion on behalf of the client. However, sometimes advocating for clients can be an involved and complex affair.

Imagine that you are a staff nurse on a surgical oncology ward. It has been a very busy morning and there is a great air of expectancy. Suddenly the consultant enters with the ward sister, followed by an entourage of staff. In the first bed, Mrs Jones is looking bemused and frightened as the consultant explains the next day's surgery: 'Don't worry . . . the growth looks a bit suspicious but we've probably got it in time. Anyway, what we'll do is cut it out and fashion a colostomy for you; that's a bag on your side which will collect motions . . . expect to be with us a week to 10 days. All the best now! Next please, sister.'

Mrs Jones looks absolutely horrified and aghast; she calls you over and asks 'What did he mean – a bag on my side? And what was that about catching it in time? I haven't got a clue what's going on or happening to me!'

How would you act as an advocate for Mrs Jones in this situation? Mrs Jones was in a very vulnerable position to begin with. The visit from the consultant has only compounded this and left her feeling totally disempowered. If you are to act as an advocate then this position has to be changed. Here are three examples of how this may be achieved:

1. Explain to Mrs Jones the nature of the operation yourself and ensure that she understands what you have said.
2. Contact the ward sister and explain that Mrs Jones is unsure and frightened about the nature of the forthcoming surgery. This is a viable alternative because the ward sister holds ultimate responsibility for the well-being of patients from a nursing perspective.
3. Approach the consultant and ask if he could explain to Mrs Jones about the nature of the surgery which is to be performed. This is a difficult thing for many of us to do; consultants are still revered by many people. As Kendrick (1992) informs us: 'We encounter certain figures, in professional practice, who hold positions of great power and authority; the image of a consultant surgeon being followed by hesitant doctors, students and nurses is a good example of this. If it inhibits us, as colleagues, we can imagine the effect it has on the patient/client.' Whilst approaching the consultant may not be well

received, a duty of care has been established with Mrs Jones which demands that consent to surgery is based on an informed consent.

Perhaps advocacy becomes of prime importance when a dying person is no longer able to make any overt statements about the care-giving process. During this chapter we have explored many concepts which can engender a sense of trust in our clients. If veracity, consent and empowerment play key roles in the care which we give to dying clients, then, when they are no longer able to take an active part in the decision-making process, at least the relationship is founded upon concepts and values which allow the nurse to have a developed insight into what direction the client would like the care giving to take. Nurses can only advocate for dying clients when trust has emerged from an acknowledgement of the importance of autonomy, individuality and freedom of choice. All of these themes are central to the ethical awareness needed in the care of the dying person, as Kendrick (1991) states: 'Ethical insight can help to break the shackles of potential power that the nurse has traditionally exerted over the patient. The result of this will be a non-judgemental partnership where the nurse may begin to approximate towards an understanding of the dying person and her/his unique needs. Death should not be veiled in a negative mystique. The nurse and the patient can do much to enhance the penultimate of life events: together they can become "partners in passing".'

A PLEA FOR ETHICS

Ethics is a challenging and rigorous discipline; it cannot give concrete, black and white answers to moral problems. Rather it provides pathways in thought which help us consider and analyse complex issues. The concepts we have examined in this chapter will help you reflect upon the ethical scenarios which arise in your own practice.

Nobody would ever hope to cover all aspects of ethical importance regarding cancer and palliative care in a single chapter. However, we have endeavoured to give a diverse and rich mix of the common ethical issues which arise in practice. It is the author's hope that this has helped to make moral theory alive and relevant to the situations which you encounter professionally.

Ethical aspects of cancer and palliative care provide a fascinating and stimulating area for applied study. Limitations of space prevent us looking at other issues, such as euthanasia, advanced directives, resource allocation and research – there is a list of selected reading after the references if you wish to consider ethics in further detail.

Tschudin (1993) argues that ethics is at the very heart of nursing; this is eloquently supported by Chadwick and Tadd (1992), who write:

Right answers in ethics are few and far between, wrong ones are devastating for all those concerned. What is important, however, is that as nurses we continually question our practice.

Ethics provides us with the 'tools' to ask these questions with reflective insight and ordered thought.

REFERENCES

Beuchamp, T.L. and Childress, J.F. (1982) *Principles of Biomedical Ethics.* Oxford University Press, Oxford.
Bok, S. (1978) *Lying: Moral Choice in Public and Private Life.* Harvester Press, East Sussex.
Chadwick, R.F. and Tadd, W. (1992) *Ethics and Nursing Practice.* Macmillan, Basingstoke.
Faulder, C. (1985) *Whose Body Is It? The Troubling Issue of Informed Consent.* Virago Press, London.
French, W.L. and Raven, C.A. (1959) *The Basis of Social Power.* University of Michigan Press, Michigan.
Gillon, R. (1986) *Philosophical Medical Ethics.* Wiley, Chichester.
Haring, B. (1974) *Medical Ethics.* St Paul Publications, Slough.
Hebblethwaite, M. (1991) Shall we pretend it isn't happening? *Journal of Advances in Health and Nursing Care,* 1(2), 75–92.
Kendrick, K. (1991) Partners in passing: the ethical aspects of nursing a dying person. *Journal of Advances in Health and Nursing Care,* 1(1), 5–25.
Kendrick, K. (1992) *People and their Rights: Enrolled Nurse Conversion Course.* Open College Press, Didsbury.
Kendrick, K. (1993) Understanding ethics in nursing practice. *British Journal of Nursing,* 2(18), 920–5.
Kubler-Ross, E. (1979) *On Death and Dying.* Tavistock, London.
Moutsopoulos, L. (1984) Truth telling to patients. *International Journal of Medicine and Law,* 3(3), 230–53.
Penner, L. (1978) *Social Psychology: A Contemporary Approach.* Oxford University Press, Oxford.
Tschudin, V. (1993) *Ethics: Aspects of Nursing Care.* Scutari Press, London.
Turner, B.S. (1987) Medical power and social knowledge. Sage, London.

FURTHER READING

Brown, J.M., Kitson, A.L. and McKnight, T.J. (1992) *Challenges in Caring: Explorations in Nursing and Ethics.* Chapman & Hall, London.
Hugman, R. (1991) *Power in Caring Professions.* Macmillan, Basingstoke.
Thompson, I.E., Melia, K.M. and Boyd, K.M. (1988) *Nursing Ethics.* Churchill Livingstone, Edinburgh.
Witts, P. (1992) Advocacy in nursing, in *Themes and Perspectives in Nursing* (eds K. Southhill, I.C. Henry and K.D. Kendrick), Chapman & Hall, London.

An introduction to hospice and palliative care

11

Alison Barnes

INTRODUCTION

Palliative care, as defined by the World Health Organization is, 'the active, total care of patients whose disease no longer responds to curative treatment and for whom the goal must be the best quality of life for them and their families'.

The word 'palliative' is derived from the Latin word *pallium*, meaning a cloak or cover. In its most literal use it refers to a person whose condition is not responsive to active treatment.

Palliative care is now a distinct specialty for both medicine and nursing; it focuses on controlling pain and other symptoms, easing suffering and enhancing the life that remains. It integrates the psychological and spiritual aspects of care, to enable patients to live out their lives with dignity, as well as offering support to families both during the patient's illness and the family's subsequent bereavement. It offers a unique combination of care in hospitals, hospices and at home. This description has been produced by the National Council for Hospice and Specialist Palliative Care Services. The council was launched in 1992 as the representative organization for palliative care services in England, Wales and Northern Ireland. Although hospice care is designed principally for people with advanced cancer, many units will admit people with other diagnoses.

DEFINITION OF TERMS

CONTINUING CARE

This refers to the care of dying patients, their families and carers; it includes medical and nursing care as well as counselling and bereavement counselling, which may continue for some time after death has occurred.

PALLIATIVE CARE

This is the active total care offered to patients with a progressive illness and their families when it is recognized that the illness is no longer curable, in order to concentrate on the quality of life and the alleviation of distressing symptoms within the framework of a coordinated service. It provides relief from pain and other distressing symptoms, integrating the psychological and spiritual aspects of care. Palliative care neither hastens nor postpones death. Its goal is to achieve the best quality of life for both patients and their families.

TERMINAL ILLNESS

This is an active and progressive disease for which curative treatment is neither possible nor appropriate and from which death is certain. The period has been defined by the National Association of Health Authorities and Trusts (NAHAT) as less than one year but could vary from a few days to many months.

REHABILITATION

In the context of palliative care, this refers to assisting patients to achieve and to maintain their maximum physical, emotional, spiritual, vocational and social potential, however limited this may be as a result of the progression of the disease.

PALLIATIVE CARE TEAM

These are specialist staff who offer advice and support to health workers in the community or hospital. The team does not take over responsibility or offer hands-on care, but is usually advisory and may comprise doctors, nurses and other professional support.

PRIMARY CARE TEAM

This consists of the team based round the general practitioner, the district nurse, health visitor, practice nurse, any therapists attached and, ideally, social workers; these will continue to provide the mainstay of support to the family even if the death should occur in hospital.

MULTIDISCIPLINARY CARE

This is the team approach to palliative care. Leadership of the team may vary according to the particular problems of the patient.

DAY CARE

A growing number of palliative care units have facilities for day patients. A full range of services is available, with opportunities to consult health care professionals and enjoy social activities. Day care often enables the patient to continue living at home.

THE HISTORY OF THE HOSPICE MOVEMENT

From the Middle Ages, Christians were welcomed on their journeys to holy sites in accommodation provided by the religious houses which became known as hospices. These resting places for pilgrims gradually came to provide care for the sick and elderly but following the dissolution of the monasteries by Henry VIII the sick and poor had nowhere to go. Eventually some of the old hospices reopened as hospitals, again providing care for the sick.

In 1842 the first facility for the care of the dying was established in France; however, most people consider that the hospice movement began in the UK.

In the middle of the nineteenth century Mary Aikenhead resurrected the name 'hospice' when, in Dublin, she founded an order of nuns called the Irish Sisters of Charity; they undertook the care of the dying. Originally the nuns provided care in people's own homes but it soon became clear that there was a need for some sort of nursing home, which was smaller and quieter than a busy acute hospital but which could provide the facilities for bedside nursing. Mary Aikenhead first gave the name 'hospice' to this special sort of home.

At the beginning of the twentieth century the Irish Sisters of Charity opened a similar home – St Joseph's Hospice – in London in 1905, and about the same time a similar home was opened by the Methodist West London Mission – St Lukes Home for the Dying Poor – which is now known as Hereford Lodge (Saunders, 1988).

THE DEVELOPMENT OF THE MODERN HOSPICE MOVEMENT

The modern hospice movement has developed in a variety of ways: some hospices have been developed within the National Health Service, some have been initiated by individual charitable groups and are known as independent or voluntary hospices, while others have been established by two national charitable organizations – Marie Curie Cancer Care and the Sue Ryder Foundation.

During the period between the end of the Second World War and the late 1960s there was a taboo against acknowledging death both in the UK and the USA. The word 'death' was seldom used; euphemisms proliferated, 'expired' or 'passed over' being preferred. During this period the active, strenuous 'high-tech' or heroic treatments were preferred.

Despite the dedication of the medical and nursing staff in hospitals, the experience of many patients and their relatives indicates that although hospitals have made great advances over the last few years in effective pain control techniques they are still unable to offer the kind of highly personalized care associated with the smaller hospice unit. There appear to be two main reasons for this failure:

1. The staff: patient ratio in hospital is lower than in the hospice which also recruits a considerable number of volunteers.
2. In hospitals there is generally a shortage of staff trained in the care of the dying, especially in the area of psychosocial care.

Gradually the social climate began to change. Antiauthoritarianism found expression in the civil rights movement; this was expressed in the health care movement as antiscience. People began to question the application of all-out life-saving technology in every instance, and they came to question the dominance of physician-led policies in the organization of health care.

The modern hospice movement in the UK began in the 1950s and the 1960s, and is usually attributed to two developments. One was the establishment of the Marie Curie Foundation and the other the creation by Dame Cicely Saunders of St Christopher's Hospice at Sydenham in 1967. Cicely Saunders' interest in terminal care dates from her meeting with a Polish refugee called David Tasma while working as a social worker in a London teaching hospital. He was dying from cancer and having discussed his needs with her, particularly for openness, he left her £500 in his will, saying 'I'll be a window in your home' (Saunders, 1993). This was the first contribution which began what was to become her life's work. Already a qualified nurse, she studied for a medical degree and on qualification went to work at St Joseph's Hospice as its first full-time medical director. Years of research on pain control and planning for the special needs of the dying led ultimately to the opening of St Christopher's Hospice. At St Christopher's the aim became not only to provide a place where effective care could be given to the terminally ill, but also where research and teaching could take place. To St Christopher's came pioneers from all over the UK and from across the Atlantic; thus St Christopher's became the catalyst and the model for hospice care, both in the UK and in the USA. From this movement many local services developed, as communities throughout the country recognized a need that was not being met by the statutory services. They began to provide services for the care of the terminally ill, particularly for people with cancer. Initially these provided rest and care but over the last 30 years they have developed into active hospices offering support, training, information and research into palliative care. This complements the services and skills of the primary health care team and National Health Service (NHS) hospitals.

The philosophy of hospice care has now spread to more than 60 countries, crossing both religious and political boundaries. Hospices and palliative care units are to be found in almost every country in the Western world, but the vast majority of people in the Third World have no access to such services. More than 9 million new cases of cancer each year are in developing countries of the world, yet only 5% of the resources for controlling cancer are spent in these countries. Consequently, in some parts of the world fewer than 20% of cancer patients enter hospital soon enough for curative treatment to be contemplated. For example, in India 80% of patients are first seen in the terminal phase of their illness (Webb, 1993).

People may also be denied access to palliative care because of political or religious ideologies; the use of morphine is still prohibited in some parts of the world and in others doctors are reluctant to use any drugs which may be interpreted as contributing to euthanasia.

At present the majority of patients in the UK die in hospital, although research has shown that the majority would prefer to die at home (Townsend *et al.*, 1990; Lovett, 1993).

MILESTONES IN THE HISTORY OF CANCER CARE

The age of reason in the development of medicine is usually identified as the eighteenth century. Before the eighteenth century no distinction was made between scientific thought and metaphysical concepts; this applied to cancer care and treatment as much as to other aspects of medical care. There were many myths about cancer at this time; most people thought it was contagious and the black bile theory prevailed. However, patterns of incidence began to emerge, and a prevalence in certain geographical locations was noted. In 1713, Ramazzini noted a higher incidence of lung cancer in nuns compared with other women. Snuff was also associated in many cases of cancer. In 1775 Percival Pott described scrotal cancer in chimney sweeps; at last, after 1000 years the black bile theory of cancer was being dispelled and surgery began to be considered as a treatment of choice.

The first known facility for treating people with cancer only was developed in Reims in France in 1740, but this had to be moved to the outskirts of the city because the residents feared that cancer was contagious. Many people consider the Middlesex Hospital in London the first cancer care institute in the UK, where a ward was set up in 1792 to study the natural history of cancer and to investigate new methods of treatment.

During the nineteenth century many facilities were developed. More radical surgery was made possible by the introduction of anaesthesia in 1846 and antisepsis in 1867. In 1851 the Cancer Hospital (now the Royal Marsden) in London was established exclusively for the treatment of people with cancer. Facilities were also developing on the other side of the Atlantic; the New York Cancer Hospital was founded in 1884, known today as the Memorial Sloan-Kettering Cancer Centre. In 1890, what is considered to be the first hospice for people with cancer in New York was set up: the St Rose's Free Home for Incurable Cancer.

At the beginning of the twentieth century, cancer was considered incurable and many people still thought it was infectious. The death rate was 90% and prevention was not a focus for attention.

In 1851 the Cancer Hospital established by Dr Marsden exclusively to treat patients with cancer was the venue for many developments in the treatment of people with cancer; later in the twentieth century it became the centre for the development of the specialization of oncology nursing in the UK and was very influential internationally. At that time the role of both doctors and nurses was seen as one of prolonging life at almost any cost by the amazing life-saving techniques that were being developed. This placed them often in complex moral and ethical positions. Stopping curative treatment and changing to palliative care is not easy, but the failure to do so may result in the lives of some people being prolonged even though they may be of doubtful quality.

The first half of the twentieth century is noted for the use of ionizing radiation in the diagnosis and treatment of cancer and for the extension of surgical procedures. The second half of the century is noted for considerable progress in the use of systemic chemotherapy coupled with an increased understanding of cell biology. There has also been a proliferation of research and considerable advances in technology. Today there is a greater recognition of the value of the prevention and early detection of cancer, with an emphasis on health education. Research has revealed some causes of cancer and changes in lifestyle may be called for to prevent some cancers.

THE DEVELOPMENT OF CANCER NURSING AND PALLIATIVE CARE NURSING AS SPECIALITIES

At the first International Conference on Cancer Nursing, held in London in September 1978, Robert Tiffany gave a paper on the delivery of nursing care in which he said, 'I believe that nurses are willing to look at their role and function. I also believe that for the provision of excellence in nursing care we need a well prepared clinical nurse supported by her colleagues in nursing research, education and management. When this collaborative spirit exists, planning the delivery of nursing care becomes an integral part of each discipline' (Tiffany, 1978). This approach holds good for any specialty but he developed his theory while working in the field of cancer care.

HOME AND HOSPITAL SUPPORT SERVICES

There are more than 400 home care teams for cancer patients in the UK, of which about 260 are free-standing community-based teams and 150 are attached to hospice in-patient units. There are about 220 hospitals with support teams or support nurses for cancer patients (St Christopher's Hospice, 1993).

DAY HOSPICES

There are currently over 200 day hospices, either free standing or attached to hospice in-patient units or teams. These provide a variety of services to patients and their relatives (St Christopher's Hospice, 1993; Faulkner *et al.*, 1993).

Palliative care nursing is not restricted to cancer care but, as 25% of all deaths are deaths from cancer, nurses are most often involved in palliative care for people with cancer. Palliative care is also important for patients with other diagnoses, particularly where there is a long terminal phase, for example in motor neurone disease or AIDS (Sims and Moss, 1991).

Cancer nursing is definitely not synonymous with palliative care nursing; as survival rates from cancer improve, nurses who specialize in cancer care are involved in looking after many patients receiving treatment who will recover from their disease. The nursing services for people with malignant neoplasms, particularly the palliative care nursing services, within the NHS, voluntary and private sectors, have developed in response to patients' needs where these are not being met in acute general wards.

As the medical specialty of oncology has developed so the specialty of cancer nursing has emerged. Yarbro (1992) uses the words of Florence

Nightingale to express the unique essence of nursing: 'Experience teaches me that nursing and medicine must never be mixed up. It spoils both . . .'. It is important to look at developments in cancer nursing separately but in relation to the general history of cancer care.

Cancer nursing in the early 1900s was primarily concerned with the bedside care and comfort of surgical patients, surgery at that time being the treatment of choice. Most patients presented with cancer at an advanced stage and encountered numerous difficulties. Nurses had to use ingenuity to overcome each individual problem, adapting and improving what equipment they had to provide good bedside care. As knowledge and treatments advanced, so cancer nursing had to adapt to the problems created by the more complex treatments. Opportunities for the development of skills and undertaking research arose and nurses extended their roles as specialists, for example in stoma care (Tiffany and David, 1990). The concept of teamwork emerged.

Cancer nursing is a unique specialty; it draws its knowledge base from physiology, psychology and sociology. It encompasses not one but a number of diseases which occur in people of all ages and both sexes. It is concerned with managing symptoms caused more frequently by aggressive medical treatment than by the disease itself.

Nursing care is provided in all settings, from the acute hospital to the day hospital, to the hospice and the patient's own home. Care is often complicated by the negative stigma that continues to surround cancer. The diagnosis is dreaded and people are often too fearful to discuss their diagnosis with other people.

Cancer or oncology nursing has progressed as the treatments and survival rates have improved. In the 1930s the convention of considering five-year end results in cancer as an indication of cure came about. At this time fewer than one in five patients was alive five years after diagnosis. During the 1940s one in four patients was alive five years after diagnosis and in the 1960s the statistics had improved to one in three. The 1980s witnessed the most significant growth in cancer survival, with half of all patients who had had a cancer diagnosis being cured.

It must be remembered, however, that there is a wide variation in survival rates, both between the type of cancer and the country in which it occurs. The five-year survival rate for people with cancer of the pancreas in England and Wales is 4%, and survival for those with cancer of the skin is 97%. In industrialized countries the overall survival rate is 50% but in developing countries survival still remains a rare event.

ORGANIZATIONS SUPPORTING CANCER NURSING

There are many organizations for nurses in cancer care; some are international, while others are organized on a continental basis or established in individual countries. There are also organizations which are multidisciplinary, and recently an organization has been formed to represent palliative care services in England, Wales and Northern Ireland; this is called the National Council for Hospice and Specialist Palliative Care Services. It enables all the providers of these services to speak with one voice and to lobby government when necessary. It acts as a vehicle for the dissemination of information.

The following groups, societies and organizations are useful sources of support and information.

International Society for Nurses in Cancer Care

- In Africa and Middle East: Israel, Namibia, South Africa.
- In Central and South America and the Caribbean: Argentina, Chile, Jamaica, Panama.
- In Europe (European Oncology Nursing Society): Austria, Belgium, Ireland, Italy, The Netherlands, Norway, Sweden, Switzerland, Turkey, the UK.
- In the Far East and Australasia: Australia, China, Japan, Singapore, Thailand.
- In North America: Canada, the USA.

This list of member countries demonstrates the very wide geographical area over which cancer nursing as a specialty has developed, but the gaps also show. In many Third World countries, palliative medicine is regarded as a luxury; when the resources are insufficient for the basic necessities of life, cancer nursing and palliative care take a low priority.

In the UK the Royal College of Nursing has a special interest group for cancer nursing; within this the Royal College's Palliative Nursing Group was formed 10 years ago to support nurses working in the comparative isolation and stressful situations of the specialty. It also provides opportunities for hospital and community nurses to share information on topics of concern. Originally the name of the group was the Symptom Control and Care of the Dying Forum but the name was changed in 1989 because palliatiation described more accurately what nurses were doing for patients.

Cancer care organizations

The World Health Organization promotes cooperation between countries and funds some medical and nursing posts. Organizations such as European Conference on Clinical Oncology and Cancer Nursing, the European Organization for Research and Treatment of Cancer, the Multinational Association of Supportive Care in Cancer, and the European Cancer Care Organization organize regular conferences, publish papers presented and serve as opportunities for the exchange of information and the promotion of good practice.

Most countries have their local groups, with many specialist groups linked to individual cancers or treatment options.

There are also Cancer Education Coordinating Groups, such as the one for the UK and the Republic of Ireland which was set up in 1982 to promote the coordination of public and professional education on the causes, effects, prevention, recognition and treatment of all forms of cancer and the care and rehabilitation of people with cancer.

There are many organizations in each country, some to ensure that professionals are educated in the care of the terminally ill, others to provide support or information to patients or carers suffering from specific cancers.

The Hospice Information Service is a national and international resource at St Christopher's Hospice which provides a link for those working in hospices with terminally ill patients and their families, as well as for members of the public. The service maintains close links with other national organizations working in this area. The main functions of the service are:

- provision of information on the nature and location of hospice and palliative care services both in the UK and overseas;
- continuing research into the activities and staffing levels of hospice and palliative care services in the UK and Ireland;
- publications: the *Directory of Hospice Care* is published annually and lists over 550 established and planned hospices and palliative care services. *Hospice Worldwide* is a regularly updated directory of overseas hospice and palliative care services in six continents;
- *Hospice Bulletin*: a news link for hospice workers.

Some of the charities also provide some financial support for patients and their families (see Chapter 17).

WHERE PEOPLE DIE

A question which often arises is, should there be a specialty for the care of the dying when death itself is a natural experience shared by everyone and an event which commonly requires the services of both nurses and doctors?

Arguably all staff should have the necessary skills and specialists would then be unnecessary. Unfortunately basic medical and nursing education has not recognized the need for death education until recently. Nursing has been slightly the better in this respect, with palliative care having been included in the registered nurse curriculum for many years. However, Wilkes (1984) reports that half the junior hospital doctors and nurses interviewed thought that their training in terminal care had been inadequate and most of the nurses felt that the wards were too busy to be a suitable place for the care of the dying.

The great majority of doctors and nurses encounter patients in the terminal phase of illness and try to become proficient in caring for them. Some are uncomfortable with this work and view it as an unwelcome part of their caseload or a failure. It is sometimes a complex moral and ethical decision to know when it is best to change from curative treatment to palliative treatment. It must be recognized that 56% of all deaths in England and Wales still occur in hospital and this figure has been increasing since the 1950s. However able the medical and nursing staff are, adequate facilities are often not available in hospitals, with little or no privacy for the patient or the family and no opportunity for the family to remain with the patient who is dying. The trend for more deaths to occur in hospital is expected to increase due to a combination of demographic, economic and social factors. This is not, however, where the patient wants to die (Lovett, 1993).

Between 1961 and 1986 the number of one-person households increased from 12% to 25%. The elderly are more likely to be living alone than any other age group, and so the option of choosing to die at home is not open to them. Even if a spouse is living he or she is likely also to be elderly and perhaps infirm and so unable to assist in the care.

Another factor which may partly explain the trend to an increase in the number of hospital deaths is the break-up of the extended family. Young adults have frequently moved away to improve employment prospects and so relatives are not nearby to help care for the patient.

There may be wide variations between urban and rural communities; small studies have shown that a person from a rural community is more likely to die at home than a person from an urban area. This distinction may be partly explained by a different attitude towards and availability of health services between urban and rural areas. People living in urban areas increasingly look to the NHS for assistance, while for many rural patients hospitals are alien territory.

However, it is interesting to note that 70% of new cancers develop in people aged 60 years or more. As the population ages, so the incidence of some cancers is likely to increase (OPCS, 1992).

THE FUNDING OF PALLIATIVE CARE SERVICES

In the UK the majority of deaths occur in acute hospitals and so it follows that the NHS bears the greatest share of the costs; 56% of all deaths and 60% of deaths from cancer in England and Wales currently occur in hospital. It has been estimated that a patient with terminal cancer will spend 90% of his or her final year at home, i.e. just 11.6 days in hospital, giving a total of nearly 5 million bed days; this represents a considerable proportion of NHS hospital resources. The reasons given for hospital admission are:

- the inability to control symptoms of disease adequately at home, for example pain, constipation or loss of apetite;
- no carer available, despite support from community nurses, social services and general practitioners; 24-hour care is possible but expensive and difficult to organize;
- lack of social service provision or sometimes the lack of knowledge that such resources are available for carers, until it is too late.

It is interesting to note that age also plays an important part in where people die. For those aged under 45 years, 53% will die in hospital, 12% in a hospice, 0.5% elsewhere (which includes psychiatric hospitals) and 33.5% at home. However, when one looks at people aged over 85 years, 52% die in hospital, 17% in a hospice, 13% elsewhere and only 17.5% at home. The problem here is that 42% of carers are over retirement age (Neale and Clark, 1992).

The funding of hospice care varies very much; the government has a declared intent to reach 50:50 funding with the voluntary sector. The scene today is very uncertain; many hospices are negotiating contracts with local health authorities for some of their patient costs but are concerned that some of the benefits that they have in the past been able to claim have been abolished. Most hospices fund-raise and are very well supported by their local communities. The 'hospice grant' has for the last few years been 'ring-fenced' money, from the Department of Health, and distributed through regional health authorities, but this is unlikely to continue. Thus contracting will become more and more important (National Council for Hospice and Specialist Palliative Care Services, 1993).

Home care services are funded by local health authorities, by the voluntary sector and sometimes by the private sector. Marie Curie Cancer Care (MCCC) has a contract with most health care providers in England, Wales, Scotland and Northern Ireland to provide home nursing services; these are funded usually 50:50 between MCCC and the local health authority.

CHARITABLE ORGANIZATIONS IN THE UK

CANCER RELIEF MACMILLAN FUND

Founded in 1911, its aim is to improve the quality of life for people with cancer and their families, at any stage of the illness and in any setting. Since then it has established 12 Macmillan cancer care units; each has between 10 and 25 beds. These were originally funded by Cancer Relief Macmillan Fund and built in the grounds of NHS hospitals. They are now all funded by the NHS. Cancer Relief Macmillan Fund provides nurses specially trained in cancer care to advise on pain and symptom control and to give emotional support to patients and their families in hospital and at home. Cancer Relief Macmillan also offers initial funding for the establishment of other specialist medical and nursing posts in the field of cancer care. Financial support for these posts may then be taken over by the NHS. Help given by the Cancer Relief Macmillan Fund includes:

- four kinds of Macmillan nurse: home care, hospital, breast care and paediatric nurses;
- the building of cancer care units as described above;
- the provision of grants for those in need;
- funding for a medical support and education programme;
- finances for other charities which provide information and self-help for people with cancer (Faulkner, 1994).

MARIE CURIE CANCER CARE

This organization was originally established in June 1948 as the Marie Curie International Memorial; the name was changed shortly after the launch to the Marie Curie Memorial Foundation. The inspiration of its originators was said to have come from a remark made by Winston Churchill that casualties from cancer were far worse than those caused by hostilities. The inaugural committee agreed the priority objectives of the foundation to be:

1. the provision of a nursing and welfare service for people in their own homes;
2. the provision of residential nursing homes;
3. the provision of grants, scholarships, fellowships or awards for the encouragement of scientific learning.

The first Marie Curie home, 'Hill of Tarvit' at Cupar, Fife, opened in December 1952. This property belonged to the National Trust for Scotland and was leased to the foundation at a peppercorn rent on condition that the ground floor remained open to the public. By 1977 the foundation had 430 beds distributed throughout the UK. As the general practitioner cover for the homes became increasingly replaced by consultant cover, so the nature of the 'homes' has altered from long-term care of people with cancer to the more rehabilitative and palliative style of hospice care. MCCC currently (1994) provides 10% of all hospice/palliative care beds in the UK and 13% of beds in the charitable/voluntary sector. MCCC today has four areas of operation:

1. 11 centres for patient care providing specialist care and advice for in- and out-patients;
2. the research institute, which investigates the causes and treatment of cancer;
3. the education department, which provides education and training for all grades of health service personnel and offers information and education to the general public;
4. the community nursing service of over 5000 nurses, caring for patients in their own homes.

These are the two most comprehensive national charities in the UK; there are, however, many other charitable organizations which concentrate on either one aspect of cancer care or research, or perhaps provide services in a restricted geographical area (Faulkner, 1993).

GAPS IN SERVICES

Wilkes (1984) in a random study of 262 deaths reports that most of the dying patients felt weak, immobile, depressed or anorexic but that a high proportion had ineffectively controlled pain, cough, dyspnoea or insomnia. The differing perception of problems by different individuals caring for the same patient reinforced the need for more integrated care and knowledge and respect for the views of those involved.

It has been suggested that the proposed form of treatment for many patients is influenced not only by straightforward medical reasons but also by the sociopsychological circumstances of patients or their wishes and the likely outcome of the therapies available, so as to enable them to die with dignity. For example: is it in the best interests of a patient suffering from a terminal malignant disease for which there is no cure, to continue to receive invasive curative therapy which may cause distress? It would be much better for the patient to change to palliative care, aimed at the relief of symptoms such as pain. We know that there are gaps in the service for patients with terminal disease in the UK but for many reasons there are even more gaps in the rest of the world.

RECENT DEVELOPMENTS IN THE UK

In the UK in 1980, a working group of the standing subcommittee on cancer of the standing medical advisory committee produced a report – *Terminal Care* – which recognized the need to provide good professional care for people terminally ill with cancer. In 1986 the Department of

Health and Social Security (DHSS) sponsored a conference under the chairmanship of HRH The Prince of Wales on palliative care. These two initiatives demonstrate the importance of the specialty of palliative care and the official recognition that this is so necessary.

In 1991, the Secretary of State for Health asked the standing medical advisory committee and the standing nursing and midwifery advisory committee to establish a joint working party with these terms of reference:

> to consider the organization of palliative care services and the measurement of their performance and to make recommendations.

Ten years had passed since the previous *Terminal Care* report and it was recognized that palliative care services were developing rapidly and very patchily. The draft report from this working party was produced at the end of 1992; the recommendations cover access to the services, education of all health service personnel and strategic planning to prevent gaps in the services.

STATE PRIORITIES

In June 1985, the heads of state of the countries of the European Community agreed in Milan on a European Programme against Cancer (European Community, 1985) and in *The Health of the Nation* (Department of Health, 1992) the UK government has also selected cancer as a target for improvement in health status, concentrating on the preventable cancers or those where life expectancy benefits from early detection.

CONCLUSION

One must look to the future. Current trends indicate a move away from residential care and a growing understanding of 'hospice' as a philosophy rather than a building. Thus experienced nurses and doctors can support patients and their families at home, where they want to be, for as long as they wish. The length of stay of patients in hospices has become shorter, with more readmissions for the control of symptoms or to give the carer or patient respite (David, 1994). As the age of the population increases there will be a need to provide more support for carers, who themselves are older (Neale and Clark, 1992), and for day care services for those living on their own.

> Those of us who live with cancer want to maximize our time; we want to feel as good as we possibly can within the limits of our illness.
> *Mara Flaherty, quoted by Anderson, 1989*

REFERENCES

Anderson, J.L. (1989) The nurse's role in cancer rehabilitation. *Cancer Nursing,* **12**(2), 85–94.

David, J.A. (1994) A comparison of admission to two hospices in the UK, in *Proceedings of the Sixth International Symposium on Supportive Care in Cancer,* New Orleans, 2–5 March 1994. Imedex USA, Alpharetta, GA.

Department of Health (1992) *Health of the Nation: A Strategy for Health in England.* HMSO, London.

European Community (1985) *Europe Against Cancer Campaign.* Commissioners of the European Community, Brussels.

Faulkner, A. (1993) Cancer centre profile: Marie Curie Cancer Care. *Journal of Cancer Care,* **2**(3), 151–63.

Faulkner, A. (1994) Cancer centre profile: Cancer Relief Macmillan Fund. *Journal of Cancer Care,* **3**(1), 47–64.

Faulkner, A., Higginson, I., Egerton, H. *et al.* (1993) *Hospice Day Care: A Qualitative Study.* Published for Help the Hospices by Trent Palliative Care Services, Sheffield.

Lovett, J. (1993) The voluntary sector provider's view, in *Needs Assessment for Hospice and Specialist Palliative Care Services,* Occasional Paper 4 (ed. M. Robbins), National Council for Hospice and Specialist Palliative Care Services, London.

National Council for Hospice and Specialist Palliative Care Services (1993) *Information Exchange,* **4**, 1–2.

Neale, B. and Clark, D. (1992) Informal palliative care. *Journal of Cancer Care,* **1**(2), 85–90.

Office of Population Censuses and Surveys (1992) *Population Data.* HMSO. London.

St Christopher's Hospice Information Service (1993) *Directory of Hospice Services in the UK and Republic of Ireland.* St Christopher's Hospice, Sydenham.

Saunders, C. (1988) The evolution of hospices, in *The history of the management of pain: from early principles to present practices* (ed. R.D. Mann), Parthenon Publishing Group, Carnforth, Lancs.

Saunders, C. (1993) Some challenges that face us. *Palliative Medicine,* **7** (suppl. 1), 77–83.

Sims, R. and Moss, V. (1991) *Terminal Care for People with AIDS.* Edward Arnold, London.

Tiffany, R. (1978) Planning the delivery of care, in *Proceedings of the 1st International Conference on Cancer Care.* Nursing Mirror, London.

Tiffany, R. and David, J.A. (1990) Management of change, in *Oncology* (ed. A. Faulkner), Scutari Press, London.

Townsend, J., Frank, H.O., Fremont, D. *et al.* (1990) Terminal care and patients' preference for place of death: a prospective study. *British Medical Journal,* **301**, 415–17.

Webb, P. (1993) Cancer Relief India. *European Journal of Cancer Care,* **2**(2), 53–4.

Wilkes, E. (1984) Dying now. *Lancet,* **ii**, 950–2.

Yarbro, C.H. (1992) Cancer nursing: the needs of today, the challenge of tomorrow, in *Proceedings of the Seventh International Conference on Cancer Nursing*, Vienna, 16–21 August 1992 (ed. C.D. Bailey) Rapid Communications, Oxford, pp. 3–5.

FURTHER READING

Clark, D. (1993) *The Future for Palliative Care: Issues of Policy and Practice.* Oxford University Press, Oxford.

Griffin, J. (1991) *Dying with Dignity.* Office of Health Economics, London.

Joint report of the Standing Medical Advisory Committee (SMAC) and Standing Nursing and Midwifery Committee (SNMAC) (1993) *Principles and Provisions of Palliative Care.* HMSO, London.

Stoddard, S. (1979) The Hospice Movement. Jonathan Cape, London.

12 Symptom control in advanced cancer

Tracey Pilsworth, Dot Pye and Anita Roberts

INTRODUCTION

This chapter gives an overview of the causes and discusses the treatment of the most common problems experienced by patients with advanced cancer. Wilkes (1984) in a survey of 262 deaths reported that the most common symptoms of terminal illness were: pain 52%, weakness 52%, dyspnoea 42% and urinary incontinence 35%. These and other difficult problems encountered in nursing patients with advanced cancer, including nausea and vomiting, constipation and non-healing wounds, are dealt with here.

It should be acknowledged that every symptom identified may not be caused by the malignant process and that making an adequate assessment is important. Symptoms can be caused by multiple factors including cancer, its treatment, general debility or unrelated pathological conditions. Even when cancer is the causal factor, symptoms may occur for different reasons and will therefore require a different therapeutic approach – for example, dyspnoea due to pleural effusion and dyspnoea related to lymphangitis. As a result, treatment may well vary from patient to patient.

When trying to control difficult symptoms it is important to establish a balance which ensures that the benefits of treatment are not outweighed by unacceptable side-effects. As cancer is a progressive disease with new symptoms appearing as it progresses, the importance of continual review and reassessment cannot be over-emphasized.

PAIN

'Pain is not a simple sensation like seeing or hearing, it is far more complex' (Twycross and Lack, 1991). Acute pain fulfils an important protective function, indicating that all is not well with our bodies; without it we would continue to damage injured tissue, for example burning a finger on a hot flame. Acute pain is brief and an end is expected. Cicely Saunders observes that pain experienced during advanced stages of cancer is of chronic nature (unlike many forms of acute pain) and has no useful function.

Pain is a subjective experience and tolerance can vary from one person to another, and, indeed vary in an individual at different times and in different circumstances. It therefore follows that, 'Pain is whatever the experiencing person says it is and exists whenever he says it does' (McCaffery, 1972).

PHYSIOLOGY

There are no specific receptors in the brain for pain. Any sensation which is intense enough can be interpreted as pain, e.g. extremes of temperature. Interpretation of pain can differ, suggesting that there are two pathways that operate so that they do not reach the conscious mind at the same rate, e.g. burning a finger on a hot iron initially gives a sharp pain, but later turns to a dull throbbing pain.

The environment or situation that the person is in at the time also allows the conscious mind to shut out pain sensation – for example: soldiers injured on the battlefield carry on fighting; a pilot carrying passengers from a crashed aeroplane only discovers he has two broken ankles himself when they are out of danger.

There have been several theories and arguments about how the brain gets its 'pain' message. In 1965 Professor Patrick Wall and Professor Ronald Melzack published a new theory which is known as the 'gate' theory and at present this is the most plausible hypothesis, having been revised again in 1977 (Wall and Melznack, 1989).

The theory is that the brain can interpret different patterns of electrical activity in the nervous system as 'pain'. It is thought that the conscious awareness of pain takes place in the area between the thalamus and the cortex. The dorsal horn acts as a gate to control messages to the brain and all sensory impulses have to pass through this gate.

There is a substance in the dorsal horn known as substantia gelatinosa. This is activated by the nerve fibres and forms the gate, transmitting the pain on upwards to the brain.

Fast nerves (alpha delta) connect directly with the hind- and the midbrain where the thalamus is situated, and as these go through the gate quickly some pain will be felt immediately (these are the nerves that are probably responsible for the reflex arc).

Slower nerves (C fibres) are responsible for deep pain sensed by the brain but take longer to get through the gate control system.

Alpha beta fibres responsible for the lighter sensation of touch and temperature also pass through the gate.

The gate may be closed, blocking transmission of pain to the brain by this lighter sensation; for example, rubbing a painful area activates transmission of tactile information, inhibiting the brain's response to the pain. If the pain is greater than other stimulation, the gate will be opened and the brain will respond to the pain.

It seems that the brain can block incoming pain sensation if the person receives sufficient alternative sensory input, for example massage, or hot and cold compresses. Thoughts, emotions and past experiences also play a part in blocking pain sensation or increasing it, which gives rise to the idea that the gate control theory is an interrelationship of physical, psychological and cognitive components, and as stated by Keela and Mobily (1992): 'The gate control theory has led to the recognition that pain can be reduced or moderated at four points'. These are:

1. the peripheral site of the pain;
2. in the spinal cord;
3. in the brain stem;
4. in the cortex.

CAUSES OF PAIN

Two-thirds of patients who have cancer suffer pain. There can be several types of pain involved. Treatments for the cancer can cause pain, for example radiotherapy burns, or chronic post-operative pain. Debility from the disease can cause aches in muscles, being unable to move from pressure. The patient may also have some other disorder present which causes pain, for example arthritis or heart disease.

Of those pains that are caused by the cancer, these sites can be numerous and have different sources:

1. **Bone pain.** This is often severe and difficult to relieve. It can be constant and is usually worse on movement or weight-bearing.
2. **Visceral pain.** Pain from the visceral organs of the body, such as liver, stomach, uterus, causing pressure and stretching-type pain, is constant and dull in nature.
3. **Nerve pain.** This is due to compression or ongoing destruction of the nerve, or a combination of both. At first compression pain can be a constant dull ache and later be accompanied by shooting pains. Pain due to the destruction of the nerve is not as common but gives a superficial burning or stinging pain. Some patients present with both types of nerve pain.
4. **Soft tissue pain.** This is sometimes due to infection, and can be a throbbing pain or painful muscle spasms. Oedema of soft tissue occurs

frequently in advance cancer caused by hypoproteinaemia, venous stasis or congestive cardiac failure. Lymphoedema is due to invasion or compression of the lymphatics.

It follows that the patient can have multiple pains needing individual treatments.

PAIN ASSESSMENT

Pain assessment is complex because the appreciation of pain is subjective and individual, affected by psychological, social and cultural factors. In addition the cancer patient may have several different pains in different parts of the body which have different causes. To help nurses in this task pain assessment charts have been developed. These can be completed by the patient alone or with assistance from the nurse. The charts use visual and verbal descriptions for the pains and a body chart to show their location. The use of pain assessment charts is described by Pritchard and Mallett (1992); their usefulness is supported by research (Walker *et al.*, 1987); the various tools have been reviewed and the fact that they are not widely used in practice lamented (Baillie, 1993).

PAIN TREATMENT

As stated above, pain is a complex experience having psychological and physical components and so more than one method of pain relief is often needed to relieve a patient's pain. After careful assessment, the most appropriate method or combination of methods is initiated with continuing multidisciplinary reassessment to ensure efficacy.

DRUGS

The most common method of pain control is the use of drug therapy. When using drugs the regime should be as simple as possible for the patient to follow. The oral route should be used (whenever possible) and pain relief depends on the drugs being given regularly, not on a p.r.n. (*pro re nata*) basis, whenever necessary. Explanation about the drugs should be given to the patient whenever possible as his or her compliance is essential; many patients have pre-conceived beliefs about drugs that need to be resolved.

Analgesics

The World Health Organization (WHO) advocates a three-step analgesic 'ladder' approach to relieve pain (WHO, 1986). This simple visual device

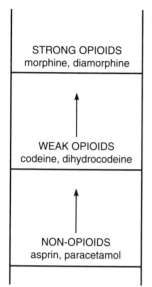

Figure 12.1 The analgesic ladder.

(Figure 12.1) was designed to encourage international consensus in pain therapy using locally available drugs. In the UK the first step would use simple analgesics such as aspirin or paracetamol regularly at four- to six-hourly intervals. If this is not sufficient to control pain a drug such as codeine or dihydrocodeine, from the next 'weak opioid' step on the 'ladder', should be selected rather than an alternative from the same group which would be no more effective. If or when this is not effective then a 'strong opioid', such as morphine or diamorphine, is prescribed.

Drugs on the first two rungs of the 'ladder' are generally given orally and for the 'strong opiates' this is also the first route of choice (Twycross and Lack, 1989). For example, morphine sulphate comes in several preparations, all with a variety of strengths:

- liquid
- fast-dissolving tablets
- slow-release tablets.

The easiest way to establish the required dose is to start the patient on the liquid form which gives relief for three to five hours. The dose will need to be titrated for each individual, using assessment and accurate records. Once the dose is established the patient's daily requirement can be calculated and given in the slow-release form, which is effective for 12 hours and is therefore only taken twice a day. This allows the patient greater freedom and ease of administration. The conversion calculation is simple: for example, the dose of liquid morphine is 10 mg four-hourly; this equals 60 mg for the day; the equivalent slow-release dose would be 30 mg twice a day.

If the patient is on slow-release morphine tablets, it is still useful for him or her to be provided with a bottle of morphine solution to take as a back-up for break-through pain. The patient should then remember or keep a diary of the amount of back-up required so that a new dosage regime of slow-release medication can be commenced.

The oral route is not always possible owing to the patient's condition or an inability to swallow. Other routes should then be considered, remembering they have individual drawbacks:

- **Sublingual.** Drugs that dissolve in the mouth through the mucosa, e.g. Temgesic. Not a route usually used as many patients with cancer suffer from dry mouths, with very little saliva to dissolve the tablet.
- **Rectal.** Many drugs come in suppository form and this route may be preferred by patients if they can insert them themselves, maintaining control over their medication regime. Some patients do not like this route, either because of discomfort or because this method is not culturally acceptable to them.
- **Parenteral route.** There are very few indications for using the intravenous route for analgesia in patients with advanced cancer.

- **Subcutaneous route.** Rather than giving repeated injections, the use of a continuous subcutaneous infusion via a syringe driver is preferred. This has an additional advantage in the community where the nurse cannot guarantee regular times for visiting the patient. There are many types of syringe driver available and the nurse should always check which type is being used to be certain the patient receives the correct dosage of drugs. There are syringe drivers now available that give the patient control for administering bolus doses of analgesia when required and these may be useful to those patients who need extra analgesia before or during painful procedures.
- **Spinal routes.** For administering analgesia these should only be considered after systemically administered analgesia has been shown to be ineffective or has intolerable side-effects. This system for the administration of drugs has to be inserted by a doctor, and the drugs must be administered by a practitioner skilled in this technique.

Side-effects

Most analgesics have side-effects, particularly in high doses. The most common of these is constipation. Laxatives should always be prescribed when using analgesics as constipation may be considered a worse symptom, causing more discomfort for the individual, than the pain suffered (see 'Constipation', below).

Co-analgesics

These are drugs that are not analgesics themselves but which relieve pain indirectly and are used in conjunction with analgesics.

1. **Non-steroidal anti-inflammatory drugs (NSAIDs).** Useful in bone pain, soft tissue infiltration, retroperitoneal pain, e.g. Froben 100 mg b.d. Some patients respond better to one NSAID than another. Therefore it can be beneficial to change one for another if they are not effective after one to two weeks. Ketorolac is suitable for parenteral use via the syringe driver.
2. **Corticosteroids.** Useful in the reduction of oedema and inflammation that surrounds a tumour, in raised intracranial pressure, nerve compression and visceral tumours, e.g. dexamethasone. Corticosteroids can have the useful side-effect of improving appetite and giving an increased feeling of well-being.
3. **Anticonvulsants.** Used for trigeminal nerve pain; can be useful for shooting or stabbing pain, e.g. carbamazepine, sodium valproate.
4. **Antidepressants.** Can be used during altered pain sensation and hypersensitivity which is the characteristic pain of nerve destruction, e.g. dothiepin, amitriptyline.

5. **Antibiotics.** The throbbing pain caused by an infected malignant ulcer or the copious purulent sputum of cancer of the lung can warrant treatment with antibiotics once a specimen has been taken for culture and sensitivity. For those patients with advanced disease, side-effects from antibiotics can cause greater distress than the problem they are being used for, and this should always be taken into consideration.

6. **Muscle relaxants.** Muscle spasm pain may be due to anxiety, tumour or nerve damage to the muscle. Diazepam may be given but can cause sedation. Baclofen is not a sedative but may have other undesirable side-effects.

RADIOTHERAPY

A single dose of radiotherapy may be indicated for localized bone pain, especially in the ribs or spine, resulting in lessening of the pain usually within 48 hours. It must be remembered that the level of analgesia used to control the pain previously may need to be reduced in consequence.

NERVE BLOCKS

Local nerve blocks may be considered where the pain is in a localized area or when other methods of pain relief have been contraindicated or have proven not to work. Injected local anaesthetic blocks may be effective for 12–18 hours. Phenol injections may be effective for 8–22 weeks, but local anaesthetic has the advantage of being discontinued if the patient finds the loss of sensation too unpleasant.

COMPLEMENTARY THERAPY

Many patients cannot find complete pain relief from conventional methods, and as the complexity of pain pathways is becoming more readily understood the use of complementary therapies has increased as a method of finding relief from pain, in conjunction with the more traditional methods of treatment.

- **Distraction** is the simple method of getting the patient to focus on something else besides the pain: reading, watching television or chatting about a favourite pastime.
- **Imagery** can be taught for the patient to use at any time; for example, if a patient enjoys fishing, he could imagine himself by the river using his senses – what can he hear, see, smell and feel? The nurse may have to

guide the patient initially but he will soon be able to take control of the sensation himself.

- **Relaxation** is often used in conjunction with imagery and can be achieved by several techniques, including yoga or simple breathing exercises; at first guided by the nurse but, again, the patient will soon be able to do this himself.
- **Aromatherapy** is the use of essential oils from plants and herbs. These oils are usually used in conjunction with massage. The oils can be either stimulating or relaxing, depending on which oil is used and the effect desired by the patient.
- **Massage** is the rhythmical stroking and kneading of the skin and muscles of the body, used to relieve aches and pains, especially where tension is present.
- **Reflexology** is a form of ancient Chinese medicine. The feet are massaged at points that correspond to different parts of the body.

Most complementary therapies require specialist training, skill and practice to be fully effective.

NURSING CARE

Just as the experience of suffering pain is unique to each patient, so too is the experience of the nurse, who brings to the situation his or her own beliefs about pain. A patient may therefore by presented in one day with different attitudes towards his pain; for example, a nurse who has herself experienced severe post-operative pain may be sympathetic, whereas a nurse who has been brought up to believe that men are strong and should be able to stand a lot of pain and 'not be a baby' may be less sympathetic. As nurses we should be aware of this and react to the patient's actual needs, not what we expect the patient to need.

Communication with the patient about pain is of the utmost importance for careful, continual assessment. The patient's cooperation is necessary to gain optimum relief with the medication used. He or she may have reservations about taking some of the drugs that may be prescribed. Discussion about treatments, how, why and when they are effective, and reasons for the pain may help patients, especially when they may feel that an increase in pain indicates a worsening of the disease.

The nurse is also responsible for correct verbal and written reporting of the patient's pain to colleagues both nursing and medical.

For care of the patient to be successful, the nurse must gain the patient's trust. All this takes time and during this period it may appear to be time wasted – this is not so; the patient who feels in control and knows about the reasons for his or her pain and the steps taken to alleviate it also has psychological relief.

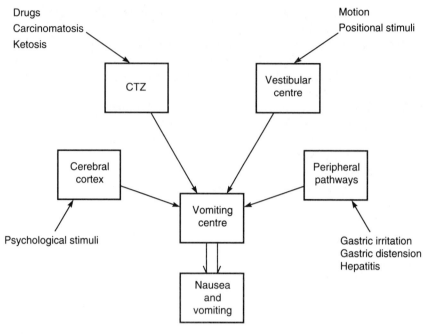

Figure 12.2   Activation pathways for nausea and vomiting.

The nurse has a responsibility to keep up to date with current research or treatments of pain and it may be applicable for him or her to take the opportunity to become proficient in some of the complementary therapies so that these treatments can be made available for patients to benefit from.

NAUSEA AND VOMITING

Nausea and vomiting are symptoms which cause enormous distress to patients with advanced cancer. Several studies have shown they are the problems patients most frequently encounter after pain (Daley and Lennard, 1991) and they occur in about one-third of patients. To facilitate the most appropriate care, the cause or mechanism responsible for nausea and vomiting has to be identified.

PHYSIOLOGY OF VOMITING

The vomiting centre is positioned in the reticular formation of the brain and receives input from:

1. The chemoreceptor trigger zone (CTZ);
2. the higher centres in the cerebral cortex;
3. the vestibular centres;
4. the peripheral pathways via the vagal nerve.

Activation of any of these sites can trigger the reflex activity that results in nausea and vomiting (Allan, 1988). Figure 12.2 shows examples of the different pathways. The CTZ is sited in the floor of the fourth ventricle and is well supplied with blood and cerebrospinal fluid. This means that emetic substances and antiemetic drugs can access the CTZ without crossing the blood–brain barrier.

CAUSES OF NAUSEA AND VOMITING

The causes of nausea and vomiting in patients who are terminally ill can usually be related to the disease, the treatment, or associated psychological distress, but is often a combination of these factors (Finlay, 1991).

Nausea and vomiting can affect patients with any type of cancer, not just those related to the gastrointestinal tract. The causes of nausea and vomiting in each of the main areas are shown in Table 12.1.

Table 12.1   The causes of nausea and vomiting

Disease		
	Gastric irritation	Gastrointestinal obstruction
	Constipation	Hepatomegaly
	Raised intracranial pressure	Squashed stomach syndrome
	Carcinomatosis	Pharyngeal stimulation
	Uraemia	Hypercalcaemia
	Hyponatraemia	
Treatment		
	Radiotherapy	Chemotherapy
	Drugs e.g. antibiotics	
	digoxin	
	carbamazepine	
	iron	
	corticosteriods	
	irritant mucolytics	
	aspirin	
Distress		
	Unpleasant sights and smells	
	Anxiety	
	Fear	

ASSESSMENT

When undertaking an assessment of the causes of nausea and vomiting, it is necessary to ascertain (Twycross and Lack, 1990):

● that the patient is actually vomiting and not just expectorating (this can be determined by applying litmus paper to the vomit);
● details of the pattern of the vomiting; for example, post-prandial vomiting occurs commonly with squashed stomach syndrome;
● evidence of raised intracranial pressure. NB: the absence of papilloedema does not always exclude raised intracranial pressure.

It may also be necessary to carry out:

● an abdominal examination;
● a rectal examination;
● a review of the current drug regime;
● a check of the patient's biochemical status; for example, plasma urea and electrolytes, plasma calcium and albumin, plasma drug levels (e.g. digoxin, carbamazepine).

Once the cause has been identified, appropriate steps can be taken to correct all reversible causes such as a cough or constipation. If nausea and vomiting persist an antiemetic needs to be considered.

CHOICE OF ANTIEMETICS

The antiemetic prescribed depends on (Twycross and Lack, 1990):

1. the cause of the nausea and vomiting;
2. the affinity with the neurotransmitter sites;
3. the preferred route of administration.

Table 12.2 illustrates some commonly used antiemetics and some indications for use.

Drugs should be given orally whenever possible. When the patient is already vomiting, it is advisable to choose an alternative route. If the patient has central access, such as a Hickman/Broviac line, this route is ideal. If there is no existing venous access, the rectal route can be used. Battery-operated syringe drivers are now widely used to administer drugs subcutaneously. This relieves patients of frequent painful injection, gives constant drug plasma levels and is technically simple.

Drugs commonly administered by a syringe driver are haloperidol, cyclizine, droperidol, metoclopramide, hyoscine and methotrimeprazine. All these drugs appear to be compatible with diamorphine for

Table 12.2   Drugs used in the treatment of nausea and vomiting

Antiemetic	Indications for use
Cyclizine	Radiotherapy to head and neck Raised intracranial pressure (RICP) Bowel obstruction Vestibular disturbances
Haloperidol Prochlorperazine Chlorpromazine Methotrimeprazine	Drug-induced vomiting Hypercalcaemia Uraemia Radiotherapy (DXT)
Metoclopramide Domperidone	Gastric stasis Oesophageal reflux
Hyoscine hydrobromide	Bonchial secretions Bowel obstruction
Octreocide	Bowel obstruction
Corticosteriods	RICP Hepatomegaly
Ondansetron Granisetron	Chemotherapy

administration by syringe driver although there have been reports of precipitation and crystallization with both cyclizine (David, 1992) and haloperidol.

Therefore, it is advisable only to infuse these drugs in low concentrations, e.g. cyclizine 25 mg/ml and haloperidol 2 mg/ml over a period of 24 hours. Metoclopramide shows evidence of degradation if infused over a period of longer than seven days (Regnard, 1987). Prochlorperazine and chlorpromazine are not suitable for subcutaneous use as they can cause skin irritation.

If an antiemetic is not working, a change of antiemetic should be considered before prescribing additional drugs. The use of corticosteroids and psychotropic drugs can also be considered. In some circumstances a single antiemetic will be unsuccessful and a combination of drugs will be necessary. Two drugs with similar actions are unlikely to be any more successful than one. However, using two antiemetics with different primary actions is more likely to give an enhanced effect.

Whilst pharmacological methods are usually necessary to control nausea and vomiting, good nursing care can do much to assist in ameliorating patients' distress.

INTESTINAL OBSTRUCTION

When nausea and vomiting are caused by intestinal obstruction it is not always possible to stop the vomiting completely. However, it is usually possible to prevent the nausea and reduce the vomiting to a level that is acceptable to the patient. It is not necessary to 'drip and suck' patients. Subcutaneous infusion of a combination of drugs, preferably via a syringe driver, will usually suffice (Twycross and Lack, 1990), for example:

- diamorphine – to control pain;
- hyoscine – to reduce colic;
- haloperidol – to prevent nausea;
- octreotide – to reduce secretions.

NURSING CARE

Provision of meals

Nurses should aim to provide small, attractively served meals which the patients want to eat. Unfortunately, many patients in hospital have to choose their meals the day before they receive them. The food they order is plated by kitchen staff who do not know how much a patient can eat. The result is that meals arrive on wards at set times with all three courses served up on the same tray! It is hardly surprising that the appetites of terminally ill patients can be non-existent and that they often push food aside. To counteract such scenarios it is vital that nursing staff involve dietitians and catering staff when planning care for terminally ill patients (Gallagher-Allred, 1991).

A choice of food is essential so that patients can avoid food which could induce nausea and vomiting. Provision should be made to store meals on the ward so that patients can eat their food when they feel like it. Only small portions should be offered, so that patients are not put off (Willans, 1980).

Taste aberration exacerbates nausea and vomiting. This can cause relatives distress when food they have lovingly prepared is rejected, and patients too often feel guilty because they are unable to tolerate the taste of the food. Situations such as this lead to an increase in anxiety, which exacerbates further the nausea and vomiting (Gallagher-Allred, 1989).

This vicious circle can be broken by nurses educating relatives about the dietary needs of the patient and advising them how to reduce taste aberrations. For example, patients with an increased threshold for sweetness can benefit from increased seasoning in their foods, and drinking cold, fizzy drinks can also be very beneficial.

Mouth care

It is essential that mouth care is offered regularly and especially after meals, to remove debris and reduce the chance of infection (Davis, 1988). Care must be given to the preparation chosen, as some patients find proprietary mouthwashes very unpleasant. Some patients may only be able to tolerate rinsing their mouths with cold water. Although not as effective as using mouthwash or toothpaste and toothbrush, it is better than no mouth care.

Patients with far advanced cancer often have ill-fitting dentures because the shape of their mouths has changed due to severe weight loss (Finlay, 1991). This can lead to sore mouths, difficulty with eating, retching and vomiting. This problem can usually be improved by referring the patients for appropriate dental treatment.

Smell

It is important that precipitating factors such as unpleasant sights and smells are identified during the nursing assessment. Many people are affected by the sights and smells that abound on hospital wards. Smells are very personal: what to one person may be a delicious aroma may be extremely nauseating to another, e.g. strong perfume, foods, cooking, air fresheners.

Mealtimes in particular can be very difficult for some patients. While screens may prevent one patient from watching another enjoying their meal, they do no prevent the sound or smell (Holmes, 1985). Side wards can provide one solution to the problem but they are not always available and patients may not want to be isolated.

Malodorous wounds can provide another potent vomiting stimulus. They are often caused by fungating tumours, which are very difficult to manage. These wounds can be tackled by giving systemic antibiotics to reduce any infection that may be contributing to the exudate.

Although often effective, antibiotics can themselves cause nausea and vomiting. An alternative method of giving these drugs is to apply them topically. Metronidazole gel has been shown to reduce odour in this way (Jones *et al.*, 1978). There are also a variety of activated charcoal dressings available which are designed to reduce odour, e.g. Actisorb (see also 'Wounds', below).

The use of complementary therapies in conjunction with traditional therapies is increasing. Aromatherapy is one therapy which can help with smells. This must be prescribed by a qualified practitioner.

Essential oils have very specific properties which can be matched to help with the problems patients are experiencing. The oils can be used topically in saline or water to irrigate fungating wounds. They can also be used effectively to alleviate nausea and vomiting.

Some essential oils can be taken orally; for example, peppermint can be very helpful for nausea. The oil can be taken in honey water by adding one drop of peppermint oil and one teaspoon of honey to one cup of water and then taken in sips every hour if necessary.

Relaxation therapy can also be beneficial in relieving nausea and vomiting. The basic principles are relatively easy to learn and can be used in almost any setting (Penson, 1991). It has been shown that if the therapist makes an audio tape using his or her voice and gives it to the patient, the benefit is increased. This is probably because the patient is familiar with the voice and can relax more easily.

Acupuncture and hypnosis are being used increasingly with drug-induced nausea and vomiting and have produced rewarding results. Homeopathic drugs can also be used to control distressing symptoms (Tschudin, 1988).

DYSPNOEA

Dyspnoea can be extremely unpleasant and frightening. It occurs in approximately 70% of patients with a bronchogenic cancer and about half of all patients with advanced cancer (Wilkes, 1984).

PHYSIOLOGY OF RESPIRATION

The respiratory centres are located in the pons and medulla of the brain. The volume of breathing is largely determined by chemoreceptors situated in the carotid artery and aortic arch, and the pattern of breathing by mechanical stimulation in the lungs relayed via the vagus nerve. Respiration is also influenced by other factors, such as:

- anxiety, fear
- anger, rage
- pyrexia
- hypercapnia
- acidosis
- profound hypoxia
- tracheobronchial irritants.

CAUSES OF DYSPNOEA

As with other symptoms, dyspnoea is often caused by multiple factors. These factors can occur as a result of the cancer, the treatment, general debility or unrelated pathology. The main causes are listed in Table 12.3.

Table 12.3   Causes of dyspnoea

Cancer	Treatment
Lymphangitis	Pneumonectomy
Superior vena caval obstruction	Fibrosis
Bronchial obstruction	Drugs e.g. bleomycin
Effusions (incl. pericardial effusion)	adriamycin
Ascites	
Abdominal distension	

Debility	Unrelated pathology
Anaemia	Chronic obstructive airways disease
Pneumonia	Heart failure
Empyema	Acidosis
Pulmonary embolism	
Atelectasis	

ASSESSMENT

Accurate assessment of the cause of the dyspnoea is vitally important. Dyspnoea which presents rapidly is often amenable to corrective therapy, e.g. infection, effusion. It is helpful to consider the following:

- Is the patient pyrexial?
- Is the patient producing sputum?
- Is the patient wheezing?

It may also be necessary to carry out:

- abdominal examination;
- chest X-ray;
- check of biochemical status, e.g. haemoglobin and white cell count, plasma, urea and electrolytes.

TREATMENT

The treatment depends very much on the cause. Whenever possible all reversible causes of dyspnoea should be treated. This very much depends on the general condition of the patient and the treatment indicated. For instance, when a patient has only a few days to live, radiation therapy for an obstructed bronchus may not be acceptable. Treatments for some reversible causes of dyspnoea are listed in Table 12.4.

Table 12.4   Treatment for reversible causes of dyspnoea

Treatment	Indications
Drugs	
Antipyrectic	Pyrexia
Antibiotics	Infections
Bronchodilators	Bronchospasm
Corticosteriods	Lymphangitis
	Bronchial obstruction
	Pericardial effusion
Diuretics	Cardiac failure
	Ascites
Digoxin	Cardiac failure
Non-drug treatments	
Abdominocentesis	Ascites
Blood transfusion	Anaemia
Radiotherapy	Bronchial obstruction
Paracentesis	Pericardial effusion
Pleural trap	Pleural effusion
Pleuradesis	

When it is not possible to treat the underlying cause symptomatic measures are necessary. These measures may also be used together with specific therapies.

Drug measures

Bronchodilators are very useful when the dyspnoea is exacerbated by reversible airway obstruction (Cowcher and Hanks, 1990). The effectiveness of bronchodilators can be assessed quickly and easily by taking peak flow measurements before and 30 minutes following treatment. Cowcher and Hanks (1990) suggest than an improvement of 15% or above indicates that the patients will derive significant benefit.

Morphine is used widely to palliate irreversible dyspnoea. The reasons why morphine relieves dyspnoea are not clear, and it would appear that there are a few mechanisms involved (Bruera *et al.*, 1990; Cowcher and Hanks, 1990). The aim of morphine therapy is to reduce dyspnoea to a level acceptable to the patient. For patients who are morphine naive a starting dose of 5 mg every four hours is usual and this can be titrated as necessary. For patients who are taking morphine for pain the dose should be increased by 50% (Twycross and Lack, 1990; Cowcher and Hanks, 1990).

Nebulized local anaesthetics such as lignocaine and bupivicaine have been used to treat dyspnoea. However, in order for these drugs to reach the alveoli, studies have shown that particles must be smaller than 0.2 nm. This can be achieved by using an ultrasonic nebulizer.

The benefits of use of benzodiazepines and phenothiazines are uncertain and studies have shown conflicting results (Cowcher and Hanks, 1990) but it would seem that benefit to some patients can be obtained because of the anxiolytic and sedative action of these drugs.

NURSING CARE

Psychological care

This symptom is very distressing and can generate a great deal of fear and anxiety, which can in turn exacerbate the symptom. In order to break this cycle a calm, reassuring attitude is invaluable. Many of the patients' fears may prove to be unfounded; however, careful explanation and continued support will help alleviate those fears that are all too realistic. Patients at home often require frequent visits to monitor progress and increase help if needed (Barnard, 1988). Both patients and their carers can derive much comfort and reassurance if they have clear and simple instructions (written if possible) telling them what to do in case of emergency.

Physical care

Careful positioning of the patient will often help. Generally patients will find the most comfortable position by themselves, often preferring to be nursed upright and well supported. If possible the patient should be encouraged to sleep on the affected side as this allows the unaffected or less affected lung to expand more fully (Robert, 1988). People who are breathless following exercise gain relief by having cold air blown on their faces. Patients who are dyspnoeic can sometimes obtain similar benefits from being in a well-ventilated room, and/or being cooled by a fan.

Nutrition and mouth care

Dyspnoeic patients often find that eating is exhausting; this can be helped by offering small, nourishing meals supplemented by dietary drinks such as Ensure and Build-up. Patients who are dyspnoeic often breathe through their mouths, which results in dryness and increased susceptibility to infection. This means that meticulous oral care is required. Fluids given in small frequent amounts will not only help combat dryness but will also replace the loss of fluid caused by rapid respiration.

Relaxation

Relaxation can be used very successfully to interrupt the cycle of anxiety and dyspnoea. When used with techniques that enhance breathing control it can increase the patient's confidence and prove to be extremely effective.

Oxygen

There is considerable debate about the use of oxygen to relieve dyspnoea. It can be useful for treating severe attacks but chronic use can increase dependence and anxiety.

CONSTIPATION

Constipation can cause much misery to dying patients. It is a very common symptom in advanced cancer and can be present in 50% of patients (Twycross and Harcourt, 1991). The treatment of constipation in advanced cancer can be more difficult than the relief of pain (Twycross and Lack, 1986).

PHYSIOLOGY OF CONSTIPATION

Nerve fibres from the autonomic branch of the nervous system supply the colon and rectum. Distension of the bowel wall stimulates the mesenteric plexus, which maintains muscle tone and initiates peristalsis and mixing contractions. Stimulation of the parasympathetic fibres increases muscle tone inside the gut, decreases tone in the sphincters and increases frequency, strength and speed of contractions. Stimulation of the sympathetic fibres results in a general decrease in peristaltic activity and an increase in sphincter tone.

Every day approximately 9 litres of fluid enters the digestive tract, approximately 2 litres is ingested fluid, the rest being secreted by salivary glands, stomach, gall bladder, pancreas and intestines. Most of this fluid is reabsorbed in the small intestine but about 1 litre enters the colon, together with undigested foodstuffs and cellular debris. The colon

Table 12.5   Causes of constipation

Disease-related	Treatment-related
Tumour affecting bowel	Drugs – opioids
Inactivity	Antiemetics
Reduced fluid intake	NSAIDs
Reduced dietary intake	Phenothiazines
Low-residue diet	Tricylic antidepressants
Dehydration	Chemotherapy – vinca alkaloids
Vomiting	
Weakness	
Inability to respond to urge to defecate	
Hypercalcaemia	
Hypokalaemia	

converts this fluid to solid stool, removing approximately 90% of the fluid by passive, osmotic absorption.

There are two main types of bowel movements:

1. segmental movements churn and mix the contents, allowing the mucosa to absorb nutrients;
2. peristaltic movements push the contents forwards.

Normally these movements are will coordinated and result in the evacuation of soft formed stools at fairly regular intervals. When the segmental movements predominate the contents are churned repeatedly but not propelled forwards, resulting in constipation (Cameron, 1992).

CAUSES OF CONSTIPATION

As with other symptoms the causes of constipation with advanced cancer can be related to the disease or to the treatment (Table 12.5).

ASSESSMENT OF CONSTIPATION

It is widely accepted in both nursing and medical literature that the normal range for bowel movement is from three stools per day to three bowel movements per week (Cimprich, 1985). Constipation is a very complex symptom and therefore using frequency of stool alone as a measurement will not usually be adequate. Other major considerations when assessing bowel functions are size, consistency and ease of passage.

It may be useful to consider:

- the presence of abdominal distension;
- the nature of bowel sounds;

- whether the stool is palpable or visible on abdominal examination;
- presence of overflow diarrhoea;
- whether the patient experiences: pain, abdominal fullness, bloating/cramping or increased flatus.

It is generally necessary to perform a rectal examination.

DRUG MANAGEMENT

Drugs used to treat constipation can be divided into different groups. The drug of choice will depend very much on the cause of the constipation. One of the most common causes of constipation in patients with advanced cancer is the use of opioid analgesia. One way that opioid drugs affect the bowel is by increasing segmental movements and decreasing peristaltic movements; this results in the faeces becoming hard and dry (Cameron, 1992). Patients taking regular opioids will therefore usually benefit from taking a stimulant laxative.

- Faecal softeners
  - docusate sodium (Dioctyl)
  - castor oil.

These act as surface wetting agents, allowing water to enter the stool, or simply lubricating the faeces. They usually take about 48 hours to have an effect.

- Bulk-forming laxatives
  - methylcellulose (Celevac)
  - ispaghula (Fybogel).

These drugs increase faecal mass, which stimulates peristalsis. They can take a few days to have an effect. They do not have any effect on hard faeces already present in the rectum.

Patients must also be able to tolerate a sufficient fluid intake to prevent an obstructing bolus being formed. It is best to avoid using bulk-forming laxatives if compression of the lumen or ulceration is suspected.

If there is a loss of colonic sensitivity, e.g. resulting from the use of opioids or vinca alkaloids, bulk laxatives may result in increased distension and discomfort without producing the necessary mechanical stimulation.

- Osmotic laxatives
  - lactulose
  - mannitol (20%).

These drugs are not absorbed from the intestines. They act by retaining or drawing water into the intestines, thus producing a liquid purge.

- Stimulant laxatives
  - senna
  - cascara
  - bisacodyl
  - danthron.

This group of drugs acts selectively on the large bowel by stimulating peristaltic movement. They should be avoided if bowel obstruction is suspected.

It has been observed that anthraquinone derivatives (e.g. senna) reverse opioid-induced constipation by directly antagonizing the effect on the large bowel without interfering with the analgesic effect. It is suggest that half a senna tablet will reverse the effects produced by 60 mg codeine and that senna should be administered in this ratio with each dose of opioid analgesic.

RECTAL MEASURES

If there is hard faeces in the rectum it is usually necessary to remove this before other measures can be successful. Suppositories such as glycerin or bisacodyl can be used or when necessary phosphate enema. If the faeces are very hard it may be necessary to use an arachis oil enema to soften the stool before using other rectal measures.

Occasionally it is necessary to perform a manual evacuation. This can be extremely distressing for the patient and sedative cover should be provided.

NURSING MEASURES

Nutrition

Much publicity has been given to the importance of eating enough dietary fibre. However, patients with advanced cancer very often have difficulty with eating a high-fibre diet because of other symptoms such as anorexia, nausea, vomiting and dysphagia. It may be possible to increase fibre content of the diet by substituting fruit juices for milky drinks, adding bran to soups and porridge, etc. If the patient can tolerate fruits, then riper, maturer fruits produce a greater effect than unripe fruit.

It is important that patients can maintain a fairly high fluid intake as this prevents fluid depletion caused by a high-fibre diet.

Some patients are unable to tolerate a high-fibre diet because of abdominal cramping, bloating and an increase in flatulence.

Dietary fibre is very complex in composition, and the physical and metabolic function of its components are not fully known. There is evidence that it may bind chemically to minerals such as iron, calcium and zinc. Therefore an excessively high-fibre diet may actually reduce available minerals and nutrients when nutritional levels are already low (Cimprich, 1985).

Exercise

Exercise increases stimulation of the bowel and the associated muscles, which may help to overcome some of the primary effects of constipation. The abdominal muscles play an important role in defecation and exercise helps to improve muscle tone. It is not necessary for the exercise to be either intense or lengthy. Simple movements such as sitting up in bed or twisting and turning in a chair can initiate changes in the mobility of the bowel (Cameron, 1992).

Environment

There are many taboos surrounding the activity of elimination, not least of which is privacy. Children learn from a very early age that elimination is a private activity. In the home, the toilet is a very private place and usually has a lockable door. When the patient becomes so ill that he or she is no longer able to get to the toilet or commode alone, difficulties often occur. Nurses and doctors begin to ask questions about their elimination habits, and to some this can be extremely embarrassing. In hospital the situation is often exacerbated as patients are obliged to use a bed-pan or commode at the bedside. Bed screens provide little privacy, as they do little to bar entry to doctors and nurses and they provide no barrier to sound or smell.

Toilet facilities should be adapted to suit the patient wherever possible; if high seats and handrails are provided patients can remain independent for as long as possible. If commodes fit over the toilet seat patients can continue to use the toilet rather than the commode at the bedside.

COMPLEMENTARY THERAPIES

Recently there has been renewed interest in the value of abdominal massage in the management of constipation. Emly (1993) describes the value of this technique in treating patients with profound disabilities and also refers to the use of abdominal massage for constipation in the elderly and for faecal leakage.

Aromatherapy can also be used to treat constipation. Tisserand (1990) suggests using 20 drops of marjoram and five drops of rose in 50 ml of base oil to be massaged into the lower back, paying particular attention to the area at either side of the spine. It should be noted, however, that massage should not be used if the patient has had recent abdominal surgery or if obstruction is suspected.

WEAKNESS

Weakness is the most common symptom experienced by those with advanced cancer. The term is used to describe many conditions and problems, and therefore in order to establish an effective line of management and treatment a careful history must be taken.

CAUSES

Drugs

A drug treatment itself may be the cause of weakness; for example, antidepressants, psychotrophic drugs or opioids.

Biochemical and haematological disorders

For example, anaemia occurs in a high proportion of patients with advanced cancer. Hypercalcaemia occurs in 10% of patients with advanced cancer (Kaye and Oliver, 1985); it is most common in primaries of the breast and bronchus.

Loss of sleep

Insomnia may be due to a number of factors all contributing to weakness; for example, emotional problems such as anxiety or depression, pain or disturbance in a noisy ward.

Altered metabolism

Metabolic changes in cancer contribute to the weakness and weight loss experienced by sufferers.

There is an increased utilization of glucose because this is the main source of energy for the tumour. The accelerated consumption of glucose also has an effect on protein and fat metabolism. The overall effect of these abnormalities is muscle wasting. Unlike the effects of starvation, where three-quarters of the weight loss is from fat and a small proportion is from muscle, in cancer patients the loss is predominantly from body muscle.

Reduced food intake

There is evidence that the altered metabolism in cancer is influenced by a reduced food intake (Bruera and MacDonald, 1988). A number of problems may cause a decreased food intake; for example, nausea and vomiting, constipation, oral thrush, loose-fitting dentures or altered taste sensation. Again, emotional factors such as depression and fear may affect appetite.

ASSESSMENT

As weakness in terminal illness may have a number of origins, a careful assessment is necessary to establish the cause for an individual case. This may involve the patient undergoing a number of investigations and procedures. A decision must be made as to how appropriate these are when considering the possible benefits and the patient's quality of life.

Drug therapy

- **Appetite stimulation.** Corticosteroids have a direct effect on appetite and are the most commonly used drug for this purpose. Some 40% of patients find benefit from this treatment.
- **Antiemetics.** Relief of nausea and vomiting contributes to an increased appetite.
- **Antidepressants and tranquillizers.** Psychological problems and insomnia may be relieved by the administration of these drugs, with a resulting increase in dietary intake.
- **Analgesia.** Pain can be a major cause of weakness due to its effects on emotion, sleep patterns and its generally exhausting nature. Appropriate analgesia is therefore important in the relief of weakness.

NURSING CARE

As diet affects the patient's degree of weakness meals are obviously an important aspect of care. For weak patients with little energy and only short concentration spans, days can be long and tedious. Meals are therefore often viewed by them as a break from the monotony. In this situation meals can help increase the patient's dietary intake and have a beneficial psychological effect.

It is important that a patient's likes and dislikes are acknowledged and that care is taken over the preparation of meals. Eating is a social activity and intake can be encouraged by company. Of course, for those who have difficulty with eating, or with swallowing and find eating with others embarrassing, a desire for privacy must be respected.

It is often helpful for patients to have a rest before a meal to ensure that they are not too tired to participate; an appetizer such as sherry may increase the appetite.

Weakness will invariably cause a decrease in the patient's activities and mobility. Care must be taken to ensure that the patient's comfort and quality of life are maintained as this occurs. For example, complications of immobility such as pressure sores must be anticipated, with assessment and preventive treatment initiated.

Progressive weakness will necessitate an increased demand for assistance in performing many activities such as washing, going to the toilet and feeding. Eventually the weakness may be so great that the patient is confined to bed and, for instance, urinary and faecal incontinence may occur.

Such deterioration in a previously independent person may cause extreme distress. This must be recognized by the practitioner with an awareness that the feelings of shame and loss of self-respect may be relieved by the manner in which assistance and care is given. Lichter (1990) recognizes that 'mobilization is the first step in motivation to enable the patient to achieve desired goals'. Thus, it is important that an optimum level of mobility for an individual is maintained for as long as possible, not only to prevent complications occurring but also to maintain the morale of the patient and relatives.

The psychological well-being of the patient must be carefully observed as the weakness creates its problems. In order to understand and accept their condition patients must be given honest explanations. Carers and relatives can work with patients to encourage acceptance of their limitations and set realistic goals. Allowing patients to discuss their situation is valuable in helping to alleviate any concerns and worries. Often alternative therapies such as massage and aromatherapy are beneficial at this time.

Weakness of some degree is inevitable for the majority of cancer patients in the advanced stages of their disease. However, many of the distressing effects can be relieved by good assessment, appropriate treatment and care.

URINARY TRACT SYMPTOMS

There are a number of urinary symptoms which may occur in the advanced stages of cancer. Often these problems can cause acute distress to the sufferer and careful appropriate management is necessary.

CAUSES

Incontinence

Lichter and Hunt (1990) found that urinary incontinence occurs in 32% of patients during the last 48 hours of life. For many it presents at a much earlier stage and some find a long period of the last months or weeks of their lives affected by this symptom, caused by the following:

- Weakness and immobility are major causes of incontinence. Loss of independence and an inability to take oneself to the toilet, to reach the urinary bottle or summon assistance will often result in incontinence.
- Urinary tract infection causing acute frequency and urgency with disturbed sensation and pain can result in incontinence.
- Constipation with faecal impaction can result in urinary incontinence either by causing an obstruction to the outflow of urine or inhibiting pelvic floor contractions.
- Many drugs have an effect on bladder function and result in urinary incontinence.
- Carcinoma of the bladder and prostate will both disrupt normal bladder functioning.
- The underlying cause of urinary incontinence is often due to damage to the delicate neurological control mechanisms which regulate the bladder; for instance, a cerebral tumour affecting the bladder centre in the cortex.
- Emotion and the psychological state can affect bladder function. Stressful situations, despair or a traumatic life event can all contribute to urinary incontinence.

Urinary retention

Retention occurs in 21% of patients with a terminal illness (Lichter and Hunt, 1990). It can be caused by the following:

- Constipation is the most common cause of retention in the elderly or debilitated. The faeces in the rectum press on the bladder, urethra and local nerves, resulting in a physical obstruction to the outflow of urine.
- A side-effect of many drugs, including phenothiazines and anti-cholinergics, can be urinary retention.
- Any tumour in the area local to the bladder, urethra and associated nerves can cause an obstruction and related retention, as can the late effects of surgery or radiotherapy in the region.

Urinary tract infection

A urinary tract infection can be asymptomatic but it can also produce many distressing problems such as incontinence, pain and fever.

- Many patients in the advanced stages of cancer will be vulnerable to infection due to their poor debilitated physical condition as a result of the disease itself, treatments or poor nutritional intake.
- The insertion of an indwelling urinary catheter creates a potential for the introduction of infection on the insertion of the catheter. Once in place infection can enter around the outside of the catheter via the urethra or up the lumen of the catheter.

Haematuria

Haematuria often causes considerable anxiety for the patient, making appropriate care imperative. There are a number of factors responsible for haematuria, such as urinary tract infection, trauma, a bladder tumour or other bleeding malignant lesions in the urinary tract.

ASSESSMENT

As assessment of the patient experiencing urinary tract symptoms should identify the cause of the problems. However, it is important to acknowledge that vigorous investigation is often not appropriate in patients with advanced cancer. Establishing and maintaining a patient's comfort is the priority at all stages of disease and therefore the following consideration should be included in the assessment:

- What is the patient's overall condition and prognosis?
- Is the patient experiencing symptoms from the problem, such as fever due to infection or pain due to retention?
- How mobile is the patient?
- Has the patient got a pressure sore which is contaminated by the urine?
- What is the patient's mental state?
- Is the patient receiving any medication which could influence bladder function?
- Is the patient constipated?

DRUG THERAPY

The causes and problems of urinary symptoms can be relieved by some drugs.

Constipation

The effects of oral aperients should be monitored in order to establish and maintain a normal bowel habit. See section on 'Constipation', above.

Urinary tract infection

An assessment should be made to establish whether the infection is causing distressing symptoms and which organism is responsible. Appropriate antimicrobials should be used to treat the infection and the patient observed carefully for side-effects of treatment such as vomiting or diarrhoea.

Haematuria

Continuous bladder irrigation with alum is useful in relieving bleeding from the bladder. To prevent symptomatic anaemia in haematuria oral iron supplements are often necessary.

Tumour obstruction

Dexamethasone may be helpful in reducing swelling in this instance.

NURSING CARE

Following a good assessment the most appropriate care to provide comfort and relief of symptoms can be prescribed.

Urinary problems are often a cause of embarrassment to the patient. Incontinence is seen as degrading and results in loss of dignity and self-respect. Thus, the way in which care is administered is very important. Norton (1986) suggests that nurses must address their own attitudes to incontinence before they can help reduce a patient's embarrassment and distress.

The environment is important for someone who is experiencing such symptoms as urinary frequency or urgency. For instance, they should have easy access to the lavatory. If their mobility is reduced, provision should be made to ensure that they have the means to call for assistance.

There is a huge range of aids and equipment to help incontinent people to manage and conceal the problem, including pads, diaper systems, penile sheaths and bed protection. Careful assessment will ensure that the most appropriate aid is used for each individual, many of whom will benefit from being involved in the choice. Norton (1986) assists this selection by giving guidelines for the criteria which incontinence aids should fulfil. They should:

● be fail-safe, i.e. contain the excreta completely and prevent leakage through to clothing or the environment at any time and under any circumstances;

- be comfortable to wear and protect vulnerable skin from soreness, chafing or pressure sores;
- be easy to use and manage by the incontinent person him- or herself, or the carer;
- disguise or control odour;
- be easily concealed under clothing, neither bulky nor noisy, and so be inconspicuous in use;
- be easy either to dispose of or wash and clean as appropriate;
- be reasonably priced and easily available.

Catheters can be of value in maintaining a patient's comfort. Fainsinger *et al.* (1992) revealed in their study that despite strictly controlled guidelines for catheter use 74% of patients still required such intervention. If there is a good indication for catheterization and it increases a patient's comfort then it should always be an option. Good catheter care, such as its insertion under aseptic conditions, use of a closed system and administration of good catheter hygiene should be observed to prevent complications occurring.

It is important that the needs of carers are also addressed. It is often very difficult for relatives to care for someone who is incontinent, not only because of the distress it causes but also the practical problems such as dealing with soiled clothes and linen. They will require support and guidance at this difficult time.

Urinary symptoms can cause acute physical problems for the person suffering from advanced cancer, together with psychological distress for both patients and their carers. There are many forms of treatment and care available at all stages of the disease which when provided in a caring, understanding manner will ensure the patient's comfort and dignity.

CONFUSION

The *Oxford English Dictionary* definition of confusion is 'throw into disorder, make unclear, bewilderment, destruction of composure'. The problems of patients with confusion can be difficult to assess and treat effectively because there are many behaviours and symptoms grouped under this one heading and all of them can have different causes or combinations of causes.

There are two basic confusional states: acute (delirium) and chronic (dementia). Acute confusion is reversible, fluctuates and is a clouding of consciousness, leading to agitation. Chronic confusion is irreversible, has a gradual onset and the consciousness is usually clear. A mixture of both can be seen in palliative care. In a study by Massie *et al.* (1983) 85% of terminally ill cancer patients were stated to suffer from delirium.

CAUSES

Two major causes of confusion can be identified in cancer patients. Direct effects – primary brain tumours and brain metastases – and indirect effects, as follows.

Drugs

Drugs used for treating pain and other symptoms may cause drowsiness; these include opioids (although this effect is unlikely if the patient has been on long-term opioid therapy), non-steroidal anti-inflammatory and corticosteroid drugs. The withdrawal of alcohol or other drugs may also cause confusion (Dunlop, 1989).

Infection

Not all patients show obvious signs or symptoms of infection and the first sign of the presence of infection may be that of confusion, especially in the elderly.

Respiratory or cardiac disease

This may have previously been known to be present but hypoxia can develop suddenly and result in confusion.

Pain from unknown trauma

The patient may have had an accident in the last few days which may have been previously undetected. For example, fracture of the neck of the femur is common in the elderly, or where bones are weakened by metastases pathological fractures can occur without the carer being aware.

Hypercalcaemia

Hypercalcaemia occurs in 5–7% of solid tumours. Confusion can be the main symptom shown by the patient (Heath, 1989).

Psychiatric illness

The patient may have a history of psychiatric illness unknown to the nurse or carer.

Problems with elimination

Constipation and urinary retention can be a cause of confusion.

ASSESSMENT

The patient may have more than one symptom and there may be several causes apparent. Assessment of the confused patient is difficult, especially as the problem can also be compounded by the anxiety of the carer to encourage an action which may be inappropriate for the type of confusion.

A careful history should be taken; this should include any previous known medical problems, including cardiac or respiratory disease, psychiatric illnesses and any trauma that has occurred recently. If possible a sample of urine should be taken to exclude infection, and a blood sample to exclude hypercalcaemia or other biochemical disturbances.

Drug therapy should be reviewed for changes in the previous few days. It is possible that some degree of confusion has been present for some time and that it has been exacerbated by changes in drugs, circumstances or conditions.

TREATMENT

If the cause of confusion can be found, then treatment should be considered although the result may not be instantaneous. A report by Bruera et al. (1992) notes that the cause of confusion can be determined for fewer than half the cases in terminally ill patients.

General supportive measures should be used, including explanations of the causes of confusion to the patient; this can lessen anxiety and worry. The presence of a relative or friend should be encouraged and attempts should be made to orientate the patient in time and place. The physical care of the patient should not be overlooked; adequate hydration and elimination need to be maintained.

Family and friends also need support at this time and it is important to maintain good communications. Explanation of the possible causes of the patient's confusion need to be given, with information on his or her management, including the use of drugs being given. Discussion of their concerns and fears and their involvement in their loved one's care will help them to be involved where appropriate.

Mutual support for the staff should be remembered; many of them will be distressed and need to know that the confusion, although it may be irreversible, can be managed.

For patients whose confusion is due to primary or secondary brain lesions, dexamethasone should be considered if not previously used.

In cases of emergency, while waiting for the results of tests to determine the specific causes of the confusion, Stiefal et al. (1992) recommend the use of midazolam to induce sedation as a safe and effective treatment for extremely agitated patients.

Drugs should only be used if symptoms cause distress to the patient and family and all possible avenues have been followed to detect the cause of the confusion:

- diazepam 5–10 mg orally or per rectum if agitated;
- haloperidol 1.5–15 mg orally or by intramuscular injection if hallucinating or paranoid and if diazepam fails to relieve agitation;
- chlorpromazine 25–100 mg orally or chlormethiazole intramuscularly if alcohol withdrawal is suspected and for very elderly patients.

The symptoms of confusion often can only be controlled by sedation. However, Fainsinger and Bruera (1992) note that Cicely Saunders stated in 1988 that this may not be the option preferred by patients and their families. Nevertheless agitated, restless patients can be a danger to themselves and to others.

Medication can only be of benefit if used appropriately as part of the overall care plan. We must consider who is going to benefit from the treatment: the patient or the staff and the family (see also Chapter 10).

Throughout, good communication is important; explanation of causes and aims of treatment should be discussed with all those involved.

WOUNDS

For those who are suffering from advanced cancer a wound may create disturbing symptoms. Foltz (1980), Sims and Fitzgerald (1985), Wells (1984) and Ivetic and Lyne (1990) all acknowledge the lack of research and published work on the management of wounds in the terminally ill, particularly in relation to fungating and ulcerating lesions. Rosen (1980) accounts for this by explaining that the condition is seen as being uncommon. Accurate data on the incidence of these wounds are lacking. However, despite the unknown incidence it is clear that the effects of a wound on the individual patient can be devastating:

> Can we begin to imagine what it must be like for a patient to see part of his body rotting and to have to live with the offensive smell of it, see the reaction of his visitors (including doctors and nurses) and know that it signifies lingering death? (Doyle, 1980)

These wounds are complex and their treatment must be adapted from the basic principles and practices generally accepted for wound care; this is necessary to alleviate and minimize distress.

CAUSES

The causes of wounds in the terminally ill may be the direct result of malignancy or be caused indirectly by treatment or general debility.

- **Direct causes.** Cancerous infiltration of the epithelium may occur at the site of the primary neoplasm or at a secondary site due to metastases.
- **Indirect causes.** Weakness and immobility resulting in pressure sores, skin breakdown following radiotherapy, surgical incisions and breakdown of wounds and stomas due to deterioration in the patient's condition are possible.

ASSESSMENT

It is essential that the wound is assessed in order to prescribe and implement the most appropriate care and to monitor progress. The assessment should not simply address the physiological state of the wound but should also include other aspects of the patient's physical and psychosocial condition.

Factors to be assessed

1. **Cause of the wound.** Can the cause be removed or relieved, for example by initiating pressure area care and using pressure-relieving aids in the case of a pressure sore?
2. **Site of the wound.** Is the site accessible to treatment, for example wounds in the vagina or mouth? Does the site interfere with other bodily activities or functions, like a sacral or glutial lesion which is contaminated during elimination or prevents the patient from sitting down?
3. **Wound dimensions.** Wound measurements should be taken and recorded on initial assessment and at regular intervals thereafter. These should include length, depth and breadth of the wound, the quantities of granulating tissue, slough and necrosis as well as the condition of the surrounding skin.

   Diagrams of the wound may be produced during the assessment, which can be facilitated by the use of dressings such as the OpSite Flexigrid or other transparent materials which allow a tracing of the wound to be made. The assessment could also include a photograph, to be kept in the record.
4. **Pain.** This should include the site, nature, intensity and frequency of pain associated with the wound, including pain caused by positioning for dressing changes. The cause of each pain should be defined; for example, infection, applications for debridement or tight bandaging.
5. **Discharge and odour.** What type of discharge is present – is it blood, serous fluid, excreta or pus? How much fluid is there; how quickly are dressings soaked? Does the wound smell, is this noticeable all the time or just when dressings are changed? Does it upset the patient or his or her visitors?

6. **Infection.** Are there any indications of pathological infection, for example inflammation, exudate, smell? All large surface wounds will have a bacterial population; this is not necessarily a problem.

TREATMENT CONSIDERATIONS IN PALLIATIVE CARE

Having assessed the wound there are a number of other factors to be considered before initiating treatment for wounds in advanced cancer.

1. **Time.** The patient's prognosis may limit the time available to produce a result. Is it realistic to consider that the wound can be healed; what can be achieved considering the prognosis? Sims and Fitzgerald (1985) reported that some of their patients survived for longer than two years in spite of extensive lesions. For these patients a good ongoing plan is very important.
2. **Comfort.** Is the wound or the treatment causing pain? Can the wound pain be reduced by treatment, or if it is increased, is it worth the pain it causes?
3. **Cost.** The cost of wound treatment in the palliative care setting should be of no greater or lesser significance than in any other area of care. However, product availability in the hospice or community setting must also be considered.
4. **Psychosocial.** Decisions on wound treatment must address psychological and social issues as well as physical problems. These include changed body image, relationships and sexuality, social isolation and the fact that the wound is a permanent reminder of illness and approaching death.

WOUND MANAGEMENT

The symptoms caused by wounds are considered here individually and some recommendations made for care. Many wounds create a number of symptoms at one time, thus treatments must be selected carefully for their effect on all the symptoms. Choice should, where possible, be based on research and a full understanding of how the treatment works. In the words of Richard Wells (1984): 'Nurses should be the prescribers of wound care and, as with all other aspects of care, such prescriptions should be based on knowledge.'

The management of wounds involves cleaning, therapeutic applications, secondary dressings and materials used to keep them in place. It is now generally accepted that the wound surface should be kept moist and be treated gently. Dressings can be soaked off in the bath or shower and the wound cleaned by irrigation or swabbing with a gloved hand rather than with forceps. Harsh fluids and antiseptics have little advantage over large amounts of water or saline when it comes to removing slough, exudate and liquefied dressings. Specific problems in the management of wounds in the terminally ill are dealt with below.

Pain

1. **Environment.** Depending on the site of the wound, positioning and environment can often contribute to the relief of pain caused by a wound; for example, the use of a pressure-relieving mattress or cushion can relieve the pain of a sacral sore or wound on the back or leg.

   Support and comfortable positioning and the encouragement of relaxation can reduce stress during dressing changes.

2. **Drugs.** Antibiotics are often considered to be inappropriate in the treatment of patients with advanced cancer. However, if a wound infection is causing pain their use should remain an option.

   The administration of appropriate analgesia following a full assessment should relieve pain experienced due to a wound, although this may not be sufficient to control pain during dressings. This pain may result in considerable distress and anxiety to the patient and family while they wait for the impending procedure. The administration of short-acting top-up analgesia is beneficial prior to or during redressing.

   For example, dextromoramide (Palfium), which can be given orally or subcutaneously, lasts for two to three hours. Nitrous oxide 50% with oxygen (Entonox) can be administered by inhalation to appropriate patients (Pritchard and Mallett, 1992).

3. **Dressings.** Occlusive dressings can reduce the amount of oxygen at the wound surface. A lack of oxygen interferes with the synthesis of inflammatory mediators such as prostaglandins which cause pain. Occlusion can therefore reduce pain, particularly if the dressing is left undisturbed. It is useful to consider the frequency of dressing change and reduce this to a minimum for patients in the terminal phase of their illness.

4. **Dressing attachment.** When the skin around the wound is sore, dressings can be held in place by garments such as cotton vests or elasticated bandages such as Netelast. This avoids repeated use of tapes.

   Foam dressings such as Silastic foam can reduce pain by supporting the wound and protecting it from further damage. Time and interference are also reduced and more time can be spent caring for the patient's psychological needs (Bale and Harding, 1987).

Necrosis and slough

1. **Surgery.** Surgical debridement of a wound can be very effective. Symptoms such as malodour and discharge can be relieved, and tissue healing commences sooner than when debridement takes place by other methods. Before a decision is made to undertake surgical debridement, careful consideration must be made of the patient's prognosis, physical condition to tolerate surgery and the overall aims of the procedure.

2. **Enzymes.** Enzymes are relatively fast debriding agents but are expensive. The most common is Varidase – a combination of streptodornase, which liquefies pus, and streptokinase, which activates fibrinolysis – it can be applied in a variety of ways:
   - injected into a necortic scab;
   - on the surface as a gauze soak;
   - into cavities or on the surface as a jelly made by reconstituting one vial with 5 ml sterile water and mixing the solution with 15 ml K-Y Jelly or Scherisorb gel;
   - for packing loosely into cavities, alginate ribbons or rope is soaked in Varidase solution.

3. **Hydrogels.** Hydrogels have a starch polymer matrix which swells to absorb moisture. Applied to necrosis or slough they act by hydrating and softening the slough, which then separates from the wound bed. This process is slow but atraumatic.

Haemorrhage

Bleeding from a wound is frightening to patient and carer alike; however, it is usually not life threatening. Regnard (1992) states: 'Haemorrhage is the cause of death in approximately 6% of patients with advanced cancer. However, in those patients catastrophic, external haemorrhage is less common than internal bleeding.' Dressings which stick should be avoided.

1. **Adrenaline.** Adrenaline is applied topically in a concentration of 1:1000 as a gauze soak. It acts as a vasoconstrictor and is usually applied to highly vascular fungating wounds.

2. **Alginates.** Alginate (seaweed) dressings have a high concentration of calcium ions; these activate the clotting cascade. These dressings also have the benefit of liquefying on the wound and can be removed by irrigation, thus reducing trauma and further bleeding.

3. **Trenoxamic acid.** This can be used topically or administered systemically; it acts by inhibiting the breakdown of fibrin.

4. **Sucralfate paste.** Applied in K-Y Jelly (one tablet dissolved in 5 ml jelly) alum binds to fibrin to prevent its removal.

Malodour

1. **Activated charcoal dressings.** An activated charcoal layer in the dressing absorbs odour and some dressings appear to absorb bacteria. In dressings with silver chemically bound to the carbon (Actisorb plus) the silver helps reduce odour by inhibiting bacterial growth in the dressing (Morgan, 1990).
2. **Antibiotics.** Infection with anaerobic bacteria is a common cause of malodour; this can be treated with metonidazole either systemically or locally as pessaries, and Metrotop, the topical gel (Newman, 1989).
3. **Alginates.** The gel formed on the wound surface when alginates are used may act as a barrier, containing the molecules responsible for the smell and preventing their passage to the external environment. Some alginates (Kaltocarb) also have an activated carbon layer.
4. **Non-conventional products.** Sugar has been used for centuries in wound care. The sugar and honey may exert an antibacterial effect by competing for the water present in the bacterial cells (Morgan, 1990).

    Live yoghurt, buttermilk and baking soda are believed to work by altering the exudate pH; this inhibits the growth of bacteria.

Exudate

1. **Hydrogels.** A starch matrix of hydrogels (Scherisorb) absorbs excess exudate and produces a moist environment over the surface.
2. **Hydrocolloids.** The hydrocolloid dressings (Granuflex, Comfeel) absorb exudate, liquefy, swell and press on the base of the wound, thus encouraging granulation.
3. **Alginates.** An alginate (Sorbsan, Kaltostat) can absorb 20 times its own weight. In so doing it liquefies and can be washed out of the wound with saline.
4. **Foam.** Foam dressings (Lyofoam, Allevyn, Silastic) absorb exudate and protect the wound. As they do not liquefy they are more useful in places where there is outside pressure which might cause leakage.
5. **Stoma products.** Where exudate is excessive and cannot be contained by dressings, stoma wafers and bags or wound managers will contain the fluid and disguise the smell. Barrier creams will be needed to protect the skin.

A wound can create many distressing symptoms and therefore the appropriate management of wounds within palliative care is necessary to improve the quality of a person's life. There are many treatments available to relieve the symptoms, some of which have been discussed here. However, new products are appearing all the time, thus the practitioner must ensure that when prescribing wound care the decisions are based on up-to-date knowledge, with an improvement in the patient's quality of life being the main objective.

CONCLUSION

The overall aim of palliative care should be to maximize the quality of the patient's life within the limits imposed by the disease. It is important that the quality of life aimed for is defined by the patient. The nursing care of patients with advanced cancer who are experiencing multiple distressing symptoms is not simple. Although often described as basic care it requires assessment, planning, intervention and evaluation by skilled and motivated staff. The multidisciplinary approach to care is the most effective way of providing a service to patients which alleviates their symptoms and reduces their distress.

Throughout, the patient is seen as an individual within the community and family. Friends and carers are part of the patient's world and as such must be part of the caring team.

REFERENCES

Allan, S.G. (1988) Emesis in the patient with advanced cancer. *Palliative Medicine*, **2**, 90–100.

Baillie, L. (1993) A review of pain assessment tools. *Nursing Standard*, 7(23), 25–9.

Bale, S. and Harding, K. (1987) Fungating breast wounds. *Journal of District Nursing*, 5(12), 4–5.

Barnard, N. (1988) Nursing the patient in the community, in *Nursing the Patient with Cancer* (ed. V. Tschudin), Prentice Hall, London.

Bruera, E. and MacDonald, R.N. (1988) Nutrition in cancer patients: an update and review of our experience. *Journal of Pain and Symptom Management*, **3**, 133–40.

Bruera, E., Macmillan, R.N., Pither, R.T. and MacDonald, R.N. (1990) Effects of morphine on the dyspnoea of terminal cancer patients. *Journal of Pain and Symptom Management*, 5(6), 341–4.

Bruera, E., Miller, M., McCallion, J. *et al.* (1992) Congestive failure in patients with terminal cancer: a prospective study. *Journal of Pain and Symptom Management*, 7(4), 192–5.

Cameron, C. (1992) Constipation related to narcotic therapy. *Cancer Nursing*, 15(5), 372–7.

Cimprich, B. (1985) Symptom management: constipation. *Cancer Nursing*, **8** (Suppl.) 1, 39–43.

Cowcher, K. and Hanks, G.F. (1990) Long term management of respiratory symptoms in advanced cancer. *Journal of Pain and Symptom Management*, 5(5), 320–30.

Daley, A.G. and Lennard, R.F. (1991) Training for palliative medicine. 1: A survey of professional opinion. *Palliative Medicine*, 5, 295–302.

David, J.A. (1992) A survey of the use of syringe drivers in Marie Curie Centres. *European Journal of Cancer Care*, 1(4), 23–8.

Davis, S. (1988) Head and neck cancer, in *Nursing the Patient with Cancer* (ed. V. Tschudin), Prentice Hall, London.

Doyle, D. (1980) Domicillary terminal care. *The Practitioner*, 224(1344), 575–82.

Dunlop, R.J. (1989) Is terminal restlessness sometimes drug induced? *Palliative Medicine*, 3, 65–6.

Emly, M. (1993) Abdominal massage. *Nursing Times*, 89(3), 34–6.

Fainsinger, R.L. and Bruera, E. (1992) Treatment of delirium in a terminally ill patient. *Journal of Pain and Symptom Management*, 7(1), 54–6.

Fainsinger, R.L., MacEacheran, T., Hanson, J. and Bruera, E. (1992) The use of urinary catheters in terminally ill cancer patients. *Journal of Pain and Symptom Management*, 7(6), 333–8.

Finlay, I. (1991) The management of other frequently encountered symptoms, in *Palliative Care for People with Cancer* (eds J. Penson and R. Fisher), Edward Arnold, London.

Foltz, A.T. (1980) Nursing care of ulcerating metastatic lesions. *Oncology Nursing Forum*, 7(2), 8–13.

Gallagher-Allred, C.R. (1989) *Nutritional Care of the Terminally Ill*. Aspen, Rockville, MD.

Gallagher-Allred, C.R. (1991) Nutritional care of the terminally ill patient and family, in *Palliative Care for People with Cancer* (eds J. Penson and R. Fisher), Edward Arnold, London.

Heath, D.A. (1989) Hypercalcaemia of malignancy. *Palliative Medicine*, 3, 1–11.

Holmes, S. (1985) Catering for the patient. *Nursing Times*, 81(28), 27–9.

Ivetic, O. and Lyne, P.A. (1990) Fungating and ulcerating malignant lesions: a review of the literature. *Journal of Advanced Nursing*, 15(1), 83–8.

Jones, P.H., Willis, A.T. and Ferguson, I.R. (1978) Treatment of anaerobically infected pressure sores with metronidazole. *Lancet*, i, 214.

Kaye, D.M. and Oliver, D.J. (1985) Hypercalcaemia in advanced malignancy. *Lancet*, i, 512.

Keela, A. and Mobily, P. (1992) Interventions related to pain. *Nursing Clinics of North America*, 27(2), 347–69.

Lichter, I. (1990) Weakness in terminal illness. *Palliative Medicine*, 4, 73–80.

Lichter, I. and Hunt, E. (1990) The last 48 hours of life. *Journal of Palliative Care*, 6, 7–15.

Massie, M.J., Holland, J. and Glass, E. (1983) Delirium in terminally ill cancer patients. *American Journal of Psychiatry*, 140, 1048–50.

McCaffery, M. (1972) *Nursing Management of the Patient with Pain*. Lippincott, Philadelphia.

Morgan, D.A. (1990) *Formulary of Wound Management Products*. Academic Pharmacy Practice Unit, Mold, Clwyd.

Newman, V. (1989) Metronidazole gel to control the smell of maloderous lesion. *Palliative Medicine*, 3, 303–5.

Norton, C. (1986) *Nursing for Continence*. Beaconsfield Publishers, Beaconsfield.

Penson, J. (1991) Complementary therapies, in *Palliative Care for People with Cancer* (eds J. Penson and R. Fisher), Edward Arnold, London.

Pritchard, A.P. and Mallett, J. (1992) *Manual of Clinical Nursing Procedures*. Blackwell Scientific Publications, Oxford.

Regnard, C. (1987) Nausea and vomiting: a flow diagram. *Palliative Medicine*, 1, 62–3.

Regnard, C. (1992) Management of bleeding in advanced cancer: a flow diagram. *Palliative Medicine*, 6, 74–8.

Roberts, W. (1988) Tumours of the chest, in *Nursing the Patient with Cancer* (ed. V. Tschudin), Prentice Hall, London.

Rosen, T. (1980) Cutaneous metastases. *Medical Clinics of North America*, 64(5), 885–900.

Sims, R. and Fitzgerald, V. (1985) *Community Nursing Management of Patients with Ulcerating/Fungating Malignant Breast Disease*. RCN Oncology Nursing Society, London.

Stiefal, F., Fainsinger, R. and Bruera, E. (1992) Acute confusional states in patients with advanced cancer. *Journal of Pain and Symptom Management*, 7(2), 94–8.

Tisserand, M. (1990) *Aromatherapy for Women*. Thorsons, London.

Tschudin, V. (1988) Complementary therapies, in *Nursing the Patient with Cancer* (ed. V. Tschudin) Prentice Hall, London.

Twycross, R.G. and Harcourt, J.M.T. (1991) The use of laxatives at a palliative care centre. *Palliative Medicine*, 5, 27–33.

Twycross, R.G. and Lack, S.A. (1986) *Control of Alimentary Symptoms in Far Advanced Cancer*. Churchill Livingstone, Edinburgh.

Twycross, R.G. and Lack, S.A. (1989) *Oral Morphine in Advanced Cancer*. Beaconsfield Publishing, Beaconsfield.

Twycross, R.G. and Lack, S.A. (1990) *Therapeutics in Terminal Cancer*. Churchill Livingstone, Edinburgh.

Twycross, R.G. and Lack, S.A. (1991) *Oral Morphine Information for Patients, Families and Friends*. Beaconsfield Publishing, Beaconsfield.

Walker, V.A., Dicks, B. and Webb, P. (1987) Pain charts in the management of chronic cancer pain. *Palliative Medicine*, 1, 111–16.

Wall, P.D. and Melzack, R. (1989) *Textbook of Pain*. Churchill Livingstone, Edinburgh.

Wells, R.J. (1984) Conroversial issues in wound care: infection control in hospital and community. *Nursing* 2(26) (Suppl.), 10–11.

Willans, J.H. (1980) Appetite in the terminally ill patient. *Nursing Times*, 76(20), 875–6.

Wilkes, E. (1984) Dying now. *Lancet*, i: 950–2.

World Health Organization (1986) *Cancer Pain Relief*. WHO, Geneva.

FURTHER READING

Cherry, D.A. and Gourlay, G.K. (1987) The spinal administration of opioids in the treatment of acute and chronic pain. *Palliative Medicine*, 1, 89–106.

Clark, A.J., Simpson, K.H. and Ellis, F.R. (1990) Continuous brachial plexus block in the management of intractable cancer pain in the arm. *Palliative Medicine*, **4**, 123–5.

David, J.A. (1986) *Wound Management: A Comprehensive Guide to Dressing and Healing*. Martin Dunitz, London.

Doyle, D., Hanks, G.W. and MacDonald, N. (eds) (1993) *Oxford Textbook of Palliative Medicine*. Oxford University Press, Oxford.

Laird, D. and Lovel, T. (1993) Paradoxical pain. *Lancet*, **341**, 241.

Stedeford, A. and Regnard, C. (1991) Confusional states in patients with advanced cancer: a flow diagram. *Palliative Medicine*, **5**, 256–61.

Thompson, J. and Regnard, C. (1992) Managing pain in advanced cancer. *Palliative Medicine*, **6**, 329–35.

Torrence, C. (1983) *Pressure Sores: Aetiology, Treatment and Prevention*. Croom Helm, Beckenham.

Twycross, R.G. and Lack, S.A. (1983) *Symptom Control for Advanced Cancer: Pain Relief*. Pitman, London.

13 Caring for the dying patient in the community

Christine Searle

INTRODUCTION

THE AUTHOR'S ANALOGY OF A PATIENT REQUIRING PALLIATIVE CARE

Imagine the National Health Service as a large busy factory with doctors, nurses, paramedics and others busily working to put back together those human beings who have come apart physically, mentally or both. As in most factories there is a conveyor belt carrying the completed product along to despatch, out into the community, to function within society as whole healthy beings.

The factory also has a second conveyor belt – 'a reject belt' – along which would travel those human beings who have been subjected to multilating surgery, horrendous chemotherapy and radiotherapy by the health service's professionals in an effort to get rid of the relentless disease. But the efforts have failed, the disease has taken over and these broken human beings travel along the reject belt feeling helpless and rejected.

Often they have been the focus of long discussions with medical or surgical teams using professional jargon and where diagnoses are given, adding to their fear and hopelessness. Most of these people will eventually return to their homes and be cared for by the significant others in their lives.

Research shows us that most people, when given the choice, would prefer to die in their own home, but instead of this deaths from terminal conditions, such as advanced cancer, still happen more frequently in a hospital or hospice. A good example is a research study by Townsend *et al.* (1990) which aimed to assess the preference of terminally ill patients with cancer for their place of final care. Townsend approached 98 patients (randomly and prospectively), of these 84 (86%) agreed to be interviewed at intervals ranging from two weeks to two months depending on their prognosis. Seventy patients died during the study and of these 59 (84%) had stated a preferred place for their final care. Given existing circumstances, 34 (58%) of these 59 wished to die at home, 12 in hospital, 12 in a hospice, and one elsewhere. 'Their own home' turned out to be the actual place for 17 (50%) who stated it to be their preferred place, whereas of the 32 patients who died in hospital 22 (69%) had stated a preference to die elsewhere. Had their home circumstances been different 41 (69%) of the 59 would have preferred to die at home, 10 (16%) in hospital, and 9 (15%) in a hospice.

The conclusion drawn from this study was that with a limited increase in community care 50% more patients with cancer could be supported to die at home, as they and their carers would prefer.

The results quoted above are typical of most of the research which has been undertaken to determine patients' preferences for their place of death and figures for the actual place that death occurred. There is an increasing trend away from the community setting towards hospitals as the place of death.

The practical aspects of nursing patients requiring palliative care until death within their own environment will differ subject to the availability of resources and the quality of professionals. There is little or no continuity in the availability of services throughout the UK. Recent government legislation is intended to improve patient care in the community by creating a new strategy between the social services and medical and nursing services. The value of this has yet to be demonstrated. However, one hopes that nursing expertise and research-based practice will allow scope for the continual development of palliative care services in the community.

This chapter will discuss the expectations of patients with a life-threatening condition such as advanced cancer who wish to remain at home until they die, the obstacles which may arise in the home setting and how the health care professional can help to prevent these.

These problems and some possible solutions will be considered from the perspective of:

- the patient who is dying;
- the significant others to that patient;
- the professional caring for the patient.

THE PERSPECTIVE OF A PATIENT WHO IS DYING AT HOME

Patterson (1977) talks about a 'crisis of knowledge of death'; this is when patients are faced with certain impending death. Often problems start at this point for patients and when, where and how the bad news or diagnosis is given will have significant implications for the patient's perception of the life that is left. In Stedeford's (1984) framework of care the most common problems of the dying person are:

- communication problems;
- direct effect of the disease and treatment;
- adjustment reactions to enforced changes in role;
- pre-existing social and psychological problems.

This framework is a useful basis for illustrating the patient's problems in relation to dying in the community.

COMMUNICATION PROBLEMS

It is important that the nurse is aware of the possible communication problems for patients and carers in the community setting. These are affected by the closeness of the family, both physically and emotionally, long-standing loyalties and grudges as well as the problems of collusion and protection. For the visiting nurse this is a minefield, particularly when having to pass on important information and instructions for care. Help in finding solutions to these problems will be found in Chapters 9 and 10.

DIRECT EFFECT OF THE DISEASE AND TREATMENT

Physical disability is as insidious as the progress of the disease and the patient may first notice this when getting about the home becomes increasingly difficult. A skilled assessment of the environment is essential (Figure 13.1).

A study of the ergonomics of the home can lead to rearrangements of the furniture and activities which can often make life easier; for example, making a bedroom downstairs so that the patient can live on one level, or providing a chemical toilet or commode will make toileting easier. Raised toilet seats and wall rails in the bathroom and on stairs give support. An assessment of each room in the house should be made and the occupational therapist be consulted as early as possible about the need for alterations and equipment. Bringing in medical comforts and aids can alter the patient's perception of his or her changing life and the disease process. It is best to introduce them before the situation becomes desparate to 'conserve the patient's energy' rather than make them feel like an invalid.

A selection of medical aids and comforts can be obtained from:

- social services;
- local hospices;

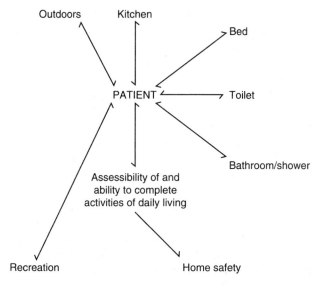

Outdoors Kitchen

Bed

PATIENT   Toilet

Bathroom/shower

Assessibility of and
ability to complete
activities of daily living

Recreation   Home safety

Figure 13.1   Areas of the environment to be assessed.

- some charity organizations provide equipment or help with finance to buy it;
- most large chemists stock a variety of medical comforts.

Maintaining patients' independence in the home can help support them physically and psychologically, maintaining their self-esteem and dignity. Much can be done to enhance the patient's independence within the home. Often, hand in hand with diminishing mobility goes an increase in pain and other physical symptoms. The control and treatment of these symptoms should be possible through the primary health care team; the control of specific symptoms is covered in Chapter 12, and specialist nurses and doctors are often able to undertake domiciliary visits to offer advice on symptom control.

Nursing patients in their own home environment lends itself to a very different philosophy of care from that in hospital. The relationship of the patient with the nurse and other professional agencies becomes territorial. The patient is the controller of the environment and this can have favourable or unfavourable implications. It should always be remembered that the patient may refuse entry to professional agencies to the home at any time. This may be only temporary due to inconvenience but some patients have real fears (hopefully irrational) about the motives for the visit.

For example, the patient may feel afraid that the intrusion of outsiders will change the status quo by advising their admission to a hospital or hospice. Once recognized, the solution to this is to safeguard the patient's needs to feel safe and in control by making sure that he or she knows there will never be undue pressure to make quick decisions about where or by whom care will be provided.

Refusal of entry can also be the result of a genuine clash of personalities. Patients cannot like every home visitor and if there is obvious antagonism between home visitor and patient it is best that another person takes on the responsibility for care, rather than persist and cause additional distress to the patient.

It must also be appreciated that the patient may resent visits at certain times. Home visitors often visit at personally inconvenient times. We should consider how many of us would like a stranger to enter the room whilst we were eating a meal or sitting there while we tried to have a telephone conversation. This can be even more irritating if we know they are anxious to 'give us an injection' or 'get on to the next patient'. The patient will respond more favourably if asked which time of day should be avoided and which would be the best for visiting. Allowing the patient to control the situation will enhance rapport and the development of a good relationship.

Patients who are dying of a life-threatening condition such as advanced cancer are extremely vulnerable even within the confines of their own home. For example, consider the feelings of Margaret, who had been diagnosed six months previously with ovarian cancer. She had deteriorated rapidly but was making that almost super-human determined effort that dying patients do, to remain as independent and 'normal' as possible. She was well supported by a loving family and an excellent palliative care team. As a Macmillan nurse herself, Margaret was aware of her physical deterioration, and symptoms such as the copious vomiting and the increasing gross oedema of both legs was slowing down her fight. One evening she was being attended by two nurses (not her usual team) and they were discussing another patient who had a similar condition to Margaret's. They mentioned that her oedema had become so gross that it took four nurses to lift her.

After they left Margaret became depressed and told her family that she would have to go into the hospital or hospice as she could not possibly be such a burden to them or the nurses (knowing herself how busy the community nurses can be). This thoughtlessness on behalf of the nurses caused distress and depression to Margaret, who desperately wanted to remain at home to die, and it took a major effort on behalf of the family and other professionals to assure her that caring for her at home would not be problematic.

This example demonstrates just how damaging a thoughtless or flippant conversation can be to the vulnerable patient who is dying at home and how it caused this women to make an irrational decision to be admitted to a hospice or hospital.

Other unfavourable situations encountered when nursing the dying patient at home rather than in hospital are often due to a lack of or the inaccessibility of resources and equipment. For example, if a patient suddenly becomes incontinent at home there is an urgent need to protect the furniture; disposable protection is not immediately obtainable. The solution is to improvise until proper equipment is available. In this situation large plastic bin liners can usually be found and these taped together will form adequate bed or chair protection of a temporary nature. Cut cardboard boxes make excellent bed cradles and book-rests. One needs to be resourceful, and equipment can often be rigged up temporarily which can make all the difference to the patient's comfort and which will allow him or her to remain at home instead of making a panic admission into a hospice or hospital. These temporary measures can also help the patient towards accepting aids which will help maintain independence. Pride may prevent the use of a Zimmer frame but having found how useful a light chair is to improve balance or getting around, the idea of a purpose-made support becomes less daunting. Patients are so vulnerable that they allow decisions to be made for them, often to take the pressure off their carers or professional helpers, and may accept admission rather than being a nuisance.

PROBLEMS ENCOUNTERED WHEN CARING FOR A DYING PATIENT AT HOME

The patient who is dying at home from advanced cancer will be passing through a series of changes, both physical and emotional. The environment – his or her home – is probably the only familiar aspect left in the patient's life at this point. To enable him or her to remain within this familiar environment until death is a right. Potential hurdles often crop up and it is the aim of the professional carer to anticipate these and avoid them (Table 13.1).

The patient who is at home, dying of advanced cancer, can feel faced with seemingly insurmountable problems which can result in inappropriate and unnecessary admission to hospital or a hospice. It should be possible for patients to die in their own home if this is their wish. The study of Townsend *et al.* (1990) indicates that the majority of patients would wish to die at home 'if circumstances were more favourable'. Favourable circumstances for home care require:

- knowledgeable support form a multiskilled team;
- access to equipment and aids;
- favourable and knowledgeable communication between the patient, professional and carer.

Patients' attitudes to themselves and their surroundings change as the disease progresses. The dilemma of the desire to remain in their familiar

Table 13.1   Problems encountered when nursing the dying patient at home and possible solutions

Possible problems	Possible solutions
Room size Furniture Toilet availability day/ night Steps/stairs Loose rugs, wires	Very careful and tactful suggestions such as moving rooms and furniture around for safety and easier access Problems with steps/stairs can be overcome by adding ramps and handrails or by changing the use of a room Sudden drastic changes in surroundings can be as disorientating as admission to hospital
Toileting	Medical comforts such as commodes, chemical toilets, raised toilet seats, handrails, female bedpans and urinals
Bathing/showering	Bathing stools can be used in showers and overtap rails used in the bath Remember that sudden drastic changes are not conducive to the patient's perception of their illness
Sitting	There are many aids available for making existing chairs easier to sit in and easier to get out of. A chair which is too low can be raised on blocks or large firm bricks. Ejector pillows can assist with getting up from a chair
Resting in the day	A well-padded, well-sprung sun-lounger can make a comfortable daytime recliner that is easily stowed away. Bean bags are a good support if positioning is difficult
Getting into bed/ Comfort in bed	Beds can be raised in the same way as chairs. Some organizations and health authorities will provide special beds. Many modern pressure-relieving mattresses can be used on the standard divan, as can over-mattress pads (Pritchard and Mallett 1992, p. 525). Here consideration must be given to the patient's partner. Whisking away the matrimonial bed of some 30 years standing to replace it with a single electrically operated all 'mod cons' can be, to say the least, traumatic
Telephone inaccessible or too quiet	Most areas in the home are able to have extra telephone points fitted and telephones can have louder ringing tones attached for those with hearing difficulties. Mobile phones can be a great asset
Concerned neighbours, friends and visitors	Concerned neighbours and friends who insist on visiting throughout the day can be tiring for the patient and this can sometimes be one of the biggest disadvantages of being at home. The patient can be advised to have a period of rest each day and the visitors can be told about this without giving offence. This type of routine will be respected and avoids stress and strain for the patient
Family collusion	If the patient and carers are not open about the diagnosis and prognosis there can be continuous added stress for both. It often causes the patient to become introverted and alienated from loved ones, family and friends. These are communication problems which may need the intervention of skilled professionals to help both patient and carer to cope

Table 13.1   contd

Possible problems	Possible solutions
Eating and drinking	Patients who are uninterested in food and eating can be persuaded to add calories by using any of the variety of high-calorie drinks which are available. There are many ways of making these attractive and more appetizing: presenting a drink in a small wine glass with cocktail decorations, rather than in the carton with a straw; small meals presented on small tea plates rather than on big dinner plates with garnishes; and the preparation of 'normal meals' which are high calorie (Shaw and Hunter, 1991); all these will hopefully stimulate the patient's interest in food. Over-anxious relatives can put pressure on patients to eat, which can exacerbate the problem. Often favourite meals which have been lovingly prepared can be rejected, causing distress to both patient and carer. Explanations for the sudden change in desire and how both disease and drugs can affect appetite are necessary to defuse the situation and help support the carer
Enteral feeding	For some individuals enteral feeding may be considered. The decision would be made with medical advice and only if overall quality of the patient's life could be enhanced by increasing calorie intake
Dehydration	Reducation in fluid intake can cause constipation and dehydration. It is helpful for the patient if small, regular drinks are encouraged. At home fluid intake is often better controlled than in hospital, where drinks are offered at set times rather than at home, where the kettle is always on the boil. Even so, gentle persuasion can be perceived as 'nagging' by the patient so carers and professionals need to use tact and diplomacy so as not to over-burden the patient, whose load is already great
Breathing	Difficulty in breathing is most frightening for the patient and onlooker, be it carer or professional. The medical cause must be diagnosed (infection, cardiac failure, pulmonary embolism, or cancer invading the lung) and the environmental causes identified (stairs, bathing, inadequate ventilation). The patient's day can be planned to avoid exertion. If oxygen is prescribed, advice about its safe use in the home (no smoking/naked lights) must be given. See Chapter 12 on symptom control. Room ventiliation is important, as is an adequate supply of pillows, reassurance, the adjustment of medical treatment and if necessary the use of anxolytic drugs

Table 13.1   contd

Possible problems	Possible solutions
Inability to continue with work, hobbies and recreation	The realization of the severity of the disease process and prognosis often hits patients when they are no longer able to work. If they have held a full-time job, salary is reduced or stops. They are left with endless time on their hands when their self-esteem as a provider or joint provider diminishes. The transition from being a well person to an invalid has the added indignity of having to rely on others to fetch carry and care. At this stage patients can be unable to recognize themselves and this unfamiliar sick role they are forced to adopt. This can cause them to become introverted. Friends, relatives and colleagues can isolate them for fear of upsetting them or saying the wrong thing; at the same time the patient is more and more frightened, anxious and possibly depressed
Inactivity	Some diversional therapy may help. This could be developed in any way that is acceptable to the individual. Day centres may help. Often it is beneficial to try and introduce some activity that the patient could perform at home, possibly related to a previous job or career, creating a purpose to the activity
Weakness	Short walks or car rides should be encouraged. If mobility is impaired so much as to prevent walking, the idea of a wheelchair may be gently introduced. The emphasis should be on a gentle introduction. To a once well person, using a wheelchair has horrid connotations
Depression, fears and anxiety	Good communications between patients and all those involved are essential to allay fears and allow the patient to begin to realize the situation and to extract from life an acceptance of the potential quality available in such undesirable circumstances
Changes in sexual relationships	Patients who have enjoyed a healthy sexual relationship with a loving partner may have to cope with difficulties. Both partners need to be encouraged to openly express any problems that arise. This is a difficult and sensitive area to share but with sensitive and understanding support solutions can be found. Margaret, the patient mentioned earlier, and her husband had enjoyed a very active physical relationship. As her condition deteriorated this changed. They were helped when the visiting aromatherapist showed her husband how to give gentle massage to her very oedematous legs with essential oils. This loving and therapeutic touching become a replacement for the sexual bonding between them
Altered body image	Patients should be encouraged to use make-up and where possible to dress as they did before they became ill
Independence	They should be encouraged to learn to manage their own stomas and to dress any small wounds. This can help them come to terms with their bodily change and help maintain their independence

surroundings versus the 24-hour professional care offered by a hospice or hospital can be an added anxiety for the patient. Most areas throughout the UK should now be able to facilitate and offer education in palliative care. Community nurses and primary health care teams are becoming more confident about caring for dying patients in the community. Nurse specialists in palliative care are being employed by local health authorities to back up and support professional carers, and support for carers can be provided by the Marie Curie Nursing Service.

THE CARER'S PERSPECTIVE OF THE DYING PATIENT IN THE HOME ENVIRONMENT

The task of nursing a chronically sick patient who is dying is physically and emotionally draining for the professional who has some degree of detachment from the patient. For the carer (in this context 'carer' includes family and significant others involved in the patient's care) there is the added burden of emotional involvement, which can manifest in a variety of guises. Last year the author experienced the loss of a close relative who had suffered for months with widespread disease. The feelings experienced during this time were that the sick relative was the fortunate one – lying there dying appeared the easier option when compared with the stress and strain of caring while trying to carry on with the demands of a busy job and family. These feelings were then overlaid by tremendous guilt. This section examines the nursing and caring of the dying person within the home environment and considers some of the situations which present both advantages and disadvantages from the perspective of the carer.

In health, living and loving are not contemplated in terms of time. When a family member is faced with death in old age or more particularly before the expected three-score years and 10, time spent with the loved one and the quality of that time left becomes all important to the carer, family and significant others involved with the patient. These people also experience the same anger, denial, guilt and depression as well as the many new and confusing emotions that the patient feels, although their perception is different. They have the added responsibilities of living, which can mean that life events still have to continue, with maybe a job, career or other family members to care for. There may be added financial strain, a cessation of social activities and hobbies and the adoption of a new role as carer of the sick. As the partner, lover, friend, son, daughter or whatever of the patient, the chances are that that relationship would not have warranted worrying over the person's eating habits, sleeping patterns, or cleaning up vomit or other bodily waste products in the past. In other words there is often only a short space of time for them to develop 'skills in nursing'. Skills of nursing and medical care which are synonymous with the hospital or institutional setting are taken on by the carer, who must adapt to this and carry out this new role in the environment of his or her own home.

With the older patient whose care giver is also elderly, extra strains and burdens are felt. After a lifetime together there are anxieties about parting and fears of 'being alone'. The physical strain for the frail elderly carer is impossible to imagine and the distress and guilt of being unable to nurse the loved one depressing.

As the patient deteriorates, the carer fights to maintain a balance between keeping his or her own life very precariously at 'the norm' and fulfilling the demands of 'this person' whose needs are considerable in physical, psychological, social and spiritual terms. To explain these complexities, the author describes the advantages and disadvantages of looking after the dying patient at home from the carer's point of view in Table 13.2.

If we weigh up the advantages and disadvantages for the carer of home nursing versus admission to the hospice or hospital, we can see that there is a shift towards the disadvantages when there is insufficient information about or access to community support to enable the carer to cope with day-to-day situations which build up into crises. This can result in a panic decision to admit the patient to a hospice or hospital. The carer needs to be well informed about the services available in the community and where to get help at all times (Chapter 17). Carers also need an understanding of the disease and the symptoms which may arise together with the knowledge that these can be controlled. Thus the best use for admission to a hospice becomes the respite which can enable the carer, after a short break, to continue nursing the patient at home.

Earnshaw-Smith (1981) speaks of a 'poorly understood illness arousing irrational fears'. It is often the scenario around the initial diagnosis, for example, 'Who broke the bad news?' and how the situation was handled. Was the care giver there with the patient or did he or she bear this news alone? These issues, if not dealt with in a way which establishes good effective communication among all those involved, can make or break the chain of events which follow.

Carers often believe that the patient will lose hope and give up on life if he or she is given a poor diagnosis or prognosis; they may ask that the patient is not told. This collusion is often used by carers as breathing space for them to take in the full extent of the situation; however, it may allow them to slip into a false sense of hope that the diagnosis may have been wrong or that a new miracle treatment will emerge to save the day. Other members of the family such as children and adolescents taking exams or awaiting job interviews may be protected by the carer, often on the instruction of the patient who doesn't want the illness to spoil the education or career opportunities for the youngsters.

The carer is invariably on the front line to receive the projected anger of

Table 13.2   Advantages and disadvantages for the carer of nursing the dying patient at home

Advantages	Disadvantages
The maintenance of control over daily routine The ability to be able to eat, sleep and continue with hobbies is easier while the patient is at home	As the patient deteriorates the daily routine changes. Sometimes work/jobs outside cease in order to provide more care
The ability to care for other family members at the same time: taking children to school, toddler and baby care at home	Other family members, due to their age, attitudes, etc. may not be able to tolerate the changes brought about by caring for the dying patient at home and family/group conflict may be present This role change and sometimes feeling of boredom and interruption of 'normal domestic routine' can leave the relative angry and resentful, which is superseded by guilt and confusion
If there is family collusion, in other words, where the carer knows the prognosis and the patient doesn't. Collusion is easier to maintain at home	Maintaining collusion can be exhausting for the carer and can alienate the patient, making him or her become introverted Communication between the whole family can become strained
The carer has a lot of control over who speaks to the patient and for how long. Other visitors such as nurses/friends can be duly primed to maintain the collusion, usually at the front door or garden gate before contact with the patient	In the home it is difficult to remain separate from other family members Emotional tension becomes high
There is more precious time which can be spent together; this can be used meaningfully by patient and carer	Sometimes the demand on the relative's time is so great that other chores, commitments or family members get left out, causing anger, guilt, resentment and confusion
Some carers like to be in control and knowledgeable anout the patient's medications and treatments	This control of drug compliance is taken over by staff in the hospital or hospice. The carers can be quite apprehensive about drugs being given to the patient in their absence.
Many carers feel more fulfilled if they can help with washing, feeding and toileting the patient. These simple tasks can be a means of expressing love between spouses and partners, which is very necessary at this devastating time	These often intimate procedures become more and more difficult at home as the patient's condition deteriorates. The carer can become nervous about them, for example getting the patient in and out of a bath or shower, or helping him or her to use the toilet, particularly at night. Being on call 24 hours a day is stressful and exhausting

the patient, whether over the food served, the wrong shopping or the laundry not being ironed satisfactorily. This, along with the heartbreaking knowledge of impending death of a loved one and the widening gap between relationships within the family, can be a huge load for any human being to carry while having to cope with his or her own emotional distress and confusion. The carer feels alone, burdened, unappreciated and exhausted.

The author believes that health care professionals can help create favourable circumstances in which the majority of patients who wish to do so can be nursed and die in their own home. The creation of these circumstances requires the knowledge, skills and attitudes of a good palliative care team. Early referral of patients to this team and their accessibility to resources such as 'hands-on' home care staff, equipment, nursing aids and medical comforts is important, although to carers the most important is access to information about the home support available to them and the patient. In most areas of the UK this information is readily available through the Marie Curie Nursing Service or local centre, the Macmillan Nursing Service and the palliative care specialist nurses appointed by local health authorities. These specialist nursing services are often hospital-based so that the hospital-to-home transition is well coordinated, enabling the primary health care team, patient and carers to have all available information at an early stage. This knowledge, together with anticipation of the patient's needs, will foster the favourable circumstances which allow the patient to die at home. Every nurse working in the community should make it a duty to develop a list of resources available in the area; this done it is easier to support dying patients and their carers at home. Use your local Yellow Pages, public library and the information in Chapter 17 to create your own resource file.

Nine guidelines for use by health and social work professionals in the development of favourable circumstances for the care of a dying person at home have been described by Jones (1992). These are as follows:

1. The professional team should be identified and accessible.
2. The team should meet to coordinate care.
3. The team should demonstrate coordinated care for the terminal stages and bereavement.
4. The team should provide time to listen, understand and analyse what patients and carers say and through this ensure that their needs are properly assessed.
5. Symptoms should be controlled.
6. Appropriate domestic, financial, moral and professional support should be provided.
7. The patient and domestic carer should feel involved in care and management.
8. The patient and carer should be taught how to help themselves.
9. The patient and domestic carer should be aware of the help that is available.

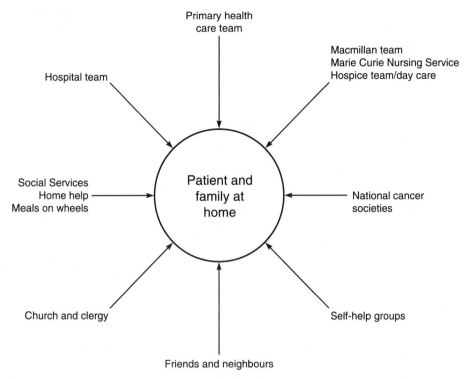

Figure 13.2   Sources of support for carers of the dying patient at home.

In point four of these guidelines the ethical issues of patients' rights and control over their care are highlighted. Professionals need to remember that they should not always assume that they know what is best for the patient, relative, carer and significant other (see Chapter 10).

Jones goes on to suggest that the last three guidelines indicate that all too often the patient and carer are not recognized as being as important as the members of the management team and that they need support in their caring role. These guidelines could provide a useful starting point when planning care to provide favourable conditions for dying at home.

Charts and records are very useful indications of progress for professionals but the author suggests that it is of little use to keep records unless the information cascades to the patient and carers in a practical and informative way.

It has been suggested by Jay (1990) that the Roy Adaptation Model of Nursing provides an adequate framework for assessment of the needs of relatives, carers and significant others, as they are constantly having to adapt. She suggests that the inadequate assessment of relatives' needs in the past may help explain why so many terminally ill patients die in an institutional setting rather than at home.

Four problem areas for carers have been identified by Hinds (1985). These are:

1. financial needs;
2. effective needs (e.g. loss of emotional closeness to the patient);
3. psychological stress of caring;
4. need for respite.

This study showed that most families could cope if care could be divided among many informal carers and also identified that 68% of relatives had anxieties over sexual relationships. However, even in a sexually enlightened society patients and carers feel this is an area badly neglected by professionals. Help with this and many other problems is available from:

- The primary health care team – doctors, nurses, social workers, physiotherapist;
- Social services – benefits, allowances, loans;
- Marie Curie Nursing Service – hands-on carers;
- Macmillan nurses – specialist advice;
- Hospice and home care teams – domiciliary visits, loans of equipment, financial help;
- Support groups – shared worries, information and education.

More information on specific support groups and help agencies will be found in Chapter 17. Figure 13.2 summarizes the support systems for patients and their carers in the community.

CARE OF THE DYING PATIENT AT HOME FROM THE PROFESSIONAL'S PERSPECTIVE

It would be reasonable to suggest that the majority of health care professionals who have decided to work with the dying do so hoping to improve the physical and psychological well-being of fellow human beings, in the same way that doctors, nurses, physiotherapists, social workers and other health care professionals working in the acute setting also see the same purpose in their activity. Reflecting on the analogy made earlier of the 'patient requiring palliative care', who is beyond the stage of being made whole, may be viewed as the outcome. Their situation may create a perception of personal inadequacy in the professional, with a sense of failure if the underlying disease has the upper hand and death is imminent.

In the past most curricula for the training of health care professionals, including doctors, nurses and social workers, have contained very little on the management of the dying or bereavement. Even police officers who are often faced with the death situation in public, are given basic theoretical knowledge but very little training for dealing with the practical aspects of death and bereavement. Religious leaders are also

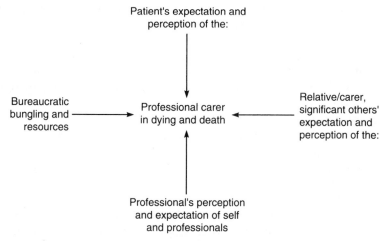

Figure 13.3   Pressures felt by the professional caring for the patient at home.

expected to deal with the dying person and their family. They have been trained in spiritual care but often find they are inexperienced when faced with the many other human complexities of death (Murray, 1991).

There has been a tremendous move towards improving the education of professionals in dealing with death and dying. The last decade has seen enormous growth in the number of books, journals, studies and research published on all aspects of palliative care, dying and bereavement. There has been an increase in awareness and in the development of knowledge and skills within the profession which has undoubtedly improved care. However, there are still large gaps, in particular in the area of community care; this, together with all the other factors mentioned in this chapter, contributes to the number of patients who eventually die in a hospice or hospital when they would have preferred to have done so in the home environment.

Figure 13.3 illustrates the demands placed on the professional carer by patients, relatives and colleagues together with the restriction sometimes felt by them because of local policies and 'red tape'.

The demands placed by the patient on the professional carer can range from ones of 'make me better', i.e. improve my situation, to 'take me out of this dying situation'. This latter demand to remove the cause of dying is an obviously impossible one to meet when imminent death is a certainty and can initially be a barrier to providing the care needed by the patient. The dying person can often be alienated by professionals. They can do this by using jargon in conversations relating to the patient's condition, by having 'over-patient' conversations with colleagues and by avoiding discussion of the diagnosis and prognosis with the patient.

When the patient is at home it is often more difficult to provide the care that the professional considers is appropriate. The patient and carer have considerably more control over decisions within their own role of doing what they consider best. Symptom control requires special expertise, knowledge and skills which the professional may not have. A conflict of roles may develop where the professional may not appreciate who is best placed to manage the patient at home. This can result in late referral and poor management, which are likely to lead to a hospice or hospital admission that could have been avoided. It is often argued that admission to an institution is for the good of the patient; however, it may often be for the benefit of the professional, thus presenting a difficult ethical dilemma.

The professional caring for the dying patient at home can often inadvertently be pressurized by carers to admit the patient to the hospice or hospital because they fear their inability to cope at home. Good planning and the early introduction of the support services will help to allay their fears, as can the offer of respite care and night nursing for when the carer feels overstressed or exhausted; thus caring can be shared and the wishes of the patient fulfilled.

The principles of hospice care can be disseminated throughout the health service so that a coordinated system of care can be based on the needs of the patient and family in the home (Wilkes, 1982).

For professionals to be able to organize and coordinate care they must have the knowledge and skills to care for a person dying of a life-threatening condition. They must have information and a knowledge and understanding of other professionals' roles, but above all they must have a defined attitude and self-perception of death and dying. The latter is probably the hardest element to develop because it comes from within the individual. The rest can be taught.

Bureaucratic intervention can result in bungling, which leads to poor communication that prevents information flowing freely between professional and professional, and between professional, patient, carer, relatives and significant others.

Clear information exchange between agencies, early referral and multidisciplinary planned care are essential for the smooth running of the service which provides good care for the dying patient in the community. Any professional visiting the patient with terminal illness for the first time should know where the patient and family stand in respect of how much information they have:

- been given
- understood
- accepted.

They should also know whether the patient and respective members of the family have the same information, and have all the relevant medical, nursing, social, spiritual and emotional information about the patient, carer and family.

Professionals needs to keep a balanced perception of their own and other professionals' roles in caring for the dying patient. No patient will be the responsibility of one person alone, so that team building is an essential part of the professional's role. Role conflict can sometimes occur and professionals can at times be very covetous of patient care; this is particularly so when caring for dying patients. Withholding information from the team is excused by undue emphasis on patient confidentiality and the egotistical buzz some professionals seem to get from feeling they are the patient's soul mate.

'Sharing the caring' and 'teamwork' should be the main aim of the professionals involved in the care of the dying patient and it is possible to achieve this in the community. Indeed working in the home setting can enhance the multidisciplinary approach to care because of the informal non-clinical atmosphere. Professionals' attitudes towards the dying patient and family will develop from their shared personal feelings as death approaches. This will be affected by the many personalities, traits and life experiences involved. It may be that some professionals will be able to recognize that they are not the best person to offer care in the dying and death situation and they will need to be professional enough to refer the case to other professionals.

A conflict of purpose may arise between professionals where the patient's situation depends on their making the best decision; for example, a general practitioner rings a hospice or hospital colleague, referring a patient for admission because of a 'crisis' in the home situation; it is difficult for the colleague to suggest that a home assessment should be made to see what can be offered to increase support and prevent admission. This could cause conflict between the colleagues and needs to be dealt with tactfully. It would be all too easy to admit the patient to the hospice before an assessment was made of the situation as a whole and the wishes of all concerned considered. A call for help is taken to mean an inability to cope and admission seems the easiest option.

In summary, when it is agreed that caring for the dying patient in his or her own home is a desirable aim, this can only be successful if the following criteria are met:

- Care is patient centred.
- Relatives/carers/significant others are well informed.
- Referral to professional carers (primary health care team and specialist nurses) is early and well-planned.
- Care is multidisciplinary.
- Key workers are identified and good communication established.
- An individual nursing assessment is made.

- Management of symptoms is comprehensive to cover total pain (physical, psychological, social and spiritual).
- Resources are mobilized.
- Plans are made for bereavement support and follow-up.

REFERENCES

Earnshaw-Smith, E. (1981) Dealing with dying patients and their relatives. *British Medical Journal,* **282**(6278), 1779.

Hinds, C. (1985) The needs of families who care for patients with cancer at home: are we meeting them? *Journal of Advanced Nursing,* **10**, 575–81.

Jay, P. (1990) Relatives caring for the terminally ill. *Nursing Standard,* **5**(5), 30–1.

Jones, R. (1992) Primary health care: what should we do for people dying at home with cancer? *European Journal of Cancer Care,* **1**(4), 9–11.

Murray, D.B. (1991) Attitudes and perceptions affecting Scottish clergy in their care of the dying. *Palliative Medicine,* **5**, 233–6.

Patterson, E.M. (1977) *The Experience of Dying.* Prentice Hall, London p. 47.

Pritchard, A.P. and Mallett, J. (eds) (1992) *Manual of Clinical Nursing Procedures.* Blackwell Scientific Publications, Oxford.

Shaw, C. and Hunter, M. (1991) *Special Diet Cookbooks: Cancer.* Thorsons, London.

Stedeford, A. (1984) *Facing Death.* William Heineman Medical Books, London, Ch. 2, p. 7.

Townsend, J., Frank, A.O., Fremont, D. *et al.* (1990) Terminal care and patient's preference for place of death: a prospective study. *British Medical Journal,* **301** 415–18.

Wilkes, E. (1982) *My Patient – My Nurse: The Practice of Primary Nursing.* Scutari Press, London.

Support for the family in bereavement 14

Val Smith

INTRODUCTION

There is an old Scottish folk-tale called 'Death in a Nut'.

Jack lived with his mother in a cottage by the sea. One morning she felt so ill that Jack was afraid she was going to die.

When gathering firewood on the shore he met an old man with a brand new scythe who asked where the cottage was. Jack knew at once that this was Death coming for his mother. So he started to fight him. He beat him over and over again and broke his scythe. Then a strange thing happened. Death became smaller and smaller until Jack held him in the palm of his hand.

Finding a hollow hazelnut at his feet, Jack popped Death into it and flung it far away out to sea. Now Death wouldn't come to his mother. She would be safe. Sure enough when he went home he found her bright and well.

Death was banished but what happened next? When Jack brought in eggs for breakfast they wouldn't break; when he dug up vegetables they couldn't be cut. In desperation for something to eat he tried to kill a cockerel but its head wouldn't come off.

In the village and all around, it was the same story. Nothing would die. It was Jack's fault and at last he told his mother what he had done.

'Jack, Jack, laddie,' she said 'ye've destroyed the only thing that keeps the world alive.'

The story ends with Jack finding the nut washed ashore and releasing Death into the world again. 'You've a lot to learn, Jack,' Death tells him. 'Without me, there's no life.'

Death is a part of life, and as the folk-tale says without death there is no life. Present-day society seems to avoid the thought of death, with a reduction in the ritual of mourning, encouraging the bereaved to 'return to normal' as soon as possible (Gorer, 1965). As nurses, in order to help family friends and relatives during bereavement it is important that we have a thorough understanding of the subject so that we are able to stand alongside the bereaved, recognizing when the grief is within normal bounds but able to identify when specialist help is needed. The resolution of grief is often not straightforward; it does not progress in a straight line but oscillates forwards and backwards at varying speeds and sometimes with the person becoming 'stuck', unable to progress to complete the mourning process.

The term **mourning** is used to indicate the process which occurs after a loss, while **grief** refers to the personal experience of loss and therefore can be influenced by the cultural and social background (Worden, 1991). **Bereavement**, however, is the state of having lost someone close through death. In the words of Marris (1986, p. vii):

> The need to grieve, therefore almost certainly derives from funda-mental aspects of our being, however its expression may become modified by social forms. Yet grieving, unlike other generic human behaviours, does not at first sight appear to be useful to the bereaved. Since it characteristically discourages him or her from at once replacing the lost relationship, it can even seem harmful. What then is its function? Grieving I argue, is a process of psychological reinte-gration, impelled by contradictory desires at once to search for the recovery of the lost relationship and to escape from painful reminders of loss.

In order to gain an understanding of the concept of loss it is important to have an appreciation of the theory of attachment. This theory is based on the work of John Bowlby (1990). He suggests that attachments are made for security and safety and that this is normal behaviour for both children and adults. When the attachment figure disappears or is threatened, an intense feeling of anxiety and threat occurs. These intense feelings are generated in the surviving family when a loved one dies. The pioneering work of Lindemann (1944) suggested that grief is a normal reaction following a significant loss. He interviewed 101 people who were recently bereaved and was able to identify many common factors (Table 14.1). Grieving is essentially a healthy and useful process which allows the individual to adapt to his or her changed circumstances. The intensity of the grief reaction can be surprising; Parkes (1986) likens it to a physical blow, with the intensity of the emotion being overwhelming.

MANIFESTATIONS OF GRIEF

Initially the bereaved are often in a state of shock following the news of death. In some, this may show as stunned silence whereas others cry or act

Table 14.1   Manifestation of grief

Feelings
Shock	Anger
Guilt and self-reproach	Anxiety
Loneliness	Fatigue
Helplessness	Sadness
Yearning	Numbness
Emancipation	Relief

Physical sensations
Hollowness in the stomach	Tightness in the chest
Tightness in the throat	Breathlessness
Weakness of the muscles	Lack of energy
Dry mouth	Sense of unreality

Thoughts
Disbelief	Confusion
Preoccupation	Sense of presence
Hallucinations	

Behaviours
Sleep disturbance	Appetite disturbance
Absent-mindedness	Social withdrawal
Dreams of the deceased	Searching
Sighing	Crying
Irritability	Restlessness
Difficulty with decision-making	
Visiting or carrying objects as a reminder of the deceased	

Lindemann (1944) and Parkes (1986).

hysterically, sometimes behaving completely out of character. Shock may last for only a few minutes or may continue for a few hours or even days. Many report feeling numb, as though the world is continuing around them but they are not part of it (Parkes, 1970).

Denial or disbelief is an immediate reaction to the news of death, with statements like 'I don't believe it' or 'There must be a mistake' commonly uttered. This, together with numbness, allows the bereaved an immediate defence against the overwhelming pain of grief (Parkes and Weiss, 1983). Denial can allow the selective forgetting of the information that has been given or a denial of the irreversibility of the situation. This could later present with involvement with spiritualism and the wish to speak to the dead person. Parkes (1970) suggests that the longer feelings of grief are inhibited the more disturbing they may be when they do finally emerge.

Within this first acute stage of grief as described by Parkes, which reaches its peak of severity within 5–14 days (Parkes, 1986), phases of yearning, searching and restlessness can be seen. This can include a preoccupation with thoughts of the dead person and the need to visit old haunts. This process was well described by Lindemann (1944, p. 142):

> The activity throughout the day of the severely bereaved person shows remarkable changes. There is no retardation of action and speech; quite the contrary, there is a push of speech, especially when talking about the deceased. There is restlessness, inability to sit still, moving about in an aimless fashion, continually searching for something to do. There is, however, at the same time a painful lack of capacity to initiate and maintain organized patterns of activity.

Anger is frequently experienced following a loss. Sometimes this anger is directed towards the doctors or nurses, or even God, because they appear most available. Often the bereaved relatives may feel their anger is inappropriate and not understand why they are experiencing it. If the anger is persistent it can lead to social isolation because the bereaved person manages to deter all helpful approaches. If, however, anger is not adequately expressed this can lead to a complicated bereavement. The anger in bereavement is similar to that expressed by the terminally ill when they are faced with their impending death. Kubler-Ross (1970) recommends that angry feelings are expressed, allowing the release of these strong emotions, and she thus encouraged her patients to yell and shout.

Guilt and self-reproach are common experiences; often doubts are expressed as to whether the correct action was taken – 'If only I had taken her to the hospital sooner' – but much of this uncertainty can be resolved with reality testing, by reviewing the course of events and examining if other actions would have been more suitable. Anxiety displays itself with feelings of insecurity, being unable to settle to any one task or difficulty with decision-making. C.S. Lewis (1961) explained this so well when he wrote, after losing his wife:

> no one told me that grief felt so like fear. I am not afraid but the sensation is like being afraid. The same fluttering in the stomach, the same restlessness and yearning.

The physical symptoms play a significant role in the experience of the bereaved, many of the sensations mimicking physical disease and accounting for additional visits to the general practitioner. Many of the thoughts and behaviours experienced by the bereaved can be unsettling or even frightening; a vagueness of manner or absentmindedness causing inconvenience, an inability to do their job or other normal everyday actions such as shopping or paying the bills. A sense of presence of the deceased and hallucinations are frequently experienced and this can be quite frightening to some, perhaps fearing that they are going mad. The knowledge that this is a common experience can be reassuring and for some the sense of presence becomes comforting (Rees, 1975).

Quite commonly people who have sustained a loss withdraw socially for a period of time, not wanting to go out and do the things that were previously enjoyed. Often this loss of interest can include not wanting to watch television or read the newspaper. Despite inactivity feelings of exhaustion and fatigue are not uncommon. Gradually as time passes most people feel able to take part in life once again and are grateful for the friends who have kept in touch, acknowledging the grief but continuing to offer invitations, even though it may have been many months before the bereaved person felt ready to accept.

Some people try and avoid reminders of the deceased and may be eager to clear away all his or her belongings and return to 'normal' as though nothing has happened. This is not usually healthy behaviour and can lead to later problems. Conversely some people are reluctant to remove anything that belonged to the deceased and may keep his or her room just as it was when the person died. Usually, as the grief progresses they are able to adjust and gradually sort out the deceased's possessions, perhaps saving one or two things of special value. Some or all of these manifestations are quite normally displayed to a varying degree by the bereaved person, but it is important to remember that grieving is unique to each individual. Some quickly readjust to their new situation, while others may take many months or years. Worden (1991) suggests that it can normally take up to two years for grief resolution following the death of a close relative. It is a subject of debate as to whether the bereaved ever fully recover; if this means a return to their former state with no residual distress, then perhaps many do not. But with the passage of time most people make adjustments and obtain enjoyment from life with only the occasional period of sadness or regret. One widow explained: 'You don't get over it; you get used to it' (Parkes and Weiss, 1983).

Worden (1991) contends that to successfully cope with a significant loss an individual must progress on a journey of mourning and on this journey there are four tasks of mourning:

1. to accept the reality of the loss;
2. to work through the pain of grief;
3. to adjust to an environment in which the deceased is missing;
4. to emotionally relocate the deceased and move on with life.

These tasks need to be accomplished for equilibrium to be re-established and the process of mourning to be completed. The tasks do not need to be completed in a specific order but for many there does seem a natural progression from a state of disorientation to reintegration. If any of these tasks remain uncompleted the grieving person becomes stuck and unable to progress, just as one might have incomplete healing of a wound.

Table 14.2   Helping the bereaved

1. Helping the survivor to come to terms with the loss
2. Identifying and allowing the expression of feelings
3. Helping to come to terms with living without the deceased
4. Allowing time to grieve
5. Explaining normal grief reactions and coping styles
6. Directing continuing support

Worden (1991).

HELPING THE BEREAVED

In order to help the bereaved Worden (1991) suggests that there are several main principles that can be followed (Table 14.2). These principles can be used when helping the bereaved person work through the four tasks of mourning.

TO ACCEPT THE REALITY OF THE LOSS

Facing the reality of the loss is the first important stage of the grief process and this reality needs to be accepted on both an emotional and an intellectual level. As indicated earlier, initially the bereaved person may be in a state of shock, not fully aware of the world around him or her. At this time of shock it is best to stay with the bereaved person unless he or she expresses a desire to be left alone. Wherever a person dies, whether it is in hospital or at home, the initial reaction of those around can have a lasting effect. A kind word or comment from a nurse or friend – 'We will miss Bert, he always had something cheerful to say' – leaves a lasting impression for the bereaved relative, a positive memory of the time of death. A cup of tea is more than just a British tradition as it allows time for reflection, something to hold on to and an opportunity to talk to a sympathetic listener. A hug or holding someone's hand if that is appropriate often says much more than actual words. In the hospital situation attending to the bereaved person in a supportive and organized manner, so that he or she knows when and how to collect the deceased's belongings and death certificate, is of great help. The bereaved are very vulnerable at this time and are not able to cope with conflicting information or detailed verbal instructions.

At the time of death it is important that the nurse is aware of any special customs that need to be performed. Some religions have important rituals that need to be conducted following death and these often involve close members of the deceased's family (Neuberger, 1987).

Over the next few days having someone around is helpful and comforting but the bereaved person may have little interest in conversation. An early step towards facing the reality of the loss is seeing the body and most relatives find this a positive experience (Cathcart, 1988). This also provides the bereaved person with the opportunity to say goodbye to the loved one and he or she may welcome the opportunity to spend a few minutes alone with the deceased.

The funeral can play an important part in the ritual of mourning (Grigor, 1986):

1. It is a public statement that the person being buried or cremated is dead.
2. It acknowledges the new status of those relatives that remain (widow, single parent, orphan).
3. For some it allows the process of 'saying goodbye' to the deceased and provides the opportunity for expression of thoughts and feelings about the deceased.
4. It brings together relatives and friends for mutual support and gives reassurance to the main mourners that the person they have lost was also significant to others.

If the ritual of mourning is avoided and friends, family and relatives are not allowed to express their sympathy and grief, this only increases their chance of denying the death as a real event (Murgatroyd and Wolfe, 1982) and thus they are unable to progress in their grief work.

TO WORK THROUGH THE PAIN OF GRIEF

The process of grief is painful but the bereaved should not be shielded from the pain, as it is needed to allow the healing following the loss to occur. The open expression of grief is helpful, with the British notion of a 'stiff upper lip' to be discouraged. Popular phrases like 'Of course she was very brave' or 'He got over it quickly and returned to normal in no time' often indicate the cultural expectations of not displaying emotion and not being given adequate time and space to grieve. When telephone calls are received and letters arrive to express sympathy it is better for the bereaved person to face these situations and be given 'permission' to express his or her emotions than feel the need to suppress them because it is socially unacceptable. The release of tears is often the first step on the road to recovery.

The practical arrangements for coping with the death must be dealt with, and a supportive friend to assist the bereaved person is of much more benefit than the well-meaning person who 'takes over' and tries to shield the bereaved from these difficult tasks. Many people claim they don't know what to say to the bereaved and therefore think it 'best' to say nothing and wait until later. Some may even cross the road to avoid coming face to face with the bereaved. This only means the bereaved person is left alone, feels rejected and wonders why he or she has not heard from a particular neighbour or friend just when some extra support would be helpful. It is not uncommon to hear of people that are told 'I know how you feel', 'It could have been worse' or 'You can always have another child.' These platitudes so often only cause added distress – how can others know how you feel? – and the thought of the future without the deceased at this early stage only seems to devalue their worth and the pain that the bereaved person is suffering. Time will heal for the majority of people but in the early stages of mourning this is totally irrelevant to the grief of the present moment. True friends can help by acknowledging the death and then offering help as appropriate over the weeks and months that follow.

TO ADJUST TO AN ENVIRONMENT IN WHICH THE DECEASED IS MISSING

In this third task of mourning the person adjusts in his or her own way, identifying the new problems ahead and exploring alternative ways of dealing with them. For many this probably occurs about three months after the loss (Worden, 1991), with the bereaved attempting to cope positively with everyday life.

Up to this time the bereaved often feels the need to talk over and over the circumstances surrounding the death. This not only helps them face the reality of the death but is a move towards adjusting to the environment in which the deceased is missing. Sometimes family and friends may want to discourage this talking, thinking that it causes unnecessary distress and may, unwisely, encourage the bereaved to hide their true thoughts. This is explained well by Parkes and Weiss (1983, p. 159):

> The repeated review by which emotional acceptance is obtained can be painful to friends and relatives, as well as to the widows and widowers themselves. Friends and relatives may urge that the review be terminated long before the widow or widower has adequately come to terms with the past. What this can mean is that after a time – often, a rather brief time – the widow or widower is left alone with the work of review.

Helping the bereaved vocalize this series of events, even if it is for the twentieth time, is part of the process of adjustment. Other important steps on this road may include visiting the place that the deceased died and the grave or site of the ashes.

When a death occurs, the family not only loses the person but also all that person had to offer and the various roles he or she had to play. When a spouse dies the bereaved may also have lost the person who paid the bills, the cook, or the car driver:

> In any bereavement it is seldom clear exactly what is lost. The loss of a husband, for instance, may or may not mean loss of a sexual partner, companion, accountant, gardener, baby-minder, audience, bed warmer and so on, depending upon the particular roles normally performed by the husband. (Parkes, 1986, p. 27)

The bereaved person has not only to cope with his or her grief but may also need to learn new skills and adjust to a completely new role in life. Here friends can be of value with practical help, to cook the occasional meal, help sort out the financial papers or offer lifts – not in an intrusive way, as many people need time and space to themselves, but in a practical and supportive manner until a period of readjustment has taken place.

Gradually over the months the bereaved person readjusts to the new situation but certain events can cause renewed and unexpected acute grief. Birthdays, anniversaries, holidays and other occasions that have special importance to that person or their family can trigger the grief reaction. Friends and relatives can best help by being aware of these events and offering time and support if this is what the bereaved person finds helpful. As part of the grief process difficulty in decision-making is common, so that the recently bereaved person should be discouraged from making major life decisions like moving house and/or changing a job. This needs to be achieved without taking away control from the bereaved person but by staying with him or her, allowing the space to fully think and talk through feelings before reaching a major decision. Mistakes have been made when a spouse has sold the house and moved to avoid painful reminders of the loved one, only to find the grief has moved with him or her and the comfort and familiarity of the old house have been left behind. For some, bereavement can lead to the use of defence mechanisms, for example regression, with feelings of helplessness and inadequacy, and the bereaved person will need to draw on all his or her coping mechanisms in order to readjust to the changed circumstance (Murgatroyd and Wolfe, 1982).

For most, however, there is a gradual readjustment when new sets of assumptions are built to replace those that have become redundant. The widow, for example, starts to think of herself as a widow (not in the negative sense of the word) as she accepts the absence of her husband and the new role she has to undertake.

TO EMOTIONALLY RELOCATE THE DECEASED AND TO MOVE ON WITH LIFE

For many people this may be the most difficult task to accomplish. They somehow let life get stuck at the time of the loss and do not allow themselves enjoyment and love after that date. Moving on emotionally does not mean stopping loving the person who has died. Rather the love is held secure and remains part of life, even helping towards viewing the future in a positive light.

Throughout the four tasks of mourning, allowing the bereaved to talk and express their feelings is of great value. The expression of guilt and anger are good examples of emotions that need the help of a non-judgemental listening ear. An effective helper will develop an open and honest relationship with the bereaved person in which they will feel secure. Being with, listening to and attending are comforting and supportive behaviours that will allow the bereaved to adjust to their new situation.

ACTIVE LISTENING

Probably one of the most important helping skills is active listening. This involves observing and interpreting both the bereaved person's verbal and non-verbal behaviour. Verbal cues are given to encourage the bereaved to continue talking without directing the conversation or offering opinions or advice. The skill of reflection is very useful during this process and can be used sensitively by the nurse to encourage the bereaved person to communicate. Reflection is a technique whereby the nurse reflects back (or mirrors) what the person has been saying. This is achieved by repeating an odd word or phrase that the bereaved person has spoken that reflects the main theme of the conversation. This technique when used appropriately indicates that the listener is attentive and encourages the bereaved person to continue talking, and it can help increase the degree of trust, while not halting the flow of conversation. It can also help clarify and bring less obvious feelings into the bereaved person's awareness. For effective helping to continue the helper will need to continue to respond accurately to the needs and cues of the bereaved person, 'staying with the person' within an environment of empathy and acceptance.

The techniques of active listening, including non-verbal and verbal cues, are explored further in Chapter 9 and in other texts (Grigor, 1986; Tschudin, 1991).

ABNORMAL GRIEF

It was suggested earlier that one of the key ways in which nurses can help bereaved families is by recognizing those people who are most at risk of having difficulty with their bereavement. Grief is a normal process and the majority cope without needing any additional professional help. Research has, however, identified that certain individuals are 'high risk' with regard to their adjustment to a significant loss (Parkes, 1975; Worden, 1991; Parkes, 1990).

FACTORS INDICATING 'HIGH RISK' FOR ABNORMAL GRIEF RESOLUTION (Parkes, 1990; Worden, 1991)

1. **A severe reaction to the loss.** The manifestation of severe distress, anger, yearning or self-reproach.
2. **An ambivalent relationship.** Where the individuals involved had ambivalent feelings towards each other, often with unexpressed hostility or in situations when the relationship was highly dependent.
3. **Circumstances surrounding the death.** Sudden deaths when there were less than two weeks to adjust to the forthcoming loss. Unnatural deaths like suicide or murder or when confirmation of the death is uncertain and the body is never found.
4. **Previous unresolved grief.** One of the complications of bereavement is unresolved grief and when a subsequent death occurs it is much harder for the bereaved person to adjust.
5. **Multiple life crises.** If the bereaved person has many additional problems or losses to cope with this may inhibit normal grief resolution.
6. **Personality factors.** People with a strong self concepts are usually better able to cope with crisis situations including bereavement by using their own coping mechanisms more appropriately.
7. **Low socio-economic status.** Although this was found to be a factor in the early period in the study of Parkes and Weiss (1983), grief resolution had returned to normal after two years for those in the low socio-economic group.
8. **Poor social support.** Those who have a close family and supportive friends cope better with bereavement. At risk would be those individuals who have recently moved house or whose family live at a distance. Probably as important as the amount of support the person receives is his or her perception of that support. Those that perceived themselves as unsupported had more problems with their bereavement.
9. **Age.** Young adults have more difficulty adjusting to bereavement than older individuals.

By having an awareness of the risk factors a better service can be offered to the bereaved. Parkes and Weiss (1983) have developed a Bereavement Risk Index which is extensively used at St Christopher's Hospice in order to predict those individuals most at risk. As a result of intervention with those in the high-risk group, their risk of an abnormal bereavement can be reduced to that for those in the low-risk group (Parkes, 1981).

ABNORMAL GRIEF REACTIONS

Occasionally nurses may come across people who are experiencing abnormal grief reactions. By recognizing when an abnormal grief reaction is present help can be given by encouraging referral to a specialist in bereavement counselling or psychiatry. These abnormal reactions include:

1. chronic grief, when the mourning is of excessive duration, with the person unable to return to normal living;
2. delayed grief, when the normal grief is inhibited or postponed, only to return with greater intensity at a future loss;
3. exaggerated grief, when the person becomes totally overwhelmed and may develop severe anxiety, depression or become dependent on alcohol or other drugs.

As suggested earlier, some grief reactions are masked by the presentation of physical symptoms, and cases have been documented when the bereaved have exhibited the same symptoms as the deceased (Worden, 1991).

Parkes and Weiss (1983) found that from their experience chronic grief is a more frequent problem and if the only intervention given is to encourage expression of grief this would be of little benefit to the individual:

> Avoidance of grief was only occasionally responsible for poor outcomes. The most frequent problem observed in our sample was not the initiation of grief but its termination. It seems unlikely that helpers who confined their activities to eliciting further expression of grief would have achieved very much with these already fully grieving widows and widowers. (Parkes and Weiss, 1983, p. 228)

The first step in helping people with abnormal grief reactions is recognizing the signs of unresolved grief.

SIGNS OF UNRESOLVED GRIEF (Worden, 1991)

1. When the person cannot speak of the deceased without experiencing intense emotion.
2. When a relatively minor event triggers an intense grief reaction.
3. When the theme of loss continually runs through a conversation.
4. When the bereaved is unwilling to move or part with material possessions long after the death has occurred.
5. When the bereaved develops similar physical symptoms to those of the deceased.
6. When radical changes are made to lifestyle following the death or

when the bereaved cuts him- or herself off from all those associated with the deceased.

7. When there is persistent depression and low self-esteem or false euphoria.
8. When the bereaved has the compulsion to imitate the deceased in an attempt to internalize him or her so he or she will never be lost.
9. Sometimes persistent self-destructive impulses can be a sign of unresolved grief.
10. When there is unaccountable sadness at certain times of the year, often associated with times shared with the deceased, such as holidays and anniversaries.
11. When there are phobias about illness or death, especially when related to the specific illness that the deceased suffered.

Occasionally the bereaved person may realize that his or her symptoms are a result of becoming stuck in the grieving process or may go to the doctor with one of the symptoms listed. Alternatively someone may notice one of the signs of unresolved grief, perhaps during a visit or during a general conversation, enabling support to be given to help the bereaved obtain specialist help.

FAMILIES

Most of the research about loss and bereavement has been carried out looking at the grief reactions of individuals, mostly spouses. Most significant losses, however, also occur within the family unit and it is therefore important to be aware of the whole family and their resultant needs. Most families function as an interactive group and seek to maintain a sense of equilibrium within their unit. Each member of the family has an influence on other members of the family and all vary in their ability to tolerate and express feelings and emotions. Some families maintain a closed style of communication where sensitive issues and the expression of emotions are avoided. Families that exhibit open communication are able to talk about these sensitive issues and express their emotions freely within the family group. The usual style of coping of each family influences how they deal with any crisis situation. Many of these coping mechanisms have been learnt over generations, with the deaths of a previous generation continuing to have a bearing on the present-day reactions. It is the families that are open in their discussions of the deceased and those that are also able to express their emotions freely who tend to cope more effectively with loss (Bowen, 1978).

The functional position and role of the deceased is important to how the remaining family members will cope with the loss. Various roles are played by different family members: the sickly one, the value setter, the scapegoat, the nurturer, etc. (Skinner and Cleese, 1983). If the deceased had a significant functional position his or her death will have a corresponding disturbance on the equilibrium of the family, with another family member being sought to fill that vacancy. Sometimes this manoeuvring of family alliances can cause considerable distress within the family.

In some families one member is identified as the 'strong one' and takes on a caretaker role for the remainder. It is this person who seems to handle the situation so well, showing little emotional distress and coping well with the challenges that are presented. It is, however, this person who does not allow him- or herself to grieve, in order to support the other members, who at a later date when confronted with a relatively minor challenge like the death of a pet or more distant friend, may experience an unexpected personal crisis (Berger, 1988). If the caretaker can be supported by others outside the family and allowed to grieve for the loss in his or her own right, that person will be able to adjust more satisfactorily. Each family member will adjust to the death in his or her own way and will each exhibit to varying degrees the manifestations of grief already described. Family therapy can have a part to play in helping dysfunctional families adjust (Worden, 1991).

For many grief does not begin when the patient dies; it starts with the diagnosis of the terminal disease and continues throughout the illness and until well after death (Weisman, 1979). During this time both the patient and relatives are attempting to come to terms with the impending loss. The classic work by Kubler-Ross (1970), written after two and a half years of listening to and learning from the stories of dying patients, presents what she describes as the five stages of adjustment to the approaching death: denial and isolation, anger, bargaining, depression, acceptance. These stages, as with grief following death, are not seen as a continuous process with the person progressing from one stage to the next, but as different reactions variously manifested in the process of adjustment.

Kubler-Ross (1970) suggests that just as the patient adjusts to the situation so must the family, and many similar emotions are experienced. Indeed during the period of terminal illness the disruption for the family may be more than that for the patient. The situation can be further complicated when relatives avoid open and free communication with the dying person. Glaser and Strauss (1966) identified four levels of communication between patients, relatives and staff: closed awareness, suspected awareness, mutual pretence awareness and open awareness. Problems arose when the patient or different family members wanted to communicate at a different level of awareness – if for example the patient adamantly denied the true situation, insisting on making elaborate plans for the future which could not be realized. This left the relatives with a real dilemma of needing to confront the patient with the reality of the situation, or to wait and cope with the additional problems once the death had occurred. It is difficulties at this time that may lead to problems later during the bereavement. If patients and their families are fully able to share during the terminal illness they are all better able to come to terms with their own grief. This period of grieving that occurs prior to the actual death is often referred to as anticipatory grief.

ANTICIPATORY GRIEF

This was first mentioned by Lindemann (1944) and he suggests that it acts as a forewarning so that survivors can begin the tasks of mourning before the actual death occurs.

Research studies on anticipatory grief have shown conflicting results as to its beneficial effect (Backer *et al.*, 1982; Sweeting and Gilhooly, 1990). Many factors affect how a person copes with loss but there is some evidence that some forewarning of death helps with the mourning process (Parkes, 1973). These results could in part be due to the fact that there is additional trauma associated with an unexpected death. On the other hand, a prolonged period of mourning also has its consequences:

> The postponement of the inevitable death often extracts a grave psychological, physiological and economic price from the patient and the family. (Allan and Hall, 1988)

One of the difficulties when considering the concept of anticipatory grief is to assume that each individual has a fixed amount of grieving to achieve and that if he or she start mourning before the person's death then there will be less afterwards. There is no evidence to support this view that normal grieving following the death will be less if it is started before the person dies. Many other factors appear to have an important bearing on the normal resolution of grief; these have been described earlier in the chapter.

One group of people who have a particularly difficult time with anticipatory grief are the parents of a terminally ill child. The child's illness is accompanied by a long series of medical treatments, hospital admission and many other stresses and strains on the family group. Many of the manifestations of grief are present throughout the illness and for some the most important recollection of the child's illness is not the death but the diagnosis which equated with death. When death finally arrives there may be a sense of relief that the suffering has ended, as well as grief at the loss of the child. Those parents that cling to denial rather than anticipatory mourning may have more problems with grief resolution once the death has occurred (Sweeting and Gilhooly, 1990).

During the terminal illness the reality of the impending death gradually dawns on the family as the patient's condition deteriorates. Often there is an awareness of the true situation, which alternates with periods of

Table 14.3   Needs of relatives of terminally ill patients

To be with the dying patient
To be helpful to the dying patient
For assurance of the comfort of the dying person
To be informed of the partner's condition
To be informed of impending death
To express emotions
To comfort and support the family members
For acceptance, comfort and support from health professionals
For hope
To be assured that the best possible care is given
To have questions answered honestly
To have as much information as possible

Hampe (1975) and Manley (1988).

denial. This denial may sometimes be manifested by the family seeking further treatments or the inappropriate use of alternative therapies. Anxiety may increase with the realization of the impending loss and because of the family's increased personal death awareness.

It is not uncommon for the family to anticipate what it will be like when the death has occurred. How will they manage? What will they do with the house? Some suggest that it is insensitive for the family to think about what will happen following the death but it is part of normal adjustment to the impending loss.

One problem that can occur with prolonged anticipatory grief is if a person withdraws emotionally too soon, long before the person has died. This upsets the relationship with the dying person, making communication in the later stages more difficult. The opposite situation may also occur when the family members draw too close and try to 'over-manage' the patient's care, not allowing the patient any autonomy or involvement in decision-making although he or she is still well able to make his or her own decisions. Sometimes this occurs to negate feelings of guilt associated with the impending loss.

The time before death can be used productively to allow family and friends to attend to personal and business matters – not only the practical issues like making a will or even arranging the funeral, but to openly express true feelings and say the things that may have remained unsaid for many years. Open expression of love or regret is very difficult but can lead to a more peaceful death for the patient and a less complicated bereavement for those surviving. People often need permission or encouragement to do this, which can be given within a supportive environment with the help of the nurse. Supporting the family during the terminal illness and helping the patient have a 'good' death is the first step in helping with the adjustment to the loss.

Table 14.3 lists the important needs identified by relatives during the terminal stages of illness, compiled from previous studies (Hampe, 1975; Manley, 1988). Once the needs have been identified steps can be taken in helping to meet them (Dracup and Breu, 1978). This can be achieved by ensuring that the relatives are fully informed, have an open and free communication with staff and are involved as appropriate with the care of the dying person. One of the strengths of the hospice movement is its emphasis on the care of the family and as a result these relatives have been shown to have fewer problems during their bereavement (Ransford and Smith, 1991).

Better bereavement should be a consequence of a better death and steps can be taken in order to reach an appropriate death. Weisman (1979) suggests that the following points are important in the move towards helping the patient have a good death:

1. Avoid avoidances.
2. Confront what can be confronted.
3. Resolve remaining conflict.
4. Trust your own sense of reality.
5. Learn to trust others.
6. Seek out and use competent help.
7. Insist on decent medical management.
8. Communicate openly.
9. Permit others to grieve.

Preparation for death can be a learning experience for both the patient and the relatives that will be left behind. Parkes and Weiss (1983) provide a good example when they describe a 60-year-old woman admitted for terminal care who confessed that she had 'spoiled' her husband.

> She had waited on him hand and foot throughout their married life and obtained satisfaction from his dependence on her. Nevertheless, she had realized, as her illness progressed, that he was quite unprepared for life as a widower. With characteristic determination she announced that since she was not going to be around much longer her husband had better learn to fend for himself. She taught him how to cook and keep house, encouraged him, and, most important of all, gradually withdrew her support from him so that, by the time she was admitted to the hospice, both of them knew that he could cope without her. (Parkes and Weiss, 1983, p. 237)

SPECIAL TYPES OF LOSS

Most of this chapter has considered loss in general terms but each type of loss does have several of its own characteristics and special problems. It is not intended to deal with these losses in any detail but they will be highlighted in order to draw attention to the unique characteristic of different types of loss.

Sudden deaths, for example accidents and heart attacks, are likely to be more difficult to grieve over (Parkes, 1975). The sense of unreality about the death may be more marked, with a longer period of numbness and nightmare visions about what happened. Often there is a strong sense of guilt, with the bereaved wishing 'If only I had been there' or 'If only I had said something different', etc. Sometimes there is the need to blame someone else, perhaps quite appropriately, but this can inhibit the grieving process. If the sudden death involves legal proceedings, which usually take time, the grief is once again delayed, stopping the family from adjusting to the loss. Often because the death is unexpected there may be unfinished business between the deceased and the bereaved person, who have not had the opportunity to say the things they wish they had said.

Suicide is a particularly difficult loss to adjust to. Not only are there the problems of a sudden death but there is also the stigma associated with suicide making it a more difficult subject to talk about. Sometimes the family are tempted to behave as though it has not really happened, thus denying their grief. Strong feelings of guilt may be present, the bereaved thinking that they should have done something to prevent the suicide. Intense anger can also occur and may be directed towards the deceased, with the survivors wondering why they had been rejected.

Miscarriages and abortions also carry their own problems. These may be associated with self-blame even when nothing could have been done to prevent the loss. Worries about the future are common, with the danger of wanting to conceive quickly before the present loss has been mourned for. Sometimes family and friends may have been unaware of the pregnancy, making it more difficult to talk about. There is a strong temptation to try and forget about the loss too soon, before the grief is fully resolved.

Sudden infant death syndrome (SIDS) has all the problems of a sudden death with particular worries about why it should have happened. Involvement with the legal system and a post-mortem, trying to establish a cause of death, contribute towards making the grief more traumatic. Sometimes particular tensions can develop between the parents as they adjust in their own way to the unexpected death. It is the practice in some hospitals, as with stillbirths and late abortions, to allow the parents to spend time with their dead baby so that they can say goodbye and this can help them adjust to the reality of the loss (Osterweis *et al.*, 1984).

A chapter of this nature would not be complete without a brief mention of some of the other losses in life that produce, to varying degrees, the grief reactions that have been described. Divorce, separation, moving house, illness and amputation to name but a few can all produce a feeling of loss. The extent of a person's reaction to these losses depends on many factors, including the person's normal coping mechanisms and that of

Table 14.4   Children's reaction to loss: type of reaction or symptom, two to six months after the loss

	Age in years	
	2–6	*6–10*
Grief reactions		
Crying	86%	85%
Sad moods, longing, grieving	73%	85%
Remembering dead father	86%	42%
Denial of death	66%	42%
Search for 'substitute father'	60%	42%
Identification with deceased father	33%	42%
Behaviour symptoms		
Separation problems from mother	73%	28%
Clinging to mother	66%	57%
Clinging to teacher	40%	14%
Aggressive behaviour	53%	57%
Temper tantrums	40%	57%
Restlessness	46%	57%
Night fears, sleeping problems	46%	0%
Concentration problems	40%	14%
Tics, 'nervous movements'	26%	42%
Rejection of strangers	26%	0%
Assuming 'adult' responsibility for mother and siblings	13%	28%

Kaffman and Elizur (1979).

their families, other crises affecting their lives that may also be present and the degree of attachment to that which has been lost. Adjustment to these losses progresses in a similar way to adjustment to loss through death, the individual's coping style and his or her support network playing an important part in the speed and extent of adjustment (Murgatroyd and Wolfe, 1982).

CHILDREN AND BEREAVEMENT

Death of a loved one experienced in childhood can have a particular significance and if the child fails to mourn adequately problems can occur in later life (Osterweis *et al.*, 1984). There has been considerable controversy about whether and at what age children are able to mourn (Worden, 1991) but the generally held view is that children do experience grief. In a study by Kaffman and Elizur (1979) of children between the ages of two and 10 years following the death of their father many features of grief are evident (Table 14.4). The stage of the child's development is significant to the reaction to loss. Even children as young as a few months of age probably respond to the separation or loss of a specific individual. They will not at this time understand the concept of death and their adjustment will be dependent on the quality of care or mothering following this time (Raphael, 1984).

SIX MONTHS TO TWO YEARS

The beginnings of grief and mourning are seen. The child is now able to form attachments to specific individuals and will therefore respond to their absence. This may be demonstrated with loud protests, anger and obvious distress which will lapse into withdrawal when the infant gives up hoping the specific person (usually the mother) will return. He or she is not yet able to understand the permanence of death but sometimes in later life may have vivid memories of 'what it felt like' at that young age.

TWO TO FIVE YEARS

By now the child's relationships are more complex and varied. He or she is able to recognize specific members of the family and has different types of relationships with each. He or she will be developing an understanding of the concept of death; its extent will much depend on the child's experience and involvement in these issues. Seeing and talking about dead insects and animals will have been helpful. Often young children find the subject of death fascinating and feel curiosity rather than the horror of the adult. Magical thinking at this age can confuse fact and fiction, the child thinking that thoughts such as 'I wish you were dead' do actually influence actions. Also to hear of someone 'dying in their sleep' or going into hospital to die can make the child afraid of sleep or hospitals. Lack of information surrounding the actual death and the family's attempts to exclude the children from what is happening, erroneously thinking they are protecting them, only adds to their confusion.

FIVE TO EIGHT YEARS

During this phase the child continues to mature and develop relationships. His or her concept of death is understood in a similar way to that of an adult. His or her newly developed super ego and sense of guilt can make the child mistakenly believe that his or her thoughts and fantasies may have caused the death. Children of this age usually realize what is happening but may resort to denial as a defence mechanism, their day-to-day behaviour appearing as though nothing has happened whereas inside they may be distressed. In some children, however, the manifestations of grief may be evident (Kaffman and Elizur, 1979). At this age children need to mourn and with a suitable opportunity will talk about their feelings, or alternatively their emotions may be displayed in the form of aggressive play (Raphael, 1984).

EIGHT TO TWELVE YEARS

As children become older their relationships develop outside the home, with more independence from their parents. They now understand how death can affect them and perceive the implications for the future following the death. Many of the behaviours and feelings already described can be displayed, children being aware of very strong emotions. This is shown in the following words of a 15-year-old boy following the death of his mother:

> I was really mad at Mom. I never blamed the taxi drivers. I don't know why, but I didn't. I just took it for granted that accidents happen and it wasn't their fault but Mom should have known better. She should have jumped back more quickly like Timmy did. Timmy was mad too – mad that he hadn't been able to pull her back. He felt helpless that he couldn't help her and that was rough. I even asked Dad, 'Do you think Mom knows she's ruined our lives?' (Krementz, 1983, p. 24)

When someone dies it is helpful if a close, loving member of the family tells the children what has happened. A death makes the children's world seem very insecure, they feel that they can no longer rely on adults always to provide safety (Jewett, 1984). The introduction of routines and reliability can help them get over this difficult phase. The tasks of mourning for children will be similar to those for the adult, although for children the loss may be reactivated much later during important life events or when they reach the same age as that of the parent when he or she died.

Commonly at the time of death children may be excluded, perhaps not told what is happening and often not allowed to attend the funeral (Pennells and Kitchener, 1990). Sometimes it is incorrectly assumed that the children are too young to understand and no clear explanations are given, so that they get a false impression about what is happening which can lead to problems later. This neglect or exclusion is frequently because the primary care giver is in acute grief him- or herself and unable to give the attention that is needed (Lopata, 1979). Children adjust better if they are informed about what is happening and have the opportunity to attend the funeral, if that is what they want. It is at this time that the family's support network of friends or the extended family can be particularly useful to reduce the child's feelings of isolation and rejection. Children need time and space and the opportunity to vocalize their feelings in order to adjust to the loss.

Younger children who sense the seriousness of the situation may need permission to 'have fun' without feeling guilty. Sometimes a child may be inappropriately expected to take on the role of a dead parent and become burdened with responsibilities he or she is not ready or able to take on (Worden, 1991).

When a child dies, this is a particularly difficult event for the family to adjust to. Both parents have lost the child but each may grieve in a different way, which can put an added strain on the marriage and provide more problems for the surviving siblings. Support that was present during a period of terminal illness should not be stopped abruptly but gradually reduced as the family adjusts (Thornes, 1988). After a child has died it may be more difficult for the family to accept the reality of the loss because it is expected that children will survive their parents. Some families react with a reluctance to deal with the child's possessions, perhaps leaving the room untouched for many years. Sometimes the siblings of the dead child are put in the difficult position of having to replace the deceased and are not allowed to develop as themselves. When there is a death in the family children may have difficulty deciding what to say to other people, not knowing how they will react. Adolescents tend to become withdrawn and grieve in private, wanting the support of their parents, who are often too upset themselves (Weitz, 1989).

Many children will experience the death of a close relative (Simmons, 1992) and therefore the support of children following bereavement is an important area to consider. Some projects have been started that provide workshops for bereaved children, including art, games, stories and discussion, in order to allow them to express their grief (Pennells and Kitchener, 1990; Burrough, 1992). Family therapy also has a role in helping all the family to adjust following a death (Black and Wood, 1989).

Like adults, when faced with loss children adjust in their own way, the majority not needing any specialized intervention provided that they are within an open and supportive environment that allows them to express and work through their own grief at their own pace. Unfortunately it is usually the case that the whole family is affected by grief, making it more difficult for the children to receive the attention and support that they need. It is here that health professionals and family friends will be able to play a valuable role.

BEREAVEMENT SERVICES

The aim of a bereavement service is to enable successful grieving to occur and to prevent whenever possible the detrimental consequences of the loss. Hospices and other specialist units usually provide a bereavement follow-up but the majority of bereaved will need to find help, if this is needed, for themselves. The service that is offered varies a great deal from one organization to another. This could include telephone follow-up, support groups, social evenings or one-to-one counselling. The extent to which these services are offered appears to depend on the resources available and the perceived importance of the services to the bereaved. Little research is available that evaluates the benefits of the majority of these services (Lattanzi-Licht, 1989). For the majority of people bereavement is a normal although painful process but no special professional intervention is required. For these people informal bereavement support is all that is needed to assist them through the tasks of mourning. Studies have shown that for the majority of bereaved people, family and friends are identified as most supportive during the process of mourning (Bowling and Cathwright, 1982; VandeCreek, 1988).

The extent of bereavement services that should be offered is open to debate. Parkes (1990) suggests that self-selection for bereavement counselling is dubious and that there appears no significant benefit when unselected counselling is offered. There is, however, considerable benefit when bereavement intervention is offered to 'high-risk' individuals (Raphael, 1977; Parkes, 1980) and one of the key roles for health professionals must be to identify this group. One danger of providing a bereavement service for everyone, apart from the cost, which is a limiting factor in many units, is the medicalization of a normal process. On the other hand, in many cases the bereaved seem unable or unwilling to ask for help at this difficult time, so unless health professionals can identify those at risk they will go unnoticed until the complications of grief become evident.

For some people self-help groups have been found to be of some value (Parkes, 1980) and in the USA widow-to-widow programmes are available. In these programmes the newly bereaved widow is contacted by another widow to offer friendship and support. In some cases contact has been sustained for several years, developing into a lasting friendship. Group sessions and group counselling can also be of benefit to some individuals, especially after the first few weeks of bereavement (Parkes, 1986).

In the UK, CRUSE offers comprehensive bereavement support for whoever wants to attend. It provides a network throughout the UK, with each local area providing a programme of events for the bereaved. This programme can include a variety of meetings, for the newly bereaved,

Table 14.5   Bereavement support organizations

The Compassionate Friends (for bereaved parents)
53 North Street
Bedminster
Bristol BS3 1EN
Tel. Bristol 0272 539639

CRUSE (for widowed people and their children)
CRUSE House
126 Sheen Road
Richmond
Surrey TW9 1UR
Tel. 081 940 4818

The Foundation for the Study of Infant Deaths (SIDS) (cot deaths)
35 Belgrave Square
London SW1X 8QB
Tel. 071 235 1721

National Association of Widows
Chell Road
Stafford ST16 2QA

The Stillbirth and Perinatal Association
37 Christchurch Hill
London NW3 1JY

---

widows, widowers, single parents with young children, social evenings, one-to-one counselling, etc. The bereaved person is able to attend whichever meeting they feel is appropriate, usually after assessment by a counsellor, and to continue as long as he or she wishes, remembering that the emphasis of the organization is to help the individual to move on through grief and not become dependent on the bereavement support that is offered.

The role of professionals in the provision of bereavement care is varied (Parkes, 1986). The tradition of most churches in the past was to visit the sick and bereaved but this has now changed. Many people are no longer church attenders, having no contact with their minister. Clergy themselves have also identified that they feel ill prepared to deal with the bereaved (Murray, 1989). Some church organizations do, however, offer valuable bereavement support in the form of 'visiting' or 'befriending', or the provision of bereavement support groups. Specialist bereavement counselling is also available for those in need from counselling services throughout the country.

Bereavement support is often a combination of professionals and volunteers. Specialists in bereavement care are not needed for the majority of individuals and families but thorough training in bereavement support is necessary for both professionals and volunteers who will be working with the bereaved (Osterweis *et al.*, 1984). Parkes (1980) pointed out how competent the bereavement volunteers at St Christopher's Hospice became after training and their initial experience. As mentioned in a previous section, preparation for death has a significant impact on the subsequent grief. Bereavement services should therefore be provided prior to death to aid a more satisfactory outcome (Parkes, 1989). The addresses of several bereavement support organizations in the UK are listed in Table 14.5.

CONCLUSION

Death is an important part of life. Although a painful experience, it is something that no one can avoid. Although grief is always the penalty for loving someone, it can for some be an opportunity to grow. This does not mean that the grief is any less during the healing process but that once that grief has resolved the person is able to move on with greater insight and understanding. For health professionals it is important that we have an awareness of normal grief reactions, an understanding of how people adjust when faced with loss and how to help with this adjustment, to identify those at high risk of having difficulty with their bereavement and the signs of unresolved grief, the special types of losses that can occur and the particular problems of children and families. By having this knowledge we will be better able to cope with grief ourselves and to offer more help and support to the bereaved person.

REFERENCES

Allan, J.D. and Hall, B.A. (1988) Between diagnosis and death: the case for studying grief before death. *Archives of Psychiatric Nursing*, 2(1), 30–4.

Backer, B.A., Hannon, N. and Russel, N.A. (1982) *Death and Dying: Individuals and Institutions*. Wiley, New York.

Berger, R. (1988) Learning to survive and cope with human loss. *Social Work Today*, 19(34), 14–17.

Black, D. and Wood, D. (1989) Family therapy and life threatening illness in children or parents. *Palliative Medicine*, 3(2), 113–18.

Bowen, M. (1978) *Family Therapy in Clinical Practice*. Jason Aronson, New York.

Bowlby, J. (1990) *Attachment and Loss*, Vol. III. *Loss: Sadness and Depression*. Penguin, London.

Bowling, A. and Cathwright, A. (1982) *Life after Death: A Study of Elderly Widows*. Tavistock Publications, London.

Burrough, A. (1992) Griefwork with children: workshop days at Pilgrims Hospice in Canterbury. *Palliative Medicine*, **6**(1), 26–33.

Cathcart, F. (1988) Seeing the body after death. *British Medical Journal*, **297**, 997–8.

Dracup, K.A. and Breu, C.S. (1978) Using nursing research findings to meet the needs of grieving spouses. *Nursing Research*, **27**(4), 212–16.

Glaser, B.G. and Strauss, A.L. (1966) *Awareness of Dying*. Aldine, Chicago.

Gorer, G. (1965) *Death, Grief and Mourning*. Camelot Press, London.

Grigor, J. (1986) *Loss: An Invitation to Grow*. Arthur James, London.

Hampe, S. (1975) Needs of the grieving spouse in a hospital setting. *Nursing Research*, **24**(2), 113–20.

Jewett, C. (1984) *Helping Children Cope with Separation and Loss*. Harvard Common Press, Boston.

Kaffman, M. and Elizur, E. (1979) Children's bereavement reactions following death of the father. *International Journal of Family Therapy*, **1**(3), 203–29.

Krementz, J. (1983) *How it Feels when a Parent Dies*. Victor Gollancz, London.

Kubler-Ross, E. (1970) *On Death and Dying*. Tavistock Publications, London.

Lattanzi-Licht, M. (1989) Bereavement services: practice and problems. *Hospice Journal*, **5**(3), 1–28.

Lewis, C.S. (1961) *A Grief Observed*. Faber & Faber, London.

Lindemann, E. (1944) Symptomatology and management of acute grief. *American Journal of Psychiatry*, **101**, 141–8.

Lopata, H.Z. (1979) *Women as Widows*. Elsevier, New York.

Manley, K. (1988) The needs and support of relatives. *Nursing*, **3**(32), 19–22.

Marris, P. (1986) *Loss and Change*. Routledge & Kegan Paul, London.

Murgatroyd, S. and Wolfe, R. (1982) *Coping with Crisis*. Open University Press, Milton Keynes.

Murray, D. (1989) The education and training of Scottish clergy in the care of the dying. *Palliative Medicine*, **4**(1), 17–23.

Neuberger, J. (1987) *Caring for Dying People of Different Faiths*. Lisa Sainsbury Foundation, London.

Osterweis, M., Solomon, F. and Green, M. (1984) *Bereavement Reactions: Consequences and Care*. National Academy Press, Washington.

Parkes, C.M. (1970) The first year of bereavement. *Psychiatry*, **33**, 444–67.

Parkes, C.M. (1973) Anticipatory grief and widowhood. *British Journal of Psychiatry*, **122**, 615–19.

Parkes, C.M. (1975) Determinants of outcome following bereavement. *Omega*, **6**(4), 303–23.

Parkes, C.M. (1980) Bereavement counselling: does it work? *British Medical Journal*, **281**, 3–6.

Parkes, C.M. (1981) Evaluation of a bereavement service. *Journal of Preventive Psychiatry*, **1**(2), 179–88.

Parkes, C.M. (1986) *Bereavement Studies of Grief in Adult Life*. Penguin, London.

Parkes, C.M. (1990) Risk factors in bereavement: implications for the prevention and treatment of pathological grief. *Psychiatric Annals*, **20**(6), 308–13.

Parkes, C.M. and Weiss, R.S. (1983) *Recovery from Bereavement*. Basic Books, New York.

Pennells, M. and Kitchener, S. (1990) Holding back the nightmares. *Social Work Today*, **21**(25), 14–15.

Ransford, H.E. and Smith, M.L. (1991) Grief resolution among the bereaved in hospice and hospital wards. *Social Science and Medicine*, **32**(3), 295–304.

Raphael, B. (1977) Preventive intervention with the recently bereaved. *Archives of General Psychiatry*, **34**, 1450–4.

Raphael, B. (1984) *The Anatomy of Bereavement*. Hutchinson, London.

Rees, W.D. (1975) Study on hallucination, in *Bereavement: Its Psychosocial Aspects* (ed. B. Schoenberg), Columbia University Press, New York.

Simmons, M. (1992) Helping children grieve. *Nursing Times*, **88**(50), 30–2.

Skinner, J. and Cleese, J. (1983) *Families and how to survive them*. Mandarin, London.

Sweeting, H. and Gilhooly, M. (1990) Anticipatory grief: a review. *Social Science and Medicine*, **30**(10), 1073–80.

Thornes, R. (ed.) (1988) *The Care of Dying Children and their Families*. NAHA, Birmingham, UK.

Tschudin, V. (1991) *Counselling Skills for Nurses*. Baillière Tindall, London.

VandeCreek, L. (1988) Sources of support in conjugal bereavement. *Hospice Journal*, **4**(4), 81–92.

Weisman, A.D. (1979) *Coping with Cancer*. McGraw Hill, New York.

Weitz, P. (1989) Adolescents and bereavement. *Bereavement Care*, **8**(2), 19–20.

Worden, J.W. (1991) *Grief Counselling and Grief Therapy*. Tavistock/Routledge, London.

FURTHER READING

Collick, E. (1986) *Through Grief*. Darton, Longman & Todd, London.

Department of Social Security (1990) *What to do After a Death*. HMSO, London.

Grigor, J. (1986) *Loss: An invitation to Grow*. Arthur James, London.

Krementz, J. (1988) *How it Feels when a Parent Dies*. Camelot Press, Southampton.

Neuberger, J. (1987) *Caring for Dying People of Different Faiths*. Austen Cornish, London.

Newett, C. (1982) *Helping Children Cope with Separation and Loss*. Harvard Common Press, Boston.

Parkes, C.M. (1986) *Bereavement Studies of Grief in Adult Life*. Pengiun, London.

Penson, J. (1990) *Bereavement: A Guide for Nurses*. Harper & Row, London.

Saunders, C. (1990) *Beyond the Horizon*. Darton, Longman & Todd, London.

Scottish Home and Health Department (1989) *What to do after Death in Scotland*. HMSO, London.

Tatelbaum, J. (1981) *The Courage to Grieve*. Heinemann, London.

Varley, S. (1992) *Badgers Parting Gift*. Harper Collins, London.

Worden, W. (1991) *Grief Counselling and Grief Therapy*. Tavistock/Routledge, London.

15 Rehabilitation: adding quality to life

Jill David

INTRODUCTION

Rehabilitation medicine generally concentrates on the physical and more severe aspects of disability, with rehabilitation centres for spinal injuries and amputees directing their efforts towards younger patients with a normal life expectancy. McLellan (1991) suggests that there are approximately 1000 individuals between the ages of 16 and 65 years in each health district 'who are unable to live at home for 24 hours or more without the help of another person'; these he refers to as 'people with appreciable dependency'. As many as 10% of our population suffer some lesser degree of disability, which, the Office of Population Censuses and Surveys reports, has a profound effect on disposable income, employment and quality of life (OPCS, 1989). It is impossible to determine how many of these people would benefit from rehabilitation or how many of them suffer as a consequence of cancer. What is certain is that the benefits of rehabilitation are difficult to measure because they are multidimensional and individual. It is hard to demonstrate cost effectiveness and as a consequence services, particularly in the community setting, are rationed.

THE PLACE OF REHABILITATION IN CANCER CARE

Advances in the treatment of cancer mean that there is a steady increase in the number of patients who survive the disease (McCaffrey, 1991). Their survival represents a continual struggle with the long-term effects of the disease and its treatment. Life for the cancer patient becomes dominated by the disease, frequent hospital visits and the sense of being taken over. The patient becomes dependent on the hospital and the health care professionals. Rehabilitation can alter this course; instead of being an 'add-on' following the completion of patients' treatment it should run a

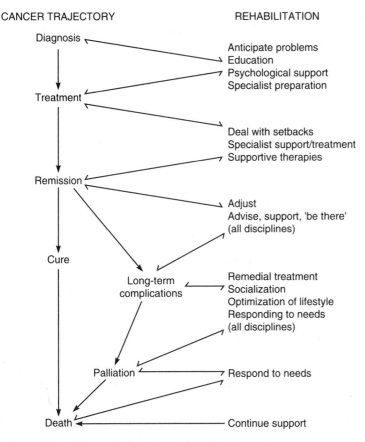

CANCER TRAJECTORY   REHABILITATION

Diagnosis
                                     Anticipate problems
                                     Education
                                     Psychological support
                                     Specialist preparation
Treatment

                                     Deal with setbacks
                                     Specialist support/treatment
                                     Supportive therapies
Remission

                                     Adjust
                                     Advise, support, 'be there'
                                     (all disciplines)
Cure
        Long-term
        complications   Remedial treatment
                                     Socialization
                                     Optimization of lifestyle
                                     Responding to needs
                                     (all disciplines)

        Palliation   Respond to needs

Death   Continue support

Figure 15.1   The relationship between rehabilitation and treatment.

parallel course supporting patients and their families from diagnosis through treatment, remission and relapse.

When asked to apply the Corbin and Strauss 'Chronic Illness Trajectory Model' to the cancer patient, Diane Scott Dorsett (1992) made her case for a recovery model. The rationale for this was that cancer is a disease where diagnosis is followed by episodes of acute treatment and periods of remission, with the possibility of cure and a normal life expectancy. On the other hand, treatment and recovery can be followed by long-term complications or periods of intermittent relapse, further treatment and ultimately death from the disease. Recovery – the basis of Dorsett's theory – is seen as multidimensional, having physical, functional, cognitive and affective dimensions. It can be strengthened by self-care and facilitated by staff. This recent model of 'cancer recovery' shares many similarities with the vision of cancer rehabilitation described by Raven in 1971: 'To minimize such effects at the time of diagnosis a plan of total care should be formulated, guidelines for it laid down, and various explanations made to assuage the patient's fears and engender the hope of future independence and a long useful life.' To be this effective rehabilitation must be considered an integral part of treatment, implemented at diagnosis and adapted to the patient's needs as they arise (Figure 15.1).

In this model, as the disease progresses new symptoms lead to further investigations, a new diagnosis, treatment or palliation and remission, which all change the patient's rehabilitation needs. Consider, for example, a patient with the original diagnosis of breast cancer, who after surgery and radiotherapy is symptom-free for several years. Her arm then begins to swell and secondary lymphoedema is diagnosed. This is a new diagnosis; it comes as a shock to a patient who considered herself cured, felt safe and had accepted her breast disfigurement. Treatment by compression bandaging is offered and her rehabilitation needs are assessed. These might be for:

- psychosocial support to cope with the new diagnosis and disfigurement;
- physiotherapy to improve arm and shoulder movement; treatment by compression bandaging, education for self-care and the teaching of manual lymph drainage techniques. In some places nurses take on lymphoedema care as an extended role following training (Benington, 1991);
- occupational therapy – to learn self-care (dressing, housework and writing skills) and have special equipment if required;
- diversional therapy (art, relaxation, outings, socialization) – to become self-sufficient, outgoing and fulfilled;
- appliance fitter – to fit an elastic sleeve and possibly advise on suitable bras and prostheses.

In addition to these services the patient might also receive support, help and advice from the dietitian, social worker and nursing staff to adjust to her changed lifestyle, cope with the threat of returning disease and to understand lymphoedema and its control. The aim of rehabilitation is to help her to become a self-caring individual with an optimum quality of life.

As survival times extend there will be an increased demand for rehabilitation services. Currently most rehabilitation services are located in hospitals and geared to the acute needs of patients following their initial treatment. Services are limited for patients in the community and may be difficult to obtain for those in the final phase of their disease. To be effective rehabilitation needs to become an integral part of cancer care, offering hope and support at diagnosis and continuing to respond to needs until the patient dies, whether that death is from cancer or not. In this way rehabilitation is a means of providing optimum functioning and the best possible quality of life.

Table 15.1   The rehabilitation team

Physiotherapist	Occupational therapist
Dietitian	Speech therapist
Chaplain	Dental hygienist
Appliance fitter	Patient education
Chiropodist	
Doctors – all disciplines	Nurses – multiskilled
Manager	

Nurse specialists in:
Breast care	Lymphoedema
Stoma care	Community liaison
Psychological support	

Support therapists:
Art therapy	Music therapy
Aromatherapy/massage	Diversional therapy

THE REHABILITATION TEAM

The modern view of rehabilitation in cancer care is that of an interacting multidisciplinary team which includes the services of many professionals together with lay staff and volunteers. In most hospitals these individuals are scattered, with allegiances to different departments, and rarely come together as a team. In the ideal situation all would be housed together with the traditional barriers and rivalries broken down. One example of this is the Marie Curie Rehabilitation Centre at the Royal Marsden Hospital, where rehabilitation comes under its own manager, is housed in one building and has its own in-patient ward (Wells, 1990; Pyle, 1993). A list of the members of the rehabilitation team is shown in Table 15.1.

Working closely with this team and meeting regularly with its members are doctors, social workers and research nurses. Many other individuals including the radiographers, hairdresser, ward clerk, domestic and catering staff, relatives, volunteers and ex-patients also make a contribution to rehabilitation. The second place where rehabilitation can be seen as a team effort is in the hospice where, because the unit is small, professionals work closely together and get to know their patients over a period of time. The services they offer are similar to those in large hospitals and are also available to day care patients who are often not able to receive rehabilitation in their own homes.

ASSESSING THE NEED FOR REHABILITATION

It has been said that at some time every patient will have some need of rehabilitation services (Raven, 1971). At the Royal Marsden Hospital dietitians state that 75–80% of patients meet the criteria for referral in their standard of care, and physiotherapists estimate that they see 75% of the patients. The demands on their skills do not come evenly from all departments. For example, dietitians see patients treated for head and neck cancers frequently and those treated for breast cancer less often or on a single occasion for general advice on healthy eating. Physiotherapists see all patients having breast surgery both pre- and post-operatively to teach a progressive exercise regime and visit wards daily to assess new patients. Referral to the rehabilitation ward in this setting was found to be uneven, some specialties referring far higher numbers of patients than would be expected. The reasons for this were in part high need for the service, for example by patients with head and neck cancers who need to learn self-care and new techniques of speech production, and require nutritional support and help in adapting to disfigurement. High referrals from other departments were usually associated with the referrers having previous good experience of the rehabilitation ward (David, 1992). These findings would support the suggestion by McLellan (1991) that 'most medical graduates are profoundly ignorant of rehabilitation medicine'. Indeed the stimulus for many referrals was the presence of a member of the rehabilitation team when the patient was being discussed.

Rehabilitators, whatever their profession, tend to work as individuals on a one-to-one basis with their clients but are in a unique position to identify problems that can be dealt with by colleagues, hence the need for collaboration and communication and the concept of teamwork in rehabilitation. As the professional most frequently in contact with patients, the nurse is in many respects a gatekeeper to the rehabilitation service and therefore needs to be able to identify how patients can benefit from rehabilitation. Rehabilitation needs can be divided into physical, psychological, occupational and social domains. The divisions between these cannot be rigid because of the interdependence of one upon the other. The primary actions of cancer and its treatments – chemotherapy, surgery and radiotherapy – are physical but their effects are seen in all domains.

1. Physical function
   - **Strength.** Loss of muscle bulk, tiredness, immobility, amputation.
   - **Nutrition.** Taste changes, loss of appetite, anorexia, malabsorption, changes in metabolism.
   - **Control.** Incontinence of bladder or bowel, movement disorders, odour, communication.
   - **Reproduction.** Sterility, mutation of germ cells, loss of desire.

2. Psychological function
   - **Changes in body image.** Mutilation, loss of function and control, alopecia, conflict with self-image and relationships.

- **Anxiety.** Fear of the unknown, of prognosis, pain and treatment, loss of income.
- **Depression.** Due to treatment, fears and anxiety.

3. Occupational function
   - **Work.** Loss of job and income, stigma of cancer.
   - **Self-care.** Need for help, insecurity, dependence on others.
   - **Finance.** Supporting self and family, loss of insurance, mortgage cover.

4. Social function
   - **Self-esteem.** Independence and confidence, worth to society.
   - **Body image.** Coping with the public and in public, stigma of cancer.
   - **Communication.** Voice changes, hearing difficulties, eye contact, emotion.
   - **Family.** Stress, loyalties, honesty.

The medical records of patients contain a lot of information which is relevant to diagnosis and treatment, while the nursing care plan contains information which enables nurses to provide quality care. Assessment for rehabilitation may need to delve more deeply into how patients function as individuals in their own environment. A balance needs to be kept between prying, suggesting problems and the need to understand the intricacy of human behaviour. Initial assessment must record problems which pre-date diagnosis; some may need to be rectified before treatment and others can affect the patient's ability to comply with cancer treatments or indicate problems which could arise later. Examples of these are shown in Table 15.2.

TOOLS FOR ASSESSING FUNCTION

Over the years many tools have been developed for the assessment of function, several of them exclusively for cancer patients. The usual stimulus for the development of a tool has been research, in particular where assessment of measurable changes in the quality of a patient's life in relation to treatment variables is required. Earlier and more well-established tools such as Karnofsky's Performance Scale (1948) were for the measurement of physical function. To supplement these it is usual to include other scales such as the Hospital Anxiety and Depression Scale (Zigmond and Snaith, 1983) to measure psychological morbidity and the Rotterdam Symptom Checklist (de Haes *et al.*, 1990) to cover symptoms. These well-established scales are necessarily short and standard, thus they prevent the patient expressing personal feelings or adding possibly useful supplementary information. This problem is well appreciated by researchers who in response have developed more specific scales to measure particular symptoms such as pain (Walker *et al.*, 1987) and nausea and

Table 15.2   Pre-existing conditions which may affect the patient's ability to cope with treatment

Physical	**Psychological**
Immobility	Depression
Malnutrition	Personality disorders
Visual impairment	Low intelligence
Age (young or old)	
Social	**Spiritual**
Unstable home	Lack of purpose to life
Financial problems	Hopelessness
Isolation	
Family responsibilities	

vomiting (Rhodes *et al.*, 1984). In the day-to-day clinical setting where a more personal approach is desirable, the use of a health diary, nutrition, pain or symptom chart is more practical. This can be completed by the patient alone or with assistance from a nurse, friend or relative. Goals can be agreed on the basis of this record, which is within the patient's control and is in itself part of rehabilitation.

See Fallowfield (1990) or Teeling Smith (1988) for further reading on quality measures and their use.

STAGES OF REHABILITATION

If we accept that rehabilitation starts with diagnosis and continues in response to the patient's needs, the four categories of rehabilitation – preventive, restorative, supportive and palliative – described by Dietz (1981) can be applied to any patient at any stage of disease and in any order. Dietz's categories and the way in which these may be interpreted in the care situation are expanded in Table 15.3. The fact that patients warrant rehabilitation at all stages of their disease is expressed by Wells (1990). He describes the three major groups into which patients' rehabilitation needs fall, regardless of their stage in the life cycle (Table 15.4), and suggests that these should apply regardless of the patient's age. This is particularly relevant because cancer is a disease predominantly affecting the elderly and it is these patients who, although surrounded by caring individuals, may be deprived of rehabilitation. For these patients the period between the end of treatment and death can be a 'long, lonely, unfulfilled and terribly wasted period of time' (Wells, 1990).

Stages in rehabilitation cannot therefore be described as a simple progression. The patient launched upon a disease trajectory finds it hard to get off. Those who are considered cured are restored and supported

Table 15.3   Interpretation of Dietz's categories in the care situation

Preventive
Reducing morbidity and disability at all times, at diagnosis, during treatment and in response to new or late consequences

Restorative
To put things right in response to disabilities caused by cancer

Supportive
To maintain through remission and lessen disability

Palliative
To attenuate disability and support to the extent of the patient's wishes

Table 15.4   Interpretation of Wells's areas of rehabilitation

Life expectancy good
Where treatment has left no disfigurement or disability
Needs: few physical services
        good counselling to prevent taking on a 'sickness role'
        health promotion

Good life expectancy
But treatment has caused physical/psychological disability or disfigurement
Needs: intensive physical rehabilitation
        intensive psychological rehabilitation
        intensive social rehabilitation

Life expectancy shortened
Treatment has failed or there has been a relapse after initial remission
Needs: full range of services
        optimal restoration of function
        continued support

through rehabilitation; those who continue to live with the threat of returning cancer can be helped to achieve a normal outlook; and those whose life expectancy is short can feel fulfilled.

REHABILITATION SERVICES

The services of many disciplines are available for the rehabilitation of cancer patients; these include the professions traditionally associated with rehabilitation, for example physiotherapy and occupational therapy. Dietitians, speech therapists and many other professionals are becoming more involved in cancer rehabilitation, as are nurses, who have developed special skills, and individuals skilled in complementary therapies. Working as a team they all respond to patients' physical, psychological and spiritual needs supporting them on the path of rehabilitation and referring them to other members of the team as needed.

THE ROLE OF TRADITIONAL DISCIPLINES IN REHABILITATION

Physiotherapy

The physiotherapist is the most clearly recognized and most widely available member of the rehabilitation team. Even so referral may not be made early enough to prevent disability. Patients anticipate disability and if not involved actively in their rehabilitation 'may soon begin to act like disabled people' (Stumm, 1988). Assessment of the patient's lifestyle and abilities, initiated before treatment, helps the therapist to work more effectively with the patient. Stumm suggests seven reasons for referring patients to the physiotherapist. These are: amputation of part of the body, loss of muscle strength, loss of joint mobility, difficulty with ambulation, lymphoedema, pain and loss of self-esteem.

- **Amputation.** Treatment offered to the patient includes preparation for the use of a prosthesis, muscle strengthening and re-educating together with training given in the use of the device. Where surgery involves the removal of or damage to muscle groups, lymph node dissection or the removal of organs (internally or externally), the effects of scarring, contraction or joint damage need to be anticipated and a regime introduced to prevent their occurrence.
- **Loss of muscle strength.** Following surgery or radiotherapy this may be associated with cramp or painful spasms which can be helped by simple isometric exercises repeated at intervals through the day. Weakness following chemotherapy responds to a gradual programme of gentle exercise to rebuild strength.
- **Loss of joint mobility.** Mobility problems may be caused by the disease or treatment. Disease causes include primary or metastatic tumours of the brain or spinal cord, bone, joint and muscle, while treatment causes might be amputation, contraction or neuropathy. Aids for walking or the use of a wheelchair together with the development of muscle strength to use them safely does much for the patient's self-esteem and independence.
- **Pain.** Pain which is related to movement, especially when due to muscle spasm, can be reduced by physiotherapy.
- **Lymphoedema.** Treatment to improve function in the affected area, together with massage, compression bandaging and elastic garments, are the current treatment choices (Badger and Twycross, 1988).

Intermittent pressure is still used in some cases. Nurses are becoming increasingly involved in lymphoedema treatment, see 'Rehabilitation nursing', below.

Physiotherapy is generally associated with curative treatment; however, many physiotherapists are treating patients in palliative care settings. In 1985 the Association of Chartered Physiotherapists in Oncology and Palliative Care was established. The role of the physiotherapist in the palliative care setting is to improve and maintain the patient's independence and quality of life. The reasons for referral are similar to those given by Stumm but relate more directly to the symptoms with which the patient presents. Lohmann (1992) suggests where help can be offered, with symptoms under the headings respiratory, neurological, orthopaedic, musculoskeletal, pain and lymphoedema. Physiotherapists stress the need for early referral and the importance of involving the patient, carer and nurse in the treatment which must often be continued in the absence of the physiotherapists. Physical therapy has psychological importance; touch is a valuable adjunct to the acceptance of an altered body image, mobility to independence, and physical well-being to a positive outlook.

Occupational therapy

Occupational therapy has suffered for too long from the image of 'basket-making'. Definitions of the profession's work stress the purposeful nature of activity, and the use of work to develop skills and enhance function. Patients are seen as whole within their environment, which may need to be adapted to enable independent functioning. Thus the purpose of activities, including 'basket-making', become relevant in the progress of the patient from dependent to independent.

The first question asked by the occupational therapist is usually 'What can you do for yourself?' and therapy follows in response to the patient's needs in terms of equipment, exercise and practice. The defined needs of the patient may be for the restoration of a skill lost, for example the ability to write. Therapy for this can also enable the patient to become independent in other areas, improved manual dexterity and the use of suitable equipment, also helping with eating and dressing.

The links between physiotherapy and occupational therapy are apparent, with borderlines blurred, particularly when there is a shortage of occupational therapists. Early referral and the anticipation of needs is particularly important when equipment has to be installed in the home because resources (money and personnel) are limited. Sadly cancer patients tend to be discriminated against, particularly where home adaptation is concerned, because their prognosis is considered to be limited.

Speech therapy

The role of the speech therapist in the rehabilitation team is most often linked to the treatment of patients with head and neck cancers. The restoration of speech and the ability to swallow for these patients involves specific exercises and in some cases the use of specialized equipment. Teaching the use and care of internally fitted valves for speech production requires a lot of time and patience from both patient and therapist. The patient will also need support and encouragement from all concerned to gain confidence in using the new method of speech.

Dental hygiene

The work of the dental hygienist is also closely linked to the treatment of patients with head and neck cancers. The patient's own teeth and the state of the mouth are assessed prior to treatment and any dental problems dealt with at an early stage. A healthy mouth is important in the prevention of infection during and after treatment and can affect the patient's well-being. Poor dental hygiene is common in the general public; many cancer patients suffer from oral problems (Jobbins *et al.*, 1992) and those debilitated by chemotherapy are vulnerable to mouth infections. Assessment of the mouth on admission is important so that early referral can be made prior to the patient developing problems.

Dietetics

Eating is a powerful sociological feature in human culture. Taking or giving food is associated with celebration, reconciliation and social gatherings, is central to family life and is seen as an essential of life. At times it is used as a weapon; famine follows war and the refusal of food (hunger strike) is used to exert pressure on government or family members. To the patient and carer alike being able to eat is equated with survival and recovery. Loss of appetite, the inability to eat and loss of weight are associated with deterioration and death; as such they cause anxiety. Malnourishment is closely associated with cancer; often loss of weight is the first indication that something is wrong and is what brings the patient to seek diagnosis.

Dietitians are consulted by the majority of cancer patients; in a recent study it was estimated that 75% of patients came within their referral criteria (David, 1992). Cancer patients become undernourished for reasons connected with both disease and treatment (Table 15.5). The recognition of weight loss (unexplained loss of 10 lbs or more) or anticipation of weight loss with traumatic treatment suggests early referral to the dietitian. Undernourishment leads to a reduced ability to cope with treatment; an established low intake or diet fads will

Table 15.5   Causes of weight loss in cancer

Treatment
Nausea/vomiting
Anxiety/depression
Tiredness
Loss of ability to eat (laryngectomy/oesophagectomy)
Loss of appetite/anorexia/taste changes

Disease
Pain
Increased demand
Altered metabolism in gastrointestinal tract disease
Cachexia

compound this problem (Hunter, 1991). Physical disability which reduces manual dexterity, and mobility problems which prevent the acquisition or preparation of food, social isolation and depression all contribute to patients' reduced intake during illness.

Other problems which can affect food intake are a dry or sore mouth, sore throat, constipation, diarrhoea, tiredness and a general lack of interest. These can be helped by tackling the underlying problems (see Chapter 12) and stimulating the interest of both patient and carer in food. *The cookbook for cancer patients* (Shaw and Hunter, 1991) and the education booklet *Overcoming Eating Difficulties* (Royal Marsden Hospital, 1989) are good sources of advice. The help of a dietitian is needed:

- when the patient has problems maintaining an adequate food intake, at this stage to monitor, give advice on healthy eating, taking small frequent meals and ways of stimulating the appetite;
- if weight loss is rapid, to advise and prescribe increased intake of foods which provide extra protein and energy. Appetite stimulants may be used and supplements such as Buildup, Ensure, Fortical or Complan may be advised, added to or between meals;
- in acute weight loss or when the patient is unable to take food by mouth, when gastrostomy or the insertion of a nasogastric tube for partial or complete enteral feeding will be needed. In extreme cases parenteral feeding will be considered.

To ensure adequate nutrition at any stage, intake must be planned and prescribed by professionals. Malnourishment does not necessarily mean that the patient is losing weight. Some conditions or treatments cause their own problems; for example, steroid treatment stimulates the appetite, making the patient always hungry. Pancreatic disease may cause a deficiency in digestive enzymes so that the patient has to take these in order to digest food. In these situations patients need the advice of the dietitian and support of the carers to ensure that they remain as fit as possible.

Alternative diets are also a cause for anxiety; these are very popular with patients who, like the public in general, are keen to try diets which promote health. Dietitians consider that these diets are generally more harmful than beneficial in nutritional terms. Alternative diets are generally strictly vegetarian and mostly eaten raw, are high in fibre, high in bulk and low in calories. This means that patients who are already suffering from a calorie deficit have no chance of catching up on weight lost, and those who find it hard to take large quantities of food cannot eat all they need. Hunter (1991) proposes that 'alternative dietary therapies are in fact forms of psychotherapy' where the individual nutrients or regimen are there as a structure on which to hang the psychotherapeutic interventions. If this is so the effect of using the technique with a sound nutritional therapy would have considerable benefit.

To ensure that patients have an adequate diet it is sensible to consult the dietitian early, before there has been a dramatic weight change. The family need to be involved so that they understand how best to help the patient, providing small, high-calorie meals rather than trying to push food when it cannot be taken. Consultation wherever possible should be direct between patient and dietitian but when this is not possible, in some community or isolated situations, the nurse will need to make the contact by telephone.

Appliance fitting

The role of the appliance fitter depends on the local situation. In many situations fitting is undertaken by the professional involved in the patient's treatment. Where one individual undertakes these duties, for example in a large hospital, a patient and resourceful individual is called for. The problems referred to the appliance fitter can be very varied, so that keeping up to date with new products and knowing the manufacturers well enough to be able to obtain unusual appliances or sizes is important. The appliances most often fitted are wigs, breast prostheses and elastic compression garments either for lymphoedema or thrombosis. Stoma products are usually supplied to the specifications of the stoma therapist.

Patients are seen at a vulnerable time and need to be able to discuss their needs in a relaxed and private situation. Often they do not know what is available, what financial assistance they can obtain or how to adjust their clothing or activities to the changes occurring. Time to talk, discuss possibilities and try out different styles is helpful.

Chiropody

The chiropodist is usually included in the team. Patients' needs for this service are variable and referrals are often for pre-existing problems. Healthy feet are a comfort to patients compromised by their illness and the removal of discomfort helps them to remain or become mobile.

Chaplaincy

In cancer the care of the patient as a whole being must include the physical, psychological and spiritual aspects of care. Of these, spiritual care is the one most frequently avoided and misunderstood. However, spiritual well-being is considered to be an essential equal contributor with physical, social and psychological well-being to a good quality of life.

The diagnosis of cancer brings with it a crisis of belief – belief in the meaning and purpose of life – and the question 'Why me?' is a frequent response to the news. The spiritual needs of people described by Cosh (1988) include the need to give and receive love, and the need for hope and creativity as well as meaning and purpose. These needs are not encompassed entirely by the religious aspects of life: therapies which restore creativity, and offer friendship and acceptance are helping the patient in spiritual terms. As Cosh points out, spiritual matters do not necessarily equate with religion, but many people fulfil their spiritual needs through formalized religion. In the hospital or hospice the chaplain is an integral part of the rehabilitation team, offering spiritual support, a listening ear and guidance to all patients regardless of their beliefs. For patients chaplains offer a way for them to reconcile themselves with their shattered expectations of life. For the other members of the team chaplains offer their specialist support and give advice when those team members have to deal with dilemmas which could not wait or when the patient does not wish to consult the chaplain directly. When nurses feel unhappy or unable to discuss spiritual issues with their patients, they should be asked who else they would like to talk to. A small research study in the USA (Highfield, 1992) has shown that the spiritual health of older patients with lung cancer was good and that those with fewer physical symptoms reported the highest levels of spiritual health. When asked who they preferred as spiritual care giver, most patients gave 'family member/friend' or 'personal pastor or rabbi' as their preference, suggesting that they preferred the support of those with whom they had an ongoing relationship.

At times of crisis many people need a thoughtful listener; in hospital the chaplain can be called on as much as a friend as a religious adviser, while at home the role may be filled by relatives and friends as well. Nurses often find spiritual questions difficult because they come 'out of the blue' and question personal values. It is a time to practise good listening and to realize that the spiritual dimension of the patient is as important to well-being as the physical and psychological.

Medicine

In the ideal situation rehabilitation and active therapy are closely linked, with rehabilitation anticipating needs and responding to them. In the real world, rehabilitation often follows when the curative aspects of medical care have been completed and the patient is not yet ready to go home. The medical input in rehabilitation will continue according to the stage of the disease; it may be active, supportive or palliative, diagnosing and treating symptoms of continuing disease as they arise. In rehabilitation the psychiatrist may be called upon to help patients cope with their return to the outside world when the changes brought about by the disease or treatment are causing them psychological problems. Research has shown that the majority of people cope well with the stresses caused by cancer but a significant number – 44% in one study – have psychiatric disorders (Derogatis *et al.*, 1983). These disorders included adjustment disorders, depression and anxiety. These crises mostly occur at times when stress would be expected to rise – diagnosis and recurrence – but for some patients symptoms persist; for example, depression is still present in as many as 25% of patients up to two years after treatment for breast cancer (Maguire *et al.*, 1978).

All patients diagnosed with a life-threatening illness are likely to suffer anxiety, stress and sadness (depression). The problem for the nurse is to recognize when the individual needs help in overcoming these normal reactions. There is no hard and fast rule as to when referral to a psychiatrist or counsellor is indicated; however, a general guide is that help is needed when the patient's ability to function normally, and his or her ability to understand and make reasoned judgements, are affected. The treatment offered may be counselling, which involves emotional support and non-directive advice in a sympathetic atmosphere (Moorey, 1988), psychological intervention including cognitive behavioural therapy to foster a 'fighting spirit' (Watson, 1983) and drug treatment, particularly for patients suffering from depression. In a number of centres and in community settings nurses trained in psychological support are available to patients and their relatives at times of stress.

Social work and patients' rights

The social work department will be involved with the patient's needs and the support of the family from diagnosis. Different pressures arise throughout treatment: financial problems due to loss of income or increased expenditure, family stress from the absence of the patient and the need to arrange visits and a multitude of other individual problems.

In the rehabilitation phase the social worker's efforts will concentrate on the patient's return home and where possible to work. In this situation they will need to advise patients of their rights and help them to resume their place in society. Many people do not know their entitlements in relation to employment or accommodation and may meekly accept termination of their employment or tenancy when hospitalized as the norm.

As vulnerable individuals, patients need the advice and support offered by experienced social workers at this time.

Complementary therapies

The public interest in 'healthy living' has founded a growth industry of health clubs and a continual stream of magazine articles on methods of achieving a beautiful body and healthy lifestyle. For patients with cancer the therapies available offer additional attention, hope, comfort and care in the busy round of treatment and hospitalization. In this supportive sense complementary therapies are increasingly accepted by the health care professions as valuable to patients in their recovery and well-being. The fact that the terms 'complementary' and 'supportive' are now more frequently used than 'alternative' to describe the treatments which are not generally offered to patients in orthodox Western medical care suggests their growing acceptance. Nurses in particular are interested in understanding and using complementary therapies with their patients. A recent survey of community nursing staff showed that 74% of them were regularly asked for information about complementary therapy and they all wanted to know more about the subject (Meldrum, 1992). The therapies most frequently asked about were aromatherapy, massage, homeopathy and stress reduction techniques. Many people believe that they benefit from complementary therapy and for some therapies research is beginning to support their beliefs.

Aromatherapy is a technique where aromatic oils of plant origin are used in gentle massage to sooth aches and pains and to enhance a feeling of well-being. The different oils, often massaged into acupuncture points, are believed to have specific effects on particular parts of the body, influencing major organs to sedate or stimulate their function. These specific treatments require experience and should only be undertaken by a trained therapist who appreciates the patient's condition; referral should be checked with the patient's medical practitioner because some patients have had reactions to the oils. Treatment is soothing and relaxing and although there is no scientific evidence for the benefits claimed for the different oils, therapists believe that they do have an effect (Dixon, 1993).

For the patient there are certainly the added benefits of personalized care: 'For that hour I was the most important person in the world'; and help for the patient to overcome problems of altered body image: 'She looked at me and touched me as if there was nothing wrong.'

Massage is an ancient, even instinctive, activity with physical and emotional expression. Kneading a painful muscle, rubbing the mother's back in labour, stroking a baby's head, the mutual stimulation between lovers, are everyday examples of the power of massage. Touching is an expression of feeling and a form of communication with meanings beyond those of words. As therapy, massage can be used at different levels. The physiotherapist will use it therapeutically to ease, stretch and strengthen muscle, improving mobility and increasing strength. In lymphoedema light massage is used to stimulate lymph nodes and enhance drainage. Nurses and aromatherapists practise more gentle massage, with slow rhythmic strokes which have been shown to relieve muscle tension and induce relaxation (Sims, 1986) as well as being incorporated into patient care to promote sleep (Holmes, 1986).

The effects of massage have been described as:

- psychological, in the reduction of anxiety and the facilitation of positive relationships;
- reflex, in inducing vasodilation and reducing muscle tension and spasm;
- mechanical, emptying lymphatics, increasing circulation, diuresis, peristalsis and skin temperature (Sims, 1986).

Although massage has proven benefits for the patient, nurses who extend their skills by learning the technique must remember that there are contraindications, for example in cellulitis where there is a danger of spreading infection, or in phlebitis where there is the risk of releasing emboli; when there are bone metastases fractures could result from even gentle massage, and when the skin is fragile further damage could be caused.

When massaging cancer patients it is always best to be gentle, use unscented oils or the patient's usual moisturizer and to avoid areas of active disease. This said, many patients enjoy massage to the hands, neck and face, finding this relaxing and non-intrusive.

Relaxation is particularly beneficial in stress management, reducing psychological arousal; it is popular as part of many exercise regimes and has long been used to help women in labour. Because of this it is widely accepted by patients who do not consider it to be 'weird or way out'. Many techniques are available, including yoga, progressive muscle relaxation and guided imagery; these can be practised alone or in groups. For those new to relaxation the group setting is a good introduction, encouraging the individual to concentrate, providing company and an adviser for techniques and comfortable positioning.

Art therapy has a well-established place in psychiatry and has more recently been found to be of value to cancer patients as a means of expressing and understanding their frustrations. Although satisfying to the patient as a creative activity, art therapy should not be seen solely as a diversion or a means of developing talent. Through art patients can fulfil many needs, exploring, expressing and questioning what is happening to their body, mind and spirit. The therapist acts as a partner, offering help when asked for, listening and discussing the art work. The art therapist works closely with the psychotherapist, who will act as a support for both patient and therapist (Connell, 1992).

Music therapy makes use of the influence of music on mood, as an expression of feelings and as a distraction. It employs the selective use of music in a planned and systematic programme to bring comfort and enhance conventional therapy. Patient and therapist work together to select music which will help the patient in different situations and with symptoms such as pain, anxiety, insomnia and depression. Music therapists also use their skills to help patients who have lost the use of language or have other communication problems, allowing them to communicate by participating in musical activities, beating a rhythm, moving to the music or joining in a song (Mandel, 1991).

Concerts and musical events are also brought to patients by the Council for Music in Hospitals. For the patient this shared experience, listening to and participating in music is a social and normalizing event in a strange environment. In the intimate setting of the day room or ward it creates a line of communication between listener and performer (Lindsay, 1993).

Creative and diversional activities are seen as an important part of rehabilitation, particularly for patients who have spent a long time in hospital or are receiving traumatic therapy. Their independence may be lost and real fears about coping in the outside world may exist. Independence, self-worth and purpose are important spiritual aspects which do not decrease as illness progresses and which should be fostered throughout life. The type of diversional activity offered will depend on the patient's character, likes and dislikes; they should not be expected to join in social activities which are contrary to their lifestyle. However, the programme of activities needs to be advertised and available. Games, books, crafts, music and television are standard activities but for patients who are confined to hospital, hospice or home, outings such as car drives, shopping trips and snacks or meals out are important as a link with normality. Stepping outside to buy a newspaper can be an important first move for patients concerned about how they look or how they can communicate. Visits from volunteers, local groups, businesses and organizations all enhance the atmosphere and create links with the local community.

The professional services and complementary therapies described above are those most often recognized as contributing to rehabilitation. Team members may make use of or call for the help of specialists in other techniques such as hypnotherapy, meditation, reflexology and spiritual healing when patients ask and it is thought they might benefit from them. Similarly some patients will attend centres whose philosophy is health enhancing and centres around organic, usually vegetarian, diets. As discussed under 'Dietetics' above the value of these centres is in enhancing the patient's ability to cope rather than in having a direct effect on the cancer.

REHABILITATION NURSING

Rehabilitation is not, as yet, recognized as a unique specialty in oncology. At ward level rehabilitation is generally seen as the responsibility of specific professions such as physiotherapy or occupational therapy. The patients whose treatment is completed but who are not fit to go home may be left to fend for themselves in a busy ward. In this situation the advantage of a low-dependency rehabilitation ward like the one in the Marie Curie Rehabilitation Centre at the Royal Marsden Hospital is apparent. Patients admitted to the ward are either transferred from the main hospital to complete rehabilitation following radical treatment or admitted from home for treatments such as compression bandaging or voice restoration. The atmosphere in the ward helps patients to attain an optimum lifestyle, with all the professional, complementary and nursing skills of rehabilitation available. In this setting ward nurses can use their skills in rehabilitation; in others nurses are increasingly extending their roles, developing specialist knowledge to treat patients with specific problems and offer advice to others about the care of their patients. Some specialties are long established and widely recognized as nursing special-ties, such as stoma care and breast care, while others like lymphoedema and psychological care are gaining recognition.

Stoma care

The stoma specialist offers ostomists counselling and expert advice on the care of their stoma, the choice of equipment, education for self-care, dealing with specific problems such as malodour, leaks and soreness, sexual advice and psychological support on a long-term basis. Most patients are seen by the specialist prior to surgery and share in planning the location of the stoma site. Post-operatively care and advice are available for the rest of the patient's life, usually on an as-needed basis. The aim of this support is to promote self-care, a positive attitude and independence (Salter, 1988). Booklets for ostomists such as those produced by Squibb (undated) help patients to realize that a normal lifestyle is possible for them along with the estimated 45 000 people in the UK who have stomas (Coloplast, 1987).

The great advantage for nurses in general is to have a specialist in stoma care available as adviser when caring for an ostomist. It is easy to get out of practice or out of date with equipment when you are not caring for patients with a stoma every day. Stoma specialists are employed in most hospital and community settings and by companies providing stoma equipment. A list of stoma care nursing services in the UK, Eire and the Channel Islands is available from the Royal College of Nursing. An update on the anatomical types of stoma, patient advice, appliances, general care and trouble-shooting can be found in the *Manual of Clinical Nursing Procedures* (Pritchard and Mallett, 1992).

Stoma specialists often combine their role with that of continence adviser, helping patients with this intimate problem through exercises to re-educate weakened muscles, teach self-catheterization, advise on the use of equipment and support, both patient and family.

Breast care

Nurses specializing in breast care support and advise patients who have cancer of the breast from diagnosis, through treatment and its after-effects. Information, support and counselling are offered on diagnosis when anxiety is high, investigations need to be explained and support offered until the results are obtained. When a number of treatment options are possible these need to be described so that the patient can make the best choice for her. The breast care specialist is usually present during consultation and is able to reinforce the advice given and answer any queries which arise. Support is offered to all patients, including those having radiotherapy, chemotherapy and hormone treatments. For those needing surgery, breast reconstruction is explained when appropriate and advice offered on prostheses, clothing and the prevention of lympho-edema. Psychological morbidity is as high as 25% in breast cancer (Maguire *et al.*, 1978); by meeting the patient at diagnosis and being a link person throughout treatment the breast care nurse is in a unique position to identify problems and refer the patient if required. There is close liaison between the breast care specialist, medical, nursing and psychological care teams, with the breast care specialist acting as a link between these groups.

Lymphoedema care

Some nurses have extended their role in breast care to include the treatment of lymphoedema and have received training in this to become part of a multidisciplinary team with doctors and physiotherapists to treat patients with lymphoedema (Benington, 1991). Although the most common site of lymphoedema is the arm and the most common predisposing condition is breast cancer, lymphoedema can affect the legs and other areas of the body when the lymphatic drainage system has been damaged. Occasionally lymphoedema occurs in people without any

Table 15.6   Lymphoedema treatment

Skin care
Assess for damage: cracks, lymphorrhoea, infection and refer for drug treatment
as necessary
Use moisturizer
Educate for self-care

Massage
Stimulate superficial lymphatics
Manual lymph drainage
Teach self massage

Compression
Bandaging
Intermittent pressure
Supply support garments
Check regularly at clinic

Exercise
Encourage normal movement
Phsyiotherapy for stiff joints
Teach exercises

history of injury to the lymphatic system; this primary lymphoedema is
believed to be the result of congenital defects in the lymphatic system. In
the cancer patient lymphoedema develops when the lymph drainage
system is blocked by scarring or fibrosis following radiotherapy or
surgery to lymph nodes or in active disease when the cancer infiltrates the
system. The development of lymphoedema often occurs many years after
initial treatment when the patients consider themselves cured. Anxiety is
added to distress as the patient considers the possible recurrence of the
disease. Prevention is obviously better than cure, and less damaging
treatments, patient education and monitoring will hopefully reduce the
occurrence in the future.

The consequences of lymphoedema can be serious; the weight and
discomfort of the swelling reduce mobility and can lead to social isolation
and depression. The pooled fluid is an ideal medium for bacterial growth
and when the over-stretched dry skin is broken cellulitis soon follows.
Many treatments have been tried for lymphoedema, including surgery to
debulk the limb, diuretics, elevation, exercise, massage, compression
bandaging and intermittent compression therapy (Hodkinson, 1992).
Practitioners today favour the methods developed by using compression
bandaging to reduce the swelling initially and then maintaining the limb
shape with elastic support garments. The principles of management, skin
care, exercise, external support and massage are described by Badger and

Twycross (1988) and apply in both active and maintenance phases of treatment (Table 15.6). Patient education for self-care is important and booklets are available to help with this (Regnard *et al.*, 1991).

The physical manifestations of lymphoedema reduce the patient's ability to perform the tasks required for daily living, such as dressing and writing, or mobility if the leg is affected. To the patient who has passed several years disease-free it is often taken as a sign of recurrence. Socially the patient can become isolated, unable to go out or not wishing to do so because they feel unsightly. Patients need to be helped to overcome these difficulties and referred to an oncology centre or hospice where specialist advice and treatment are available. Many patients suffer for years without treatment, often because they or their doctors do not know that treatment is possible.

Psychological care

A diagnosis of cancer has a dramatic impact on the patient. Feelings of fear, anger, sadness and disbelief are common; most patients will cope with these in their own way and most nurses will be able to support them through these feelings. However, in the ward setting it may be difficult for the nurse or patient to work them through to a satisfactory conclusion. In some centres oncology nurses with training in psychology work with psychiatrists to provide a support service for patients who have problems which they cannot cope with or find it difficult to express. The stage of referral depends on the individual situation and will usually follow discussion between the ward or out-patient staff and the psychological support team, although some patients are self-referring.

Therapy will involve an agreement between patient and therapist for a number of sessions with defined aims. As the patient regains control further aims may be agreed or support offered.

Community liaison

Cancer treatment often involves repeated hospital admissions and journeys to the hospital for treatment or check-ups while living at home. Liaison between professionals in the hospital and the community is essential to the patient's well-being. The responsibility for passing on care information rests with the nurse in charge of the patient's care, and updates of the patient's status are as important when coming from the community nurse to the hospital on admission as going to him or her on discharge. Many hospitals now have nurses who specialize in community liaison and have referral documents which detail the patient's treatment and current care requirements (Houlton, 1988). Such documentation is valuable to community nurses, who are thus prepared for the tasks to come and can plan their day appropriately. For the patient it means that the nurse who visits appreciates his or her situation and is able to continue the treatment as planned.

The nurse's role in rehabilitation

If rehabilitation is recognized as an integral part of care in all phases of the cancer illness, then the nurse must play a key role in rehabilitation. As teachers of self-care, listeners, counsellors and coordinators they contribute to the patient's return to society and help to optimize their lifestyle. As specialists they have taken on roles which extend their nursing input to individual patient groups and supply support, expertise and information to their colleagues.

Nurses working in isolated situations have particular responsibilities for ensuring that their patients receive rehabilitation services. They can be resourceful, developing their own skills in areas such as teaching relaxation and attending counselling or aromatherapy courses. They can also build up their own library of resources, including information on local services, relaxation tapes, booklets for patients and lists of local help for patients and carers. Knowing where to find out information and forming networks with specialists is far more useful than trying to retain all the information as an individual. For the patient the nurse then becomes a coordinator of the multidisciplinary rehabilitation team (Anderson, 1989).

THE ROLE OF REHABILITATION

The role of rehabilitation is to assist the patient in the journey to independence. This can be by using specialist skills or by enhancing and complementing those of other therapists. At diagnosis patients are seen as cases for treatment and become dependent on the system for treatment; they are undressed, deskilled and part of a strange community. Rehabilitation has other aims for the patient, seeing an individual who wants independence, a purpose to life and an independent existence in spite of the constraints of illness. Rehabilitation can shift detrimental effects of cancer on health by improving the quality of life (Figure 15.2). Because the aim of rehabilitation is to help patients achieve an optimum quality of life, rehabilitation is as appropriate for the elderly and patients in palliation as it is for the young and patients having curative treatment. In the palliative care setting as well as in any other, rehabilitation should be patient led and will include all the therapies described at an appropriate intensity for the individual patient. Some people may question the need to rehabilitate when life expectancy is limited; there are ethical and financial dilemmas but few will question the right to an optimum quality of life.

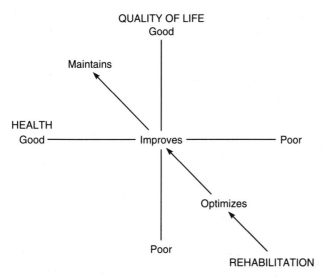

Figure 15.2   The influence of rehabilitation on health and quality of life.

Every living human being, no matter how sick, possesses a finite life expectancy, and something can be done to improve the quality of that remaining time to live. (Gunn, 1984)

REFERENCES

Anderson, J.L. (1989) The nurse's role in cancer rehabilitation. *Cancer Nursing*, **12**(2), 85–94.

Badger, C. and Twycross, R. (1988) *Management of Lymphoedema*. Sir Michael Sobell House, Oxford.

Benington, G. (1991) Nursing management of lymphoedema. *Nursing Standard*, **6**(7), 24–7.

Coloplast Ltd (1987) *Ostomy and Ostomy Patients: An Introductory Guide for Nurses*. Medicine Group (UK), Oxford.

Connell, C. (1992) Art therapy as part of a palliative care programme. *Palliative Medicine*, **6**, 18–25.

Cosh, R. (1988) Spiritual issues in cancer care, in *Oncology for Nurses and Health Care Professionals*, Vol. 2 (eds R. Tiffany and P. Webb), Harper & Row, Beaconsfield.

David, J.A. (1992) *A study of Rehabilitation in a Specialist Oncology Centre*. Marie Curie Cancer Care Report, London.

de Haes, J.C.J.M., van Knippenberg, F.C.E. and Neijt, J.P. (1990) Measuring psychological and physical distress in cancer patients: structure and application of the Rotterdam symptom checklist. *British Journal of Cancer*, **62**, 1034–8.

Derogatis, L.R., Morrow, G.R., Fetting, J. *et al.* (1983) The prevalence of psychiatric disorders among cancer patients. *Journal of the American Medical Association*, **249**, 751–7.

Dietz, J.H. (1981) *Rehabilitation Oncology*. Wiley, New York.

Dixon, L. (1993) The gentle touch. *Cancer Nursing Society News Letter*, **2**(1), 5.

Dorsett, D.S. (1992) The trajectory of cancer recovery, in *The Chronic Illness Trajectory Framework* (ed. P. Woog), Springer, New York.

Fallowfield, L. (1990) *The Quality of Life: The Missing Measurement in Health Care*. Souvener Press (A & E) Ltd, London.

Gunn, A. (1984) *Cancer Rehabilitation*. Raven Press, New York.

Highfield, M.F. (1992) Spiritual health of oncology patients. *Cancer Nursing*, **15**(1), 1–8.

Hodkinson, M. (1992) Lymphoedema: applying physiology to treatment. *European Journal of Cancer Care*, **1**(2), 19–23.

Holmes, P. (1986) Fringe benefits. *Nursing Times*, **82**(22), 20–2.

Houlton, E.J. (1988) The cancer patient in the community, in *Oncology for Nurses and Health Care Professionals*. Vol. 2: *Care and Support* (eds R. Tiffany and P. Webb), Harper & Row, Beaconsfield.

Hunter, M. (1991) Dietary therapies for cancer: challenging the alternatives. *European Journal of Cancer Care*, **1**(1), 27–9.

Jobbins, J., Addy, M., Bagg, J. *et al.* (1992) A clinical trial of chlorhexidine oral spray in terminally ill cancer patients. *Palliative Medicine*, **6**, 299–307.

Karnofsky, D.A., Abelman, W.H., Carver, L.F. and Burchenal, J.H. (1948) The use of nitrogen mustard in the palliative treatment of carcinoma. *Cancer*, **1**, 634–53.

Lindsay, S. (1993) Musical care. *Nursing Standard*, **7**(19), 20–1.

Lohmann, C. (1992) The role of the physiotherapist. *Palliative Care Today*, **2**, 26–7.

McCaffrey, D. (1991) Surviving cancer. *Nursing Times*, **87**(32), 26–30.

McLellan, D. (1991) Rehabilitation. *British Medical Journal*, **303**, 355–7.

Maguire, G.P., Lec, E.G., Bevington, D.J. *et al.* (1978) Psychiatric problems in the first year after mastectomy. *British Medical Journal*, **i**, 963–5.

Mandel, S.E. (1991) Music therapy in the hospice: 'Musicalive'. *Palliative Medicine*, **5**, 155–60.

Meldrum, R. (1992) Complementary therapies: what nurses need to know. *Primary Health Care*, **2**(9), 6.

Moorey, S. (1988) The psychological impact of cancer, in *Oncology for Nurses and Health Care Professionals*. Vol. 2: *Care and Support* (eds R. Tiffany and P. Webb), Harper & Row, Beaconsfield.

Office of Population Censuses and Surveys (1989) *Survey of Disability in Great Britain*. HMSO, London.

Pritchard, A.P. and Mallett, J. (eds) (1992) *Manual of Clinical Nursing Procedures*. Blackwell Scientific Publications, Oxford.

Pyle, L. (1993) Rehabilitation at the Royal Marsden Hospital. *Journal of Cancer Care*, **2**(1), 29–32.

Raven, R.W. (1971) The concept of cancer rehabilitation and its implications, in *Symposium on the Rehabilitation of the Cancer Disabled* (ed. R W. Raven), Heinemann, London.

Regnard, C., Badger, C. and Mortimer, P. (1991) *Lymphoedema: Advice on Treatment*. Beaconsfield Publishers, Beaconsfield.

Rhodes, V.A., Watson, P.M. and Johnson, M.H. (1984) Development of a reliable and valid measure of nausea and vomiting. *Cancer Nursing*, **7**(1), 33–41.

Royal Marsden Hospital Patient Education Group (1989) *Overcoming Eating Difficulties*. Royal Marsden Hospital, London.

Salter, M. (1988) *Altered Body Image*. Scutari Press, London.

Shaw, C. and Hunter, M. (1991) *Special Diet Cookbooks: Cancer*. Thorsons, London.

Sims, S. (1986) Slow stroke back massage for cancer patients. Occasional paper. *Nursing Times*, **82**(13), 47–50.

Stumm, D. (1988) Living with cancer: rehabilitation, in *Oncology for Nurses and Health Care Professionals*. Vol. 2: *Care and Support* (eds R. Tiffany and P. Webb), Harper & Row, Beaconsfield.

Squibb Surgicare (undated) Booklets: *Understanding Colostomy, Understanding Ileostomy, Understanding Urostomy*. Squibb Surgicare, Hounslow.

Teeling Smith, G. (ed.) (1988) *Measuring Health: A Practical Guide*. Wiley, Chichester.

Walker, V., Dicks, B. and Webb, P. (1987) Pain assessment charts in the management of chronic cancer pain. *Palliative Medicine*, **1**, 111–16.

Watson, M. (1983) Psychological intervention with cancer patients: a selected review. *Psychological Medicine*, **13**(1), 839–46.

Wells, R.J. (1990) Rehabilitation: making the most of time. *Oncology Nursing Forum*, **17**(4), 503–7.

Zigmond, A.S. and Snaith, R.P. (1983) The hospital anxiety and depression scale. *Acta Psychiatrica Scandanavica*, **67**, 361.

Further reading

Denton, S. (1991) Nursing patients with breast cancer, in *Oncology for Nurses and Health Care Professionals*. Vol. 3: *Cancer Nursing* (eds R. Tiffany and D. Borley), Harper Collins, London.

Downie, P.A. (1978) *Cancer Rehabilitation: An introduction for Physiotherapists and the Allied Professions*. Faber & Faber, London.

Harvey, J. (1988) Nutrition, in *Nursing the patient with cancer* (ed. V. Tschudin), Prentice Hall, New York.

Tiffany, R. and Borley, D. (eds) (1991) *Oncology for Nurses and Health Care Professionals*. Vol. 3: *Cancer Nursing*. Harper Collins, London.

Tiffany, R. and Webb, P. (eds) (1988) *Oncology for Nurses and Health Care Professionals*. Vol. 2: *Care and Support*. Harper & Row, Beaconsfield.

Young, M.E. and Quinn, E. (1992) *Theories and Principles of Occupational Therapy*. Churchill Livingstone, Edinburgh.

16 Educational opportunities in cancer care

Eileen Gape

INTRODUCTION

The nurse caring for patients with cancer can choose to function primarily on the technical level, i.e. administering medications, performing procedures, assessing the patient's physical status and moving rapidly from one task to another, and indeed a high level of technical competence is necessary; but this alone is not sufficient. The nurse also needs to be an analytical problem solver, a creative seeker of new ways of achieving a high quality of life for the patient with cancer.

Nursing is a unique discipline, completely separate and different from medicine. A doctor does not have the knowledge or skills necessary to practise nursing, any more than a nurse has the knowledge and skills to practise medicine. The nurse–patient relationship is as important as the doctor–patient relationship, not subordinate to it.

Doctors and nurses, however, should not be rivals; they should function interdependently. Very little in health care can be achieved by a single person or a single discipline. Communication, mutual respect and cooperation are necessary to provide quality patient care. It is the cancer patient who experiences the greater loss if this relationship does not exist (Burns, 1982).

How then can the nurse identify the necessary knowledge and practical skills to achieve a high quality of life for the patient with cancer?

The Advisory Committee on Training in Nursing (Commission of the European Communities, 1988) recommends that pre-registration education should include:

1. prevention, detection and diagnosis of cancer;
2. identification of the problems of patients with cancer and specific responses to their needs;

3. administration of anticancer therapy programmes;
4. participation in rehabilitation of the patient with cancer;
5. participation in the terminal stages of the illness;
6. care of the family of the patient with cancer.

It is further recommended that students, together with other professionals concerned, should actively participate in action programmes against cancer, collaborate in informing and educating the general public about the positive benefits of prevention, screening and detection, and the early treatment of cancerous conditions.

The need for continuing education by post-registration nurses was also addressed by the Advisory Committee (Commission of the European Communities, 1988). It was recognized that continuing education can be varied in its form and content and frequently overlaps with in-service training. Continuing education is seen as planned educational activities ranging from formal, organized teaching to private, distance learning designed to build upon pre-registration training and post-registration experience to maintain and enhance the individual's knowledge and professional skills. By contrast, in-service training is seen as consisting of activities intended to assist nurses to maintain and improve their competence in carrying out their professional role and responsibilities specific to the expectations of the employer.

The recommendations of the committee concluded that the continuing education/training programmes for all nurses should:

1. update acquired knowledge, reinforce specific aspects and stimulate and promote reflection on nurses' actual professional experience with cancer patients;
2. cover relationships and personal and ethical issues nurses have to face in their work with patients who have cancer as well as the necessary theoretical information on pathology, diagnostic and therapeutic methods;
3. use a flexible approach both to the conditions of access to courses and to the structure of such courses.

It was further recognized that advanced training would also be necessary for some nurses and it was recommended that this should:

1. be at the highest appropriate level;
2. incorporate theoretical medical knowledge together with a knowledge of human relationships and the acquiring of skills in managing teams of nurses responsible for patients with cancer;
3. involve the nurses in research work in the field of cancer nursing, the nurse being encouraged to publish his or her work;
4. following completion of high-level training, ensure that the nurse continues to take part in relevant research and fulfils an advisory role

in the departments concerned with providing specialist training for nursing staff.

Despite these recommendations of the Advisory Committee in respect of pre-registration and the need for continuing education for all nurses in cancer care, nurses are frequently concerned that they do not have sufficient knowledge and skills to achieve the high quality of life they strive to attain for their patients (Commission of the European Communities, 1988).

Corner and Wilson-Barnett (1992) in a study of newly registered nurses (i.e. within six months of first registering as a registered general nurse with the UKCC) found that they rated themselves as most competent in giving physical care to patients with cancer as well as feeling competent in communicating generally with these patients. However, they rated themselves as being less competent in more specific areas of communication and psychological care, e.g. helping patients come to terms with the fact they have cancer, dealing with an uncertain future and talking about death and dying with the patient. They rated themselves the least competent in teaching the early detection of cancer, and prevention of cancer was another area in which they felt they lacked competence.

This is a sad reflection on the abilities of nursing at a time when the Department of Health is promoting the reduction of ill-health and death from four cancers, i.e. cervical, breast, skin and lung, by promoting the necessary changes in individuals' lifestyles, e.g. diet and smoking, together with improving the uptake in breast and cervical cancer screening (*The Health of the Nation*, 1992). It also raises doubts as to the effectiveness of nurses in their abilities to implement the European Commission's 'Europe Against Cancer' initiative which aims to reduce by 15% the number of deaths from cancer in Europe by the year 2000 by promoting, amongst other measures, a simple 10-point code to aid prevention and early detection.

How then do nurses acquire the knowledge and practical skills necessary within cancer nursing? Fortunately within the UK there are many varied opportunities for the development of these. It is not possible to give a definitive guide to these opportunities but what follows is an overview of several possible methods of development that could be utilized by nurses in varying circumstances.

DISTANCE LEARNING

In distance learning the tutor and the student rarely if ever meet and students learn from packages (Keane, 1989). Arguably the Open University is the most renowned proponent of this learning method. They have produced many courses at a variety of levels, e.g. certificate, diploma and degree. Some courses have a built-in assessment scheme which may be optional (usually at an additional cost) or compulsory.

The use of other than written supplementary material may be incorporated into the package, i.e. audio cassette tape, video or in some cases television programmes which are integral to the course. As some of these programmes may involve early-morning or late-night transmissions, the possession of a video recorder can be most helpful!

Several distance learning packages may be found useful by nurses, including:

- Reducing the Risk of Cancers Course, code P578X;
- Health and Disease Course, code U205;
- Research Methods in Education and the Social Sciences Course, code DE304
- Death and Dying Course, code K260.

More details and a full list of courses are available from The Open University, Walton Hall, Milton Keynes MK7 6AA.

OPEN LEARNING

Open learning is different from distance learning in that it seeks to meet the varied requirements of individual students by enabling them to decide what, where, when and how they learn (Lewis, 1986). It encourages individuals to take responsibility for their learning. Two major developments in this field have been the Nursing Times Open Learning Programme and the Royal College of Nursing's Nursing Update.

The Nursing Times Open Learning Programme which commenced in 1991, was not designed solely for enrolled nurses' conversion, but so that its two-year programme should also provide varied, stimulating material for all nurses (Davidson, 1991). It focuses on three main areas, i.e. research, management and professional development. The course is flexible in that the user can follow one component, e.g. research, if that is the area most in need of developing by the user.

The course material is published weekly in the *Nursing Times*, the perforated sections can be taken out, allowing the user to use the material and work through it at his or her own pace. Further information is available from Nursing Times, 4 Little Essex Street, London WC2R 3LF.

1991 also saw the launch of the Royal College of Nursing (RCN) update programme. This consists of a series of television programmes (broadcast in the very early morning), with each broadcast being supplemented with distance learning material. The written material, published in the *Nursing Standard*, identifies learning objectives and offers complementary activities, e.g. participants may be asked to utilize a library to read about the subject in more depth (Casey, 1991).

Nurses have the option to choose which learning units are applicable to their area of practice and also the option to be assessed. Assessment is in two stages and a fee is charged for this. The first stage of assessment is by means of a written question paper and answer sheet which must be returned for marking within three months of publication.

The second stage of assessment is a practice assessment to be assessed by a peer (of the same or a higher grade than the student) and will follow guidelines set down by the RCN. This assessment must be carried out within three months of the notification of a 'pass' result of the first-stage assessment (Wells, 1991). For further information contact IANE, Royal College of Nursing, 20 Cavendish Square, London, W1M OAB.

In 1993 Marie Curie Cancer Care launched an open learning package for nurses in cancer care. Cancer Care Nursing is a flexible programme designed for registered nurses who want to undertake a course to diploma level. On completion of the programme and assessments, successful students are awarded the Marie Curie Diploma in Cancer Care. This is equivalent to 72 credits from Humberside College of Health at Higher Education Diploma level. These credits may be used as a component part of a full Higher Education Diploma, which requires a total of 120 credits (see 'Credit accumulation and transfer' below). For further information write to Cancer Care Nursing Diploma, Marie Curie Cancer Care, Education Department, 17 Grosvenor Crescent, London SW1X 8QJ.

RECORDABLE QUALIFICATIONS

Since 1983 the National Boards for Nursing, Midwifery and Health Visiting has been responsible for approving courses of which some can be recorded on the professional register of the United Kingdom Central Council for Nurses, Midwifery and Health Visiting (UKCC). The four boards for England, Wales, Scotland and Northern Ireland have sought to take full account of the needs of the profession and the service required in each country, while ensuring standards are met. This has resulted in each country establishing its own framework of continuing education.

SCOTLAND

The National Board for Nursing, Midwifery and Health Visiting for Scotland (NBS) instituted its framework in 1985 with the introduction of Professional Studies One and Two modules, which lead to the award of the NBS Diploma in Professional Studies. Professional Studies One comprises modules which are generic in nature and cover the major areas of study of technology and science, moral, legal and political issues that relate to nursing. Examples of these modules include:

- Infection – Prevention and Control
- Interpersonal Relationships
- Learning, Teaching and Counselling
- Management of Nursing Practice in Terminal Care
- Management of Pain.

Professional Studies Two is intended to enable the nurse to develop knowledge and competence in a specific area of practice while not losing contact with the broader issues and developments within the profession. Examples of these modules are:

- Nursing Care of Terminally Ill Patients and Carers
- Attitudes to Death and Dying
- Nursing Care of a Patient Requiring Chemotherapy
- Nursing Care of a Patient Requiring Radiotherapy
- Understanding and Managing Pain
- Continuing Care in Advanced Disease
- Symptom Control in Advanced Disease
- Foundation Skills in Nursing People with Cancer
- Nursing the Adult with Specific Cancers.

The NBS Diploma in Professional Studies is awarded on completion of six modules:

- Professional Studies One – three modules
- Professional Studies Two – three modules.

Nurses can, however, complete either Professional Studies One (three modules) or Professional Studies Two (three modules) if they so wish. The NBS will forward the details of nurses who are awarded the diploma to the UKCC to have the award recorded on the nurse's record (NBS, 1991). Currently the three modules of Professional Studies One should be of an equal length and undertaken in a minimum of 27 weeks, exclusive of leave. However, the three modules need not be taken consecutively. The same conditions apply to Professional Studies Two. Further information and details of these and other courses can be obtained from the National Board for Nursing, Midwifery and Health Visiting for Scotland, 22 Queen Street, Edinburgh EH2 1JX.

WALES

The Welsh National Board for Nursing, Midwifery and Health Visiting (WNB) outlined its framework for the Development of Professional

Practice in 1989. This modular scheme is built around a common core that includes all the elements of professional practice:

- Conceptual Frameworks for Nursing, Midwifery and Health Visiting
- Health Promotion
- Professional Issues
- Interpersonal Skills
- The Understanding of Research
- Clinical Management
- Practice Issues
- Teaching and Assessing.

A Certificate in Professional Practice is awarded for two modules: the common core and two further modules focusing on clinical practice (WNB, 1994). Examples of certificate modules include:

- Assessment and Management of Pain
- Rehabilitation
- Cancer Nursing
- Care of the Elderly
- Care of the Dying Patient and the Family
- Working with Families
- Basic Counselling Skills
- Palliative Care Nursing
- Applied Nutrition in Health Care
- Breast and Cervical Screening
- Teaching, Assessing and Supervision.

A Diploma in Professional Practice is awarded for a further four diploma-level modules focusing on the broader aspects of professional practice (WNB, 1994). Examples of diploma modules include:

- Health Promotion
- Advances in Cancer Nursing (Radiotherapy and Chemotherapy)
- The Application of Research to Practice
- Women's Health
- Leadership and Resource Management.

Each module (certificate/diploma) will normally extend over a period of 12–15 weeks, with a commitment of 120 hours study per module. The certificate must normally be completed within five years, whereas there is no time limit for the completion of the diploma. Both the Certificate and Diploma in Professional Practice are recordable with the UKCC.

ENGLAND

In 1991 the English National Board for Nursing, Midwifery and Health Visiting (ENB) unveiled its 'Framework for Continuing Professional

Education' and also the 'Higher Award'. Ten key statements form the basis of the new framework, i.e. the nurse will:

- ensure professional accountability and responsibility;
- aim for clinical expertise with a specific client group;
- use research to plan, implement and evaluate strategies to improve care;
- encourage multidisciplinary team working and building;
- develop flexible and innovative approaches to care;
- use health promotion strategies;
- facilitate and assess development in others;
- handle information and make informed clinical decisions;
- set standards and evaluate quality of care;
- instigate, manage and evaluate clinical change.

The ENB through the introduction of the professional portfolio will help practitioners to record their continuing education in relation to the 10 key statements and gain recognition for courses they have attended (Maggs, 1991). Current courses available include:

- ENB 237   Oncology Nursing for Registered Nurses
- ENB 240   Paediatric Oncological Nursing for RSCN
- ENB 243   Oncology Nursing for EN
- ENB 931   Care of the Dying Patient and the Family.
- ENB 285   Continuing Care of the Dying Patient and the Family

The ENB through a system of credits will enable nurses who wish to achieve the Higher Award, which is a professional qualification at degree level and is expected to be completed within five years (Thompson, 1991). Further information is available from ENB Careers, PO Box 356, Sheffield S8 OSJ.

NORTHERN IRELAND

The National Board for Nursing, Midwifery and Health Visiting for Northern Ireland also recognizes that it must ensure that nurse education is responsible and relevant to the needs of patients, clients, practitioners and employers (DHSS, 1991). Courses currently available include Oncological Nursing for RGNs (237). The structure of continuing education in Northern Ireland is currently changing and the national board published its new framework in January 1993. This incorporates three stages, with the national board awarding a certificate, diploma and advanced diploma in professional studies (National Board for Nursing, Midwifery and Health Visiting for Northern Ireland, 1993). Further information is available from the National Board for Nursing, Midwifery and Health Visiting for Northern Ireland, RAC House, 79 Chichester Street, Belfast BT1 4JE.

CREDIT EXEMPTIONS

Each national board, through its respective framework, is striving to ensure that nurses have the maximum opportunities for continuing professional development. However, they also acknowledge that many nurses have already completed or are intending to complete courses outside of the boards' frameworks. The national boards have therefore devised accreditation systems and will consider awarding credit exemptions within their frameworks.

For example, a nurse who has undertaken ENB/WNB 237 (Oncological Nursing for Registered Nurses) and who then decides to enter the WNB Framework for Professional Practice could be awarded two credits: one for common core and one at certificate level. They would therefore enter the framework at diploma level. Further details are available from each national board (see previous addresses).

Alongside this system of credit exemptions the national boards are also looking at credit transfer between other awarding bodies, e.g. universities, polytechnics and the former Council for National Academic Awards (CNAA). This scheme is known as the Credit Accumulation and Transfer Scheme or more popularly as CATS. Scotland has a similar scheme, i.e. the Scottish Credit Accumulation and Transfer (SCOTCAT).

CREDIT ACCUMULATION AND TRANSFER SCHEME

The CATS scheme was developed by the now defunct CNAA to provide a flexible system designed to give people credit for their learning achievements. Its basic principle is that provided the learning can be adequately and appropriately assessed it can be considered for credit towards an academic award (McManus, 1991). This then further allows for the 'credit' to be transferred when the student attends other courses or other institutions, thereby avoiding the need for the student to repeat learning as these changes occur. It will also allow the students to be exempted, i.e. credit exemption, from particular parts of courses, again avoiding repetitious learning.

There are three levels of CATS in the current CNAA system:

- Level one = 120 credits = first year of a degree = certificate;
- Level two = 120 credits = second year of a degree = diploma;
- Level three = 120 credits = third year of a degree = degree (honours).

NB: These levels are cumulative, therefore to obtain a diploma it would be necessary to have 120 credits at level one as well as the 120 necessary at level two.

An agreement between the CNAA and ENB in 1989 (CNAA, 1989) has resulted in many nurses, midwives and health visitors being able to gain this academic credit for both pre-registration and post-registration courses, e.g. it is expected that ENB 237 will result in an award of 30 credits at level one.

Each national board is utilizing the CATS system in some way, e.g. the ENB for its Higher Award requires a nurse to achieve:

- 120 credits at level one;
- 120 credits at level two;
- 120 credits at level three.

On fulfilment of these requirements the nurse will be awarded an honours degree together with the ENB's professional qualification of the Higher Award (Maggs, 1992).

In Wales the WNB have negotiated credit transfer for the Diploma in Professional Practice with the University of Wales and in principle with the Open University. Further information is available from each national board. In addition to accrediting formal courses, the CATS scheme also allows for the accreditation of prior experiential learning.

ACCREDITATION OF PRIOR EXPERIENTIAL LEARNING (APEL)

Learning can occur through many routes and in nursing can involve drawing on personal experiences; for example, nurses who had surgery themselves can use this experience to help them understand the anxieties patients may also experience and develop a strategy for helping them through this process. APEL therefore encourages nurses to reflect on meaningful learning and identify their personal qualities, skills and knowledge (Hull, 1992).

There are three basic stages involved for nurses who wish to use APEL:

1. The students must claim that they have gained experiences which are worthy of academic credit and produce the evidence of their 'learning'.
2. Assessment and verification of this evidence.
3. The award or credit for the learning against the course to be undertaken.

It is the student's responsibility to initiate a claim for credit and to provide the evidence. Evidence can be direct or indirect and come from a variety of sources.

Direct evidence reflects nurses' own work, i.e. anything they have produced themselves or been primarily responsible for, for example:

- samples of patient documentation – care plans, etc.;
- teaching material;
- personal profile demonstrating reflective practice.

Indirect evidence could include:

- certificates, statements of completion, or record of attendance of other courses;
- proof of attendance at study days, conferences, etc.;
- appraisals or individual performance reports from managers.

The assessment process is obviously easier if the evidence offered by nurses is clear and concise. Also nurses need to be aware of problems regarding confidentiality if, for example, patients' care plans are to be used in evidence (WNB, 1992).

Nurses are not particularly renowned for maintaining professional profiles, but with the advent of APEL, to make the best of continuing education opportunities the documenting of learning experiences and reflection on these is a necessity.

PROFESSIONAL PROFILES

James (1991) suggests that 'reflective practice' is a way in which professionals learn and that there exists three levels of reflection:

1. The technical – reflection is concerned with improving efficiency and effectiveness, the concern being to ensure that the intended objectives are achieved, e.g. a lesson brought about the intended learning outcome.
2. The educational – reflection considers the appropriateness of the purpose and objectives of the learning experience, i.e. is this the most appropriate topic to be learning at this time and is what I have learnt suitable for me?
3. The moral and ethical – where the values that underpin practice and the conflicts of such values within particular professional activities are considered.

Profiles in the initial stages of professional development can assist nurses to identify the experiences which have contributed to their learning as well as identifying the impact they have made within their working environment. It can also help nurses to identify their future learning needs as well as recognizing their responsibilities to extraprofessional activities, e.g. their families, leisure activities and interests. Thus students can in consultation with others:

- identify their own learning needs;
- set their own learning programmes;
- monitor and evaluate their own development.

Professional profiles can take several forms, and to assist nurses national boards have developed profiles which are available for purchase. However, the importance of writing cannot be over-emphasized as at some stage in profiling it is necessary to write about practice and experience. Tripp (1987) and Holly (1989) have demonstrated how writing about an experience is a powerful enhancer of learning from that experience. It is important that the writing is not just a description of events but is a critical and analytical reflection of the experience. Profiling can then contribute to the APEL process and enable many learning experiences to be accredited, including courses/study days organized by non-awarding bodies, e.g. the Marie Curie Foundation and other cancer agencies.

THE MARIE CURIE MEMORIAL FOUNDATION (MCMF)

The MCMF has established an education department which holds courses all over the UK in response to local needs. In addition it has also demonstrated its commitment to improving the care of cancer patients through education by the appointment of several nurse teachers who are based at the Marie Curie Centres, which are situated throughout the UK. These centres are able to provide educational opportunities for local nurses as well as in some centres offering courses to nurses throughout the UK.

COURSES

One of the most popular courses has been the three-day course 'The Care of the Patient with Cancer' for trained nurses working in general hospitals or the community. These courses have usually incorporated:

- prevention;
- diagnosis and the treatment of cancer;
- communication skills;
- palliative care;

- statutory and voluntary support for cancer patients and their families.

However, the education department will adapt courses to ensure that local needs are met. These courses are held at various venues throughout the four countries of the UK.

Other courses currently offered by the education department include:

- **Courses in palliative care.** These are more advanced two- to three-day courses on the continuing care of cancer patients and incorporate symptom control, communication, psychological, spiritual and bereavement care.
- **Screening course for practice nurses.** This includes training in taking cervical smears and carrying out breast and pelvic examination. The course is of five days – two two-day modules and a follow-up day.
- **Chemotherapy study day for district and community nurses.** This is an introduction to cytotoxic drugs and their side-effects, nursing care and care of central lines.
- **Administration of cytotoxic drugs.** This three-day course is for nurses involved in reconstitution and administration of cytotoxic drugs.
- **Communication with the seriously ill.** A three-day course with a fourth follow-up day for health care workers intended to develop and extend their communication and counselling skills.
- **Occupational health nurses training.** To provide knowledge and skills for prevention and screening of cancer in relation to work-place initiatives.

In addition the MCMF education department organizes conferences on specific topics related to cancer and cancer care as well as arranging individually designed courses for organizations and groups (MCMF, 1992). Further information is available from Education Department, Marie Curie Cancer Care, 17 Grosvenor Crescent, London SW1X 8QJ.

INTERACTIVE VIDEO

An exciting innovation developed by the MCMF is the interactive video learning package *Cancer Patients and their Families at Home*. Despite its title it is suitable for all nurses who work with cancer patients, irrespective of the environment in which the patient is nursed. The system incorporates a video disc on which real-life situations involving doctors (general practitioners), nurses, cancer patients and their carers are recorded. In addition there are sections which consist of an interactive learning programme. The package is arranged in chapters and includes pain diagnosis, pain management, nausea and vomiting, other symptoms, and excellent chapters dealing with, for example, bad news, awkward questions, common emotions and coping with these emotions.

The system has the flexibility of being suitable for use by small groups as well as by individuals. The package is available for purchase but for individuals the cost is probably prohibitive. However, all of the 11 Marie Curie Centres in the UK have this system. Nurses wishing to use this learning resource can obtain further information by contacting either the education department (see previous address) or by contacting their nearest Marie Curie Centre.

DIPLOMA IN PALLIATIVE NURSING

This is another exciting innovation by the foundation and developed at the Marie Curie Centre, Penarth (Wales). This year-long course consists of a combination of distance learning and residential weekends. It is open to nurses who have a minimum of three years post-registration experience of which one year must have been in cancer nursing. Further details can be obtained from Education Centre, Holme Tower Marie Curie Centre, Bridgeman Road, Penarth, S. Glam. CF6 2AW.

NATIONAL BOARD APPROVED COURSES

Some Marie Curie centres are able to offer approved courses, e.g. ENB 931, or are approved as a clinical area for students on approved courses, e.g. ENB 931 (England), Professional Studies Two Module (Scotland), WNB modules (Wales). Nurses wishing to undertake national board approved courses at Marie Curie Centres should contact their local centre for further details.

CANCER RELIEF MACMILLAN FUND

Cancer Relief also has a very active commitment to education and organizes study days, workshops and conferences throughout the UK on a wide range of issues concerning cancer care. Further information can be obtained from Cancer Relief Macmillan Fund, 15–19 Britten Street, London SW3 3TX.

HELP THE HOSPICES

Courses supported by Help the Hospices include the Maguire/Faulkner courses on communication and counselling skills, as well as the teaching of these skills. Further information is available from Help the Hospices, BMA House, 34–44 Britannia Street, London WC1X 9JG.

ROYAL COLLEGE OF NURSING

Members of the college have the opportunity to become members of special interest groups at no additional cost. The Cancer Nursing Society and the Palliative Nursing Group are two such special interest groups. The special interest groups send regular newsletters to their members as well as organizing study days and annual conferences. Study days and the annual conference are open to non-RCN members. Members, however, usually attend at a reduced fee.

SPECIALIST HOSPITALS/HOSPICES

In addition to the aforementioned educational opportunities, the International Directory of Cancer Nursing Educational Experiences and Professional Organizations (Sanville *et al.*, 1990) lists several hospitals/ hospices within the UK which offer a wide variety of courses to nurses. These include the following:

- The Royal Marsden Hospital and Institute of Cancer Research, Fulham Road, London SW3 6JJ.
- Weston Park Hospital, Whitman Road, Sheffield S10 2SJ.
- Christie Hospital and Holt Radium Institute, South Manchester School of Nursing, Mauldeth House, Mauldeth Road West, Manchester M21 7RL.
- North Down College of Nursing, The Ulster Hospital, Duonald, Belfast, Northern Ireland. (Course placements undertaken at the Northern Ireland Radiotherapy and Oncology Unit, Belvoir Park Hospital, Belfast.)

The above list, taken from the directory, is not exhaustive and readers are advised to contact their local cancer hospital/hospice for details of their educational programmes. Some useful addresses for England and Wales are:

- St Christopher's Hospice, 51–59 Lawrie Park Road, Sydenham, London SE26 6DZ.
- Sir Michael Sobell House, Churchill Hospital, Oxford OX3 7LJ.
- South Wales Oncology and Radiotherapy Hospital, Velindre Hospital, Velindre Road, Cardiff CF4 7XL.

DRUG COMPANIES/MEDICAL SUPPLIERS

Many companies/suppliers produce educational material and it is impossible to list here all that is available. Nurses are advised to contact the companies that supply their products for further information. However, two useful learning aids are as follows.

MAC-PAC

This is a medical education computer program which enables doctors and nurses to increase their knowledge of the management of pain and symptoms of patients with advanced cancer. It has been produced by Napp Laboratories on behalf of the Cancer Relief Fund. There is the original program which focuses on the management of the patient at home, and the 1992 program which focuses on the hospital patient. In addition Napp has produced a distance learning pack together with a 'game' to test your skill.

The Mac-Pac Computer Challenge, as the computer system is known, is available from the Napp analgesic representatives. There is no need for any equipment to be provided as the representative will supply the computer and all necessary software. Further information is available from Napp Laboratories, The Science Park, Cambridge, CB4 4GW.

GRAESBY

Many nurses will recognize the name of Graesby as the manufacturers of what is arguably the most widely used range of syringe drivers within the UK. For those nurses who need to familiarize themselves with this equipment, Graesby have produced a wide range of educational material including a VHS video, *Getting on with Life*, which outlines the uses and setting up of the company's syringe drivers. Further information is available from Graesby Medical Ltd, Colonial Way, Watford, Herts, WD2 4LG.

POST-REGISTRATION EDUCATION AND PRACTICE (PREP)

In writing about education and cancer nursing it is not possible to evade the issue of PREP. While the necessary legislation has not yet been passed at the time of writing, it would seem a certainty that nurses will soon have to demonstrate professional updating, incorporating a minimum of five days of study in order to re-register every three years.

It is not yet known exactly what will actually constitute 'updating' but amongst the opportunities described above there should be the chance for all nurses to enhance their professional development within cancer nursing. 'Study' is not necessarily attending a study day.

CONCLUSION

Learning can happen in a variety of ways, in a variety of settings. Some of the ways outlined above will be more readily available to some nurses than others. The education needs of the 'part-timers' are often especially difficult to meet as these nurses are often balancing child care with work commitments, as well as the opposition they may face from employers over funding and study leave (Nazarko, 1991).

The variety of learning opportunities included in this chapter have ranged from self-directed to formal learning, assessed to non-assessed and certificate to degree level. If we are to uphold the belief of the European Oncology Nursing Society (1989, p. 6) that

> every patient with cancer has the right to the best available treatment, care and support . . . and that . . . educational opportunities equip nurses to act as a resource to patients and their families. Informed nurses also have the responsibility to provide information to the public about cancer, its prevention and treatment

cancer nurses will avail themselves of the opportunities available to them.
Happy learning.

REFERENCES

Burns, N. (1982) *Nursing and Cancer*. Saunders, London.

Casey, N. (1991) A project comes alive. *Nursing Standard*, 6(1), 19–20.

Commission of the European Communities (1988) *Advisory Committee on Training in Nursing: Report and Recommendations on Training in Cancer*. European Community Brussels.

CNAA (1989) *Press Release 89/7*. CNAA, London.

Corner, J. and Wilson-Barnett, J. (1992) The newly registered nurse and the cancer patient: an educational evaluation. *International Journal of Nursing Studies*, 29(2), 177–90.

Davidson, L. (1991) Open for all. *Nursing Times*, 87(5), 46–7.

DHSS (Northern Ireland) (1991) *A strategy for Nursing, Midwifery and Health Visting for Northern Ireland*. DHSS, Belfast.

European Oncology Nursing Society (1989) *A Core Curriculum for a Post Basic Course in Cancer Nursing*. Haigh & Hochland, Manchester.

Holly, M.L. (1989) Reflective writing and the spirit of enquiry. *Cambridge Journal of Education*, 19(1), 71–80, cited in James (1991).

Hull, C. (1992) Experience counts. *Nursing Times*, **88**(23), 36–7.

James, C. (1991) *Personal Professional Profiles: A Personal View*. Paper presented to the Open Learning Conference, Kensington Town Hall, University of Bath.

Keane, P. (1989) Open Learning: meeting educational needs. *Senior Nurse*, **9**(2), 12–14.

Lewis, R. (1986) *Open Learning*. Open University, Milton Keynes.

Maggs, C. (1991) Framework for futute needs. *Nursing Times*, **87**(14), 55–6.

Maggs, C. (1992) CATS: your question answered. *Nursing Times*, **88**(23), 34–6.

McManus, M. (1991) Credit accumulation and transfer schemes. *Nursing Standard*, **6**(7), 28–30.

MCMF (1992) *Diary*. Marie Curie Cancer Education, MCMF, London.

National Board for Nursing, Midwifery and Health Visting for Northern Ireland (1993) *The Structure of Professional Education*. NBNI, Belfast.

National Board for Nursing, Midwifery and Health Visiting for Scotland. (1991) *Continuing Education for the Nursing Profession in Scotland*. NBS, Edinburgh.

Nazarko, L. (1991) Outclassed and uneducated. *Nursing Standard*, **6**(6), 54.

Sanville, U.J., McCorkle, R. and Deininger, H. (1990) *International Directory of Cancer Nursing Educational Experiences and Professional Organizations*. National Cancer Institute, London.

The Health of the Nation (1992) Government White Paper, HMSO, London.

Thompson, A. (1991) A framework for updating. *Nursing Standard*, **6**(6), 19.

Tripp, D.H. (1987) Teachers journals and collaborative research, in *Educating Teachers, Changing the Nature of Pedagogical Knowledge* (ed. J. Smyth), Falmer, London, cited in James (1991).

Wells, J. (1991) Assessment. *Nursing Standard*, **6**(1), 20–1.

Welsh National Board (1994) Newyddion. WNB, Cardiff.

Welsh National Board (1991) *Newyddion: WNB News*. WNB, Cardiff.

Welsh National Board (1992) *The Accreditation of Prior Learning*. WNB, Cardiff.

17 Where to get help

Jan Viret

The patient's charters, both national and local, set down the rights and standards that individual patients may expect from the National Health Service. These include access to a general practitioner and through him or her to an extensive primary care team of knowledgeable health professionals with back-up networks of further local resources. This chapter aims to outline these local resources and a wide range of possible regional and national sources of information and support; for access either when more is needed by an individual, or when the system does not seem to be working to the patient's advantage.

From the moment a diagnosis of cancer is suspected, whole new areas of needs are exposed, both for the individual person and for family and carers. These range from the need for a clear initial medical diagnosis, information about the diagnosis and the implications that this may have for the future, to the treatment options and the resources of support and information that may be needed to make decisions about these options. Care needs will range from the physical and practical to psychological needs for support and adjustment to the disease and to social, financial and spiritual needs.

For each person to come to terms with what is happening to him or her and to remain in control of his or her life, timely and appropriate information and support is needed, which may come from specialist consultants and associated professional health workers, the general practitioner and primary health care team, together with their resources and networks. A local hospice or palliative care team may be a useful resource and a member of the primary health care team may know who is the appropriate person to contact there. Help may also be needed from social services; voluntary agencies and self-help groups may also provide invaluable information and support. The Citizens' Advice Bureau (the telephone number of which can be found in the local telephone directory) may be able to give useful advice about what is available locally and where appropriate help may be found.

One of the key features of recent White Papers and legislation is that patients should receive a seamless service, where health, social services and social security combine to assess and meet complex health, social and financial needs. Local community care plans were implemented in each locality (local authority as lead agency working with the district health authority, family health service authority and voluntary sector) in April 1993, to assess, plan and provide appropriate combined health and social care.

GENERAL PRACTITIONER SERVICES

The general practitioner (GP) and primary health care team give care to the patient within the family setting. They can also be a source of information, advice and support on all aspects of health care; different members of the team have specific areas of interest, knowledge and expertise, and may be a valuable resource. In addition, health centres can provide more general information about cancer prevention, health promotion and screening services, also about local groups and networks, voluntary services and local helplines that may be useful. Few health centres have a direct link with social services or social security offices; telephone numbers and addresses of these may be found in the local telephone directory.

PATIENT RIGHTS

The White Papers *Working for Patients* and *Caring for People* stress the importance of patient choice. GPs have to provide a patient leaflet stating the services they offer to help patients choose a GP. The method of changing a GP has become easier and without prejudice (forms may be obtained from the practice the patient wishes to care for him or her). Patients have the right to referral to a consultant acceptable to them when the GP thinks it necessary, and to be referred for a second opinion if GP and patient agree that this is desirable. For some patients specific and detailed information is necessary to exercise choice in making these decisions, and this information may need to be obtained from multiple sources.

Patients have the right to see information in computerized health records, but record holders may withhold information they think is harmful to the patient. The same rights apply to manual records written after 1st November 1991. Parents have the right to see their children's records if the child is too ill, young or has a learning disability and could not understand them. Patients have the right to see reports written by the doctor for an employer or insurance company (unless the doctor decides the patient could be harmed by it). The patient may refuse to allow an employer or other agency to see the report or may wish to add comments.

Doctors must not pass on confidential information without the patient's consent, except to other professionals involved in treatment or to close relatives, except in specific circumstances outlined in law.

A free health care information line has been set up, where calls will be routed to regional information services. Queries will be answered on a whole range of issues including waiting list times. The national number is 0800 665544 and the call is free. Some district health authorities and local provider units have set up their own information telephone line, which is available to the general public as well as health professionals to answer queries, particularly those relating to local health services.

MAKING A COMPLAINT

Where a patient is dissatisfied with the service offered by any part of the National Health Service or social services and wishes to comment or complain, information should be provided by each health authority and local authority as to how to do this. The Community Health Council, whose telephone number may be found in the local directory, will give advice and may take on an advocacy role in some instances. If the patient is still not satisfied, he or she may complain to the Health Service Commissioner for England, Church House, Great Smith Street, London SW1 (tel. 071 276 3000). Normally this must be done within a year. The Health Service Commissioner cannot deal with doctors' decisions about diagnosis and treatment.

SOCIAL SECURITY BENEFITS

Information about the many benefits to which patients and carers may be entitled is most readily available through a medical social worker or through the local social security office or benefits agency.

There is a national free telephone line (0800 666 555) for free and confidential advice on all social security benefits, which is open Monday to Friday, 0930–1630. This information is also available in Chinese (0800 252 451), Punjabi (0800 521 360), Urdu (0800 289 188) and Welsh (0800 289 011). If information or confidential advice for people with disabilities or carers is required, there is a free-phone benefits enquiry line (BEL), on 0800 882200 between 0900 and 1630, Monday to Friday, in English.

Leaflets giving information about different benefits may be obtained from the social security office or benefits agency, post office or health centre. If they are unavailable or a large quantity is required, order them through the Leaflets Unit, PO Box 21, Stanmore, Middlesex HA7 1AY, or Health Publications Unit, No. 2 Site, Heywood Stores, Manchester Road, Heywood, Lancashire OL10 2PZ.

Social security benefits beginning April 1992 include the Disabled Living Allowance and the Disabled Working Allowance.

DISABLED LIVING ALLOWANCE (DLA)

If a patient has an illness or disability and needs help with personal care or with getting around and is under 66 years of age, he or she could be entitled to this allowance. It replaces the Attendance Allowance and Mobility Allowance for this age group. The Attendance Allowance is still available for those over 65 years of age. To get the DLA, people must normally have needed help for three months, and must be likely to need help for a further six months or more. For people not expected to live longer than six months because of an illness, special rules apply. They do not have to wait three months and they qualify for help with personal care automatically, even if no help is needed.

DISABLED WORKING ALLOWANCE

This is a benefit which provides a top-up for people who can work, but whose illness or disability limits their earning capacity. For more information, contact the local social security office or ring the benefit enquiry line. A claim pack is available through the social security office, post office or telephone 0800 100 123, a free-phone line open 24 hours a day, seven days a week.

EMPLOYMENT RIGHTS

Those people who have a progressive, disabling disease, for example cancer, and who may be restricted either by disease or its treatment, can have problems with employment. All normal rights and protections of employment apply (Wages Act 1986). Where employees have problems, either concerning the level of work that is possible, or if they are limited in the hours they are able to work, they may obtain help from the occupational health department or personnel department at their place of work. In addition a social worker or the local Department of Social Security or benefits agency will provide information about the rights and benefits to which each individual may be entitled. The self-employed and those who have queries about contributions to National Insurance can obtain advice and information from the Contributions Agency of the Department of Social Security (telephone number to be found in the local directory). The Citizens' Advice Bureau has access to legal advice and other resources that may provide additional help.

In addition there are some services specifically designed for disabled people looking for employment. Following a Consultative Document, these are under review by the Department of Employment and are run by the Employment Service (an executive agency in the Employment Department Group). They used to be run by the Manpower Services Commission. In 1992, placement, assessment and counselling teams (PACTs) took over the functions of the Disablement Advisory Service, disablement resettlement officers (DROs) and employment rehabilitation teams.

Training is the responsibility of the department's Training, Enterprise and Education Division (TEED). Delivery of training, within departmental guidelines, is undertaken by training and enterprise councils (TECs), and in Scotland by local enterprise companies (LECs).

PROFESSIONAL NURSING RESOURCES

1. Networks of specialist nursing services may be available. Most districts have a clinical nurse specialist for palliative care (sometimes a Macmillan nurse), breast care and stoma care who may be based in the acute unit, the community unit or a local hospice.
2. Nursing societies and associations: national or local. Many are specialist groups run under the auspices of the Royal College of Nursing. These include palliative care, oncology, stoma care and breast care. More information can be obtained from the Royal College of Nursing (071 409 3333). Where groups do not have this formal affiliation, information may be obtained from the local specialist nurse.
3. Library facilities, specialist nursing and professional cancer and palliative care journals are available or obtainable.

HEALTH PROMOTION UNITS

Local health promotion units may be based in purchaser or provider units in the health authority. Some environmental health officers, based in district council offices, may also have a health promotion role. Health promotion units provide advice, consultancy, training, liaison with other agencies and resources for the promotion of positive health and the prevention of ill-health. There is support for the local unit from the Health Education Authority to work towards locally defined targets based on the White Paper *The Health of the Nation* and on local needs.

AIDS AND EQUIPMENT

Arrangements for the provision of aids and equipment may be complicated and specific to each district. If there is a local helpline, information concerning local services and networks may be readily available. Resources may be known to the primary health care team and may include the acute unit where treatment has been given, the surgical appliance office, community services, community rehabilitation services, social services, the local hospice unit or palliative care team, the local branch of the Red Cross or other voluntary agencies.

REFERENCE BOOKS AND BOOKLETS

These books are examples of what is available. It is not a comprehensive list.

1. Patient information booklets on the implications of living with cancer, specific cancers, forms of treatment and side-effects are available free to patients and their families and at a small charge to health professionals. Publication lists are available from BACUP, Publications Department, 3 Bath Place, London EC2 3JR; The Royal Marsden Hospital; and Haigh & Hochland, International University Booksellers, The Precinct Centre, Oxford Road, Manchester M13 9QA.
2. The *Directory of Hospices in the UK and Republic of Ireland* – updated each year. Published by The Hospice Information Service, St Christopher's Hospice, 51–59 Lawrie Park Road, Sydenham, London SE26 6DZ (tel. 081 778 9252).
3. *Directory of Cancer Support and Self-Help* (1993) – details of over 400 support groups (free). CancerLink, 17 Britannia Street, London WC1X 9JN (tel. 071 833 2451); and 9 Castle Terrace, Edinburgh EH1 2DP (tel. 031 228 5557).
4. *The Handbook of Community Nursing* – updated each year; gives details of community nursing services, social services, nurse specialists and liaison nurses (free). Published by: The Newbourne Group, Headway Home and Law Publishing Group Ltd, Greater London House, Hampstead Road, London NW1 7QQ (tel. 071 388 3171). Regional and district health authorities may produce their own health directory.
5. *People who Help* – a 'Professional Nurse' booklet (revised edition 1992); a guide to voluntary and other support organizations and self-help groups concerned with health and social care. Cost £4.95 (1994). Published by: Clive Whitfield, Profile Productions Ltd, 70 Elthorne Avenue, London W7 2JW.

6. *Disability Rights Handbook* – a guide to rights, benefits and services for all people with disabilities and their families. This is updated each year in May, but further bulletins are published quarterly to update information in the handbook and to cover other related topics. Cost of the handbook £7.95 (1994) (reduced cost for those receiving benefit); bulletins £11.25 (1994); reduction for purchasing the complete set. Published by The Disability Alliance, Educational and Research Association, 1st Floor East, Universal House, 88–94 Wentworth Street, London E1 7SA (tel. 071 247 8776). For details of leaflets giving information of social security benefits see above.

GOVERNMENT POLICY DOCUMENTS ON HEALTH AND SOCIAL CARE

1989   White Paper, *Working for Patients*
        White Paper, *Caring for People*
1991   Patients' Charter
1992   White Paper, *The Health of the Nation*, the strategy of health for England.

THE NHS AND COMMUNITY CARE ACT, 1990

The Act was implemented in three stages:

April 1991
1. Purchaser/provider split in the NHS, including setting up NHS Trusts and GP fund-holding arrangements. All services are now provided through contracts.
2. The replacement of family practitioner committees with new health authorities – family health service authorities (FHSAs) for the family practitioner services (GPs).
3. Independent inspection units in social services departments (SSDs).
4. Formal complaints procedures in SSDs.

By April 1992
5. Publication of Community Care Plan for 1992–3 by local authorities in association with health and voluntary agencies.

April 1993
6. Separation of purchaser/provider functions in SSDs.
7. Introduction of assessment and case management in SSDs.
8. Transfer of social security resources to local authorities for purchasing social care in nursing homes and residential settings.

CONTACT ADDRESSES

Special services offered by various organizations:

Phone information helpline	A
Information on request	B
Financial and/or practical help	C
Counselling/emotional support	D
Self-help/support group	E
Hospice care	F
Home nursing care	G

Age Concern (National Council on Ageing)

B

1268 London Road, London SW16 4EJ
Telephone: 081 679 8000
WALES: 4th Floor, 1 Cathedral Road, Cardiff CF1 9SD
Telephone: 0222 371566
SCOTLAND: 54A Fountainbridge, Edinburgh, EH3 9PT
Telephone: 031 228 5656

Offers support for older people and those who care for them. Local groups provide services such as day centres, lunch clubs and transport visiting schemes. Information leaflets available.

Association to Aid the Sexual and Personal Relationships of People with a Disability (SPOD)

A   B   D

286 Camden Road, London N7 OBJ
Telephone: 071 607 8851

Provides practical information and emotional support for people who are disabled and need help with sexual and personal relationships. List of publications and information sheets. Workshops to facilitate learning for professionals.

BACUP

A   B   D

121–123 Charterhouse Street, London EC1M 6AA
Information: 071 613 2121
Outside London: 0800 181199 (free)
Administration: 071 696 9003
Counselling: 071 696 9000

Helps patients, families and friends to cope with cancer. Trained cancer nurses provide information, emotional support and practical advice by telephone or letter. A range of free publications and a newspaper are available. One-to-one counselling service in Greater London.

Breast Cancer Care

A   B   C   D   E

15–19 Britten Street, London SW3 3TZ
Helpline: 071 867 1103
Administration: 071 867 8275
Freephone: 0500 245345
SCOTLAND: Suite 2/8, 65 Bath Street, Glasgow G2 2BX
Helpline: 041 353 1050
Administration: 041 353 0539

A free service of practical help and advice, information and support to women concerned about breast cancer. Volunteers who have had breast cancer themselves assist the staff in providing emotional support, nationwide. Breast Cancer Care complements medical and nursing care.

Bristol Cancer Help Centre

A   B   D

Grove House, Cornwallis Grove, Clifton, Bristol, BS8 4PG
Telephone: 0272 743216

Provides a complementary approach to cancer aimed towards the whole person rather than just the disease. Therapy, support and education at the centre combine to stimulate positive attitudes, self-healing and self-help. Information is available from the centre.

British Association for Counselling

A   B   D

1 Regent Place, Rugby CV21 2PJ
Telephone: 0788 578328

BAC members are individuals and organizations concerned with counselling in a variety of settings. The information office publishes directories listing counselling services and will refer enquirers to an experienced local counsellor, free of charge. Send SAE with enquiries.

British Colostomy Association

A   B   D

15 Station Road, Reading, Berkshire RG1 1LG
Telephone: 0734 391537

Information and advisory service, giving comfort, reassurance and encouragement to patients to return to their previous active lifestyle. Emotional support is given on a personal and confidential basis by helpers who have long experience of living with a colostomy. Free leaflets and list of local contacts available. Can arrange visits in hospitals or at home on request.

Cancer Aftercare and Rehabilitation Society (CARE)

A   B   D   E

21 Zetland Road, Redland, Bristol BS6 7AH
Telephone: 0272 427419

Provides social and emotional support for people with cancer and their families and friends through a national network of branches. Telephone and personal counselling by trained counsellors. Offers a telephone link service for people with cancer to be put in touch with one another.

Cancer Relief Macmillan Fund

A   B   C   F   G

Anchor House, 15–19 Britten Street, London SW3 3TZ
Telephone: 071 351 7811
SCOTLAND: 9 Castle Terrace, Edinburgh, EH1 2DP
Telephone: 031 229 3276

Supports and develops services to provide skilled care for people with cancer and their families. Macmillan nurses; Macmillan units for in-patient and day care; financial help through patient grants. Services usually part of the NHS. Information on Macmillan services available on request. Patient grant applications through community, hospital and hospice nurses, social workers and other care professionals.

CancerLink

A   B   D   E

17 Britannia Street, London WC1X 9JN
Telephone: 071 833 2451
SCOTLAND: 9 Castle Terrace, Edinburgh EH1 2DP
Telephone: 031 228 5557

Provides emotional support and information in response to letter and telephone enquiries on all aspects of cancer, from people with cancer, families, friends and professionals working with them. Resource to over 370 cancer support and self-help groups throughout Britain, and helps people who set up new groups. Various free publications available.

Carers' National Association

A   B   E

29 Chilworth Mews, London W2 3RG
Telephone: 071 724 7776

Offers information and support to people caring for relatives and friends. Can put carers in touch with local sources of information and help. Lobbies government, both local and national, on behalf of carers. Offers a range of free leaflets.

CLIC UK

A   B   C   D   E   F   G

CLIC House, 11–12 Fremantle Square, Cotham, Bristol BS6 5TL
Telephone: 0272 244333

Aims to help young people under 21 years who have any form of cancer or leukaemia, and their families. Provides free 'home from home' accommodation adjacent to paediatric oncology units (nine homes at present). Support home care nursing team in the south-west, and provides welfare grants.

Compassionate Friends

A   B   D   E

53 North Street, Bedminster, Bristol BS3 1EN
Telephone: 0272 539639

A self-help group of parents who have lost a son or daughter of any age, including adult. Quarterly newsletter, postal library, range of leaflets. Personal and group support. Befriending, rather than counselling.

Counsel and Care for the Elderly

B   C

Lower Ground Floor, Twyman House, 16 Bonney Street, London NW1 9PG
Telephone: 071 485 1566

Advice service for elderly people, their relatives and professionals, information leaflets, grants to help people remain in or return to their homes.

Crossroads Care: Association of Crossroads Care Attendant Schemes

C

10 Regent Place, Rugby, Warwickshire CV21 2PN
Telephone: 0788 573653
WALES: Watton Chambers, The Watton, Brecon
Telephone: 0874 623090
SCOTLAND: 24 George Square, Glasgow G2 1EG
Telephone: 041 226 3793

Provides care attendants who come into the home to give the carer a break; 180 autonomous schemes throughout England, Scotland and Wales.

CRUSE: Bereavement care

A   B   D

Cruse House, 126 Sheen Road, Richmond, Surrey TW9 1UR
Telephone: 081 940 4818
Bereavement line: 081 332 7227
WALES: Bryn Tirion, Churchill Close, Llanblethian, Cowbridge, S. Glam. CF7 7JH
Telephone: 0446 775351
SCOTLAND: 18 South Trinity Road, Edinburgh EH5 3PN
Telephone: 031 551 1511

Helps any bereaved person by providing counselling individually and in groups by trained counsellors. Local branches. A telephone helpline is available. Advice on practical problems and social contact. Training course for professionals and counsellors. Publications list available.

Dial UK (Disablement Information and Advice Lines)

A

Park Lodge, St Catherine's Hospital, Tickhill Road, Balby, Doncaster DN4 8QN
Telephone: 0302 310123

80+ autonomous organizations varying in size and the facilities they offer. Can offer telephone information and advice on any aspect of disability.

Disability Information Trust

B

Mary Marlborough Lodge, Nuffield Orthopaedic Centre, Windmill Road, Headington, Oxford OX3 7LD

Comprehensive information booklets giving details of equipment for disabled people can be purchased from the trust. Examples include communication, gardening, walking aids, clothing and dressing.

Disabled Living Foundation

B

380–384 Harrow Road, London W9 2HU
Telephone: 071 289 6111
SCOTLAND: Disability Scotland, Princes House, 5 Shandwick Place, Edinburgh EH2 4RG
Telephone: 031 229 8632

National resource for information on aids and equipment for people with a disability.

Family Fund

C

Joseph Rowntree Memorial Trust, PO Box 50, York YO1 1UY
Telephone: 0904 629241

Run by the Joseph Rowntree Memorial Trust on behalf of the government to give financial help in the form of grants to families of 'severely handicapped' children. Aid is given through the fund's own social worker.

Help the Aged

A B D

16–18 St James's Walk, London EC1R OBE
Telephone: 071 253 0253 (Mon.–Fri. 0900–1730)
Senior Line: 0800 289404 (free Mon.–Fri. 1000–1600)
SCOTLAND: 53 Black Friar Street, Edinburgh EH1 1BN
Telephone: 031 556 4666
Winter Warmth: 0800 838587 (October to March, free)

Fund-raising charity that supports simple, practical projects that bring care and contact to elderly people at home and abroad; also provides an advice service for elderly people, their relatives, carers and friends.

Hodgkin's Disease Association

A B D

PO Box 275, Haddenham, Aylesbury, Bucks HP17 8JJ
Telephone: 0844 291479
Helpline: 0844 291500 (0900–2200, every day)

Provides information and emotional support for lymphoma (Hodgkin's disease and non-Hodgkin's lymphoma) patients and their families. Literature and videos available. National network of helpers with experience of the disease, with whom enquirers may be linked, usually by telephone.

Hospice Information Service

A B

Hospice Information Service, St Christopher's Hospice, 51–59 Lawrie Park Road, Sydenham, London SE26 6DZ
Telephone: 081 778 9252

The Hospice Information Service publishes a directory of hospice services which provides details of hospices, home care teams and hospital support teams in the UK and the Republic of Ireland. For copies of the directory or details of local services, write or telephone.

Institute for Complementary Medicine

B

PO Box 194, London SE16 1QZ

Can supply names of reliable practitioners of various kinds of complementary medicine, such as homeopathy, relaxation techniques and osteopathy. Also has contact with support groups. Please send SAE for information, stating area of interest.

Institute of Family Therapy

D

43 New Cavendish Street, London W1M 7RG
Telephone: 071 935 1651

The institute's Elizabeth Raven Memorial Fund offers free counselling to families who have suffered a bereavement within the past 12 months, or those with seriously ill family members. Works with the whole family. While the service is free, voluntary donations to the fund are accepted to help other families.

Let's Face It

A B D E

Christine Piff, 10 Wood End, Crowthorne, Berks RG11 6DQ
Telephone: 0344 774405

A contact point for people with facial disfigurement. Provides a link for people with similar experiences. Telephone and letter contact; meetings for self-help or social contact.

Leukaemia Care Society

A B C D E

PO Box 82, Exeter, Devon, EX2 5DP
Telephone: 0392 464848 (24-hour answering machine)

Promotes the welfare of people with leukaemia and allied blood disorders, and helps relieve the needs of their families. Offers family caravan holidays, friendship and support through voluntary area secretaries throughout the UK. Limited financial assistance. Membership, newsletter and series of publications are free.

Malcolm Sargent Cancer Fund for Children

C D

14 Abingdon Road, London W8 6AF
Telephone: 071 937 4548

Can provide cash grants for parents up to the age of 21 with cancer, to help pay for equipment, travel, fuel bills, etc. Apply through medical social worker; Malcolm Sargent social workers work in many paediatric oncology units.

Marie Curie Cancer Care

A B C F G

28 Belgrave Square, London SW1X 8QG
Telephone: 071 235 3325
SCOTLAND: 21 Rutland Street, Edinburgh EH1 2AE
Telephone: 031 229 8332

Nursing care available in 11 Marie Curie Centres throughout the UK. Admission criteria and information from the individual matrons. Day care, home care and bereavement care may be available. Day and night nursing can be provided in the patient's home, through the Marie Curie Community Nursing Service, administered and partially funded by the local health authority, but free at point of delivery. Welfare grant schemes; applications through the district nursing service.

National Association of Laryngectomee Clubs

A   B   D   E

Ground Floor, 6 Rickett Street, Fulham, London SW6 1RU
Telephone: 071 381 9993

Information booklet. Promotes the welfare of laryngectomees within the UK. Encourages the formation of clubs with objective of assisting rehabilitation through speech therapy, social support and monthly meetings. Advises on speech aids and medical supplies. Offers a referral service.

National Council for Hospice and Specialist Palliative Care Services

B

59 Bryanston Street, London W1A 2AZ
Telephone: 071 611 1153/1216/1225

The National Council brings together all those working in the field. It is made up of national cancer charities, professional organizations, regional representatives and observers from the Scottish Partnership Agency for Palliative and Cancer Care and the Department of Health.

National Council for Voluntary Organizations (NCVO)

A

26 Bedford Square, London WC1B 3HU
Telephone: 071 636 4066

Can give information about voluntary organizations in your area.

National Self-Help Support Centre

E

26 Bedford Square, London WC1B 3HU
Telephone: 071 636 4066

A voluntary organization that has a database of local and national groups for specific illnesses and disabilities.

Neuroblastoma Society

A B D E

'Woodlands', Ordsall Park Road, Retford, Nottingham DN22 7PJ
Telephone: 0777 709328

Information and advice by telephone or letter for patients and their families. Provides contact where possible with others who have experienced the illness for mutual support. Provides funds for British medical research into improving the treatment of neuroblastoma.

Oesophageal Patients Association

A B D

16 Whitefields Crescent, Solihull, West Midlands B91 3NU
Telephone: 021 704 9860

Leaflets, telephone advice and support, before and during treatment. Visits, where possible, by former patients to people with oesophageal cancer.

Retinoblastoma Society

B D

The National Coordinator, c/o Academic Department of Paediatric Oncology, St Bartholomew's Hospital, West Smithfield, London EC1A 7BE
Telephone: 071 600 3309

Links families in the same situation and area to give moral support and practical help. Creates an opportunity for parents to exchange information and share experiences.

Save Our Sons (SOS)

A B D

Tides Reach, 1 Kite Hill, Wooton Bridge, Isle of Wight PO33 4LA
Telephone: 0983 882876 (evenings preferred)

Information and emotional support for men and boys with testicular cancer. Advice given by qualified nurse, who will listen and offer help where possible. Leaflet on self-examination techniques available. Send SAE.

Sue Ryder Foundation

D F

Cavendish, Sudbury, Suffolk CP10 8AY
Telephone: 0787 328052

International organization; cares for disabled and sick people of all ages. Six homes in England specialize in cancer care offering respite care, long-term care, day centres, domiciliary nursing service, advice and bereavement counselling.

Urostomy Association

A B D E

Central Office, 'Buckland', Beaumont Park, Danbury, Essex CM3 4DE
Telephone: 0245 224294

Assists patiens before and after surgery with counselling on appliances, housing, work situations or relationship problems, to enable patients to resume as full a life as possible. Branch and house meetings held. Can arrange hospital and home visits by former patients on request.

Women's Health

A B

52 Featherstone Street, London EC1 8RT
Health enquiry: 071 251 6580

Provides information for women in a supportive manner, helping women to make informed decisions about their own health.

Women's Nationwide Cancer Control Campaign

A B D

Suna House, 128–130 Curtain Road, London EC2A 3AR
Helpline: 071 729 2229 (Mon.–Fri. 0930–
                                     1630)
Cervical screening information
tape: 071 729 5061 (24-hour)
Breast awareness information
tape: 071 729 4915 (24-hour)

Provides information and emotional support on breast checks, smear tests and colposcopy.

WALES

Tenovus Cancer Information Centre (Wales)

A   B   D

Cancer Information Centre, 142 Whitchurch Road, Cardiff
Administration: 0222 619846
Helpline: 0800 526527 (Mon.–Fri. 0900–
                                             1700)
Answering machine at other times
Screening Programme Organizer: 0222 619846

An information, support and counselling service for people with cancer
and their families. Cancer helpline manned by a trained cancer nurse.
Contact also by letter or personal visit to the drop-in centre. Bilingual.
Information on health promotion is provided; Tenovus mobile health
screening unit for women, run by an all-female team, operates throughout
Wales.

Wales Council for Voluntary Organizations

A

Llys Ifor, Crescent Road, Caerphilly, Mid Glamorgan CF8 1XL
Telephone: 0222 869224

Can give information about voluntary organizations in Wales.

SCOTLAND

Counselling Information Scotland

A   B   D

Clive Powell, Scottish Health Education Group, Woodburn House,
Canaan Lane, Edinburgh EH10 4SG
Telephone: 031 452 8989

Contact in Scotland for British Association for Counselling.

Scottish Council for Voluntary Organizations

A

18–19 Claremont Terrace, Edinburgh EH7 4QD
Telephone: 031 556 3882

Can give information about voluntary organizations in Scotland.